T0313702

Laryngeal Cancer

Clinical Case-Based Approaches

Rogério A. Dedivitis, MD, PhD, FACS
Professor
Department of Head and Neck Surgery
University of São Paulo School of Medicine
São Paulo, Brazil

Giorgio Peretti, MD, PhD
Professor and Chief
Department of Otorhinolaryngology–Head and Neck Surgery
University of Genova
Genova, Italy

Ehab Hanna, MD, FACS
Professor and Vice Chairman
Department of Head and Neck Surgery
The University of Texas MD Anderson Cancer Center
Houston, Texas

Claudio R. Cernea, MD
Associate Professor and Chairman
Department of Head and Neck Surgery
University of São Paulo School of Medicine
São Paulo, Brazil

212 illustrations

Thieme
New York • Stuttgart • Delhi • Rio de Janeiro

Acquisitions Editor: Timothy Y. Hiscock
Managing Editor: Prakash Naorem
Director, Editorial Services: Mary Jo Casey
Production Editor: Shivika
International Production Director: Andreas Schabert
Editorial Director: Sue Hodgson
International Marketing Director: Fiona Henderson
International Sales Director: Louisa Turrell
Senior Vice President and Chief Operating
   Officer: Sarah Vanderbilt
President: Brian D. Scanlan

Library of Congress Cataloging-in-Publication Data
Names: Dedivitis, Rogério A., editor. | Peretti, Giorgio, editor. |
Hanna, Ehab Y., editor. | Cernea, Claudio R., editor.
Title: Laryngeal cancer : clinical case-based approaches / Rogério A.
   Dedivitis, Giorgio Peretti, Ehab Hanna, Claudio R. Cernea.
Other titles: Laryngeal cancer (Dedivitis)
Description: New York : Thieme, [2019] | Includes bibliographical
references and index. |
Identifiers: LCCN 2018046970 (print) | LCCN 2018047807 (ebook)
| ISBN 9781684200023 | ISBN 9781684200016 (hardback) | ISBN
9781684200023 (e-book)
Subjects: | MESH: Laryngeal Neoplasms—surgery | Laryngectomy—
methods | Salvage Therapy—methods
Classification: LCC RC280.T5 (ebook) | LCC RC280.T5 (print) | NLM
WV 520 | DDC 616.99/422—dc23
LC record available at https://lccn.loc.gov/2018046970

Important note: Medicine is an ever-changing science undergoing continual development. Research and clinical experience are continually expanding our knowledge, in particular our knowledge of proper treatment and drug therapy. Insofar as this book mentions any dosage or application, readers may rest assured that the authors, editors, and publishers have made every effort to ensure that such references are in accordance with **the state of knowledge at the time of production of the book.**

Nevertheless, this does not involve, imply, or express any guarantee or responsibility on the part of the publishers in respect to any dosage instructions and forms of applications stated in the book. **Every user is requested to examine carefull**y the manufacturers' leaflets accompanying each drug and to check, if necessary in consultation with a physician or specialist, whether the dosage schedules mentioned therein or the contraindications stated by the manufacturers differ from the statements made in the present book. Such examination is particularly important with drugs that are either rarely used or have been newly released on the market. Every dosage schedule or every form of application used is entirely at the user's own risk and responsibility. The authors and publishers request every user to report to the publishers any discrepancies or inaccuracies noticed. If errors in this work are found after publication, errata will be posted at www.thieme.com on the product description page.

Some of the product names, patents, and registered designs referred to in this book are in fact registered trademarks or proprietary names even though specific reference to this fact is not always made in the text. Therefore, the appearance of a name without designation as proprietary is not to be construed as a representation by the publisher that it is in the public domain.

© 2019 Thieme Medical Publishers, Inc.

Thieme Publishers New York
333 Seventh Avenue, New York, NY 10001 USA
+1 800 782 3488, customerservice@thieme.com

Thieme Publishers Stuttgart
Rüdigerstrasse 14, 70469 Stuttgart, Germany
+49 [0]711 8931 421, customerservice@thieme.de

Thieme Publishers Delhi
A-12, Second Floor, Sector-2, Noida-201301
Uttar Pradesh, India
+91 120 45 566 00, customerservice@thieme.in

Thieme Publishers Rio de Janeiro,
Thieme Publicações Ltda.
Edifício Rodolpho de Paoli, 25º andar
Av. Nilo Peçanha, 50 – Sala 2508,
Rio de Janeiro 20020-906 Brasil
+55 21 3172-2297

Cover design: Thieme Publishing Group
Typesetting by DiTech Process Solutions, India

Printed in USA by King Printing Company, Inc.   5 4 3 2 1

ISBN 978-1-68420-001-6

Also available as an e-book:
eISBN 978-1-68420-002-3

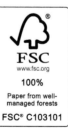

FSC
www.fsc.org
100%
Paper from well-managed forests
FSC® C103101

I would like to dedicate this book to my multiprofessional teams at Hospital das Clínicas of the University of São Paulo School of Medicine and at Santos City—Santa Casa da Misericórdia and Ana Costa Hospitals and UNILUS and UNIMES Universities.

Rogério A. Dedivitis

I would like to dedicate this book to my wife, C. Smussi, MD, and to my multiprofessional team at Policlinico San Martino of the University of Genoa, School of Medicine.

Giorgio Peretti

This book is dedicated to my family for the joy and blessing they bring to my life; my parents who encouraged me to follow my dreams; my fellows, residents, and students who continue to teach me; and my patients, whose endurance, resilience, and faith continue to amaze me.

Ehab Hanna

I would like to dedicate this book to my wife, Selma S. Cernea, MD, and to my multiprofessional team at Hospital das Clínicas of the University of São Paulo School of Medicine.

Claudio R. Cernea

Contents

Contents

Foreword

During the past several decades, the attention of those treating cancer of the head and neck has been drawn to the epidemic of human papillomavirus (HPV)-related cancers of the oropharynx. This book, *Laryngeal Cancer: Clinical Case-Based Approaches,* is devoted to the treatment of cancer of the larynx and is a timely, well-organized, and comprehensive addition to the literature in our specialty. One of the most appealing aspects of this book is that it is written in a "case report" style. While case reports are frowned upon in journals, it is a very efficient, familiar, and compelling teaching technique because it reflects how we first learn about case management beginning with our Physical Diagnosis Course in medical school. This book addresses the management of each stage of cancer of the larynx, describing in detail both the surgical and the nonsurgical approaches.

The reader will benefit from using this book as it is written in a personal, easy-reading case report style including a description of the surgical techniques, which includes "Tips" and "Traps" meant to keep the surgeon—and the patient—out of trouble. The discussion is limited to important issues. The chapters are richly illustrated and referenced. The book is quite contemporary, including chapters on the use of the surgical robot, reconstructive techniques, and targeted therapy for advanced cancer.

I know and have a great deal of respect for all of the distinguished Editors who are all professors in top-tier universities. Dr. Hanna is Co-Editor of Cancer of the Head and Neck and Dr. Cernea is Co-Editor of Pearls and Pitfalls in Head and Neck Surgery. The contributing authors, most of whom I know personally, are from the United States, Brazil, Europe, and India.

Eugene N. Myers, MD, FACS, FRCS, Edin. (Hon)
Distinguished Professor and Emeritus Chair
Department of Otolaryngology
University of Pittsburgh School of Medicine
Pittsburgh, Pennsylvania

Foreword

In this excellent and exhaustive volume, an important group of renowned authors from all over the world describe the essential treatment options for laryngeal cancers. With abundant illustrations and lucid narrative, they take readers through each process, step by step, provide tips and highlight traps, and ponder outcomes and consequences.

The book is an indispensable addition to each head and neck surgeon's library.

A. R. Antonelli, MD
Full Professor of Otorhinolaryngology–
Head and Neck Surgery
Past Chair of the Department of
Otorhinolaryngology
University of Brescia
Brescia, Italy

Preface

The goal of this text is to gather the expertise of distinguished specialists around the globe with high interest in laryngeal cancer. It intends to comprehensively cover the diverse primary subsites of laryngeal cancer, stages of the disease, and various treatment modalities based on real clinical cases. Thus, the chapters focus on lesions with similar characteristics but treated by means of different approaches. As a result, besides otolaryngologists–head and neck surgeons, other specialists are also very well represented here, including radiation and medical oncologists, and others interested in the management of laryngeal cancers. Pathologists, radiologists, speech pathologists, and all professionals who deal with laryngeal disorders will also find this text useful and informative.

Most of the chapters are based on a clinical case, with the treatment approach and the outcome presented. The case is then discussed in detail with particular focus on the treatment adopted, the rationale for choosing a particular treatment, and the outcome. Pearls and pitfalls of management are also presented.

The diagnosis and treatment of laryngeal cancer have been ever evolving. A century ago, stroboscopy, narrow-band imaging, and other diagnostic tools were not available. Similarly, innovative treatment approaches have evolved with focus on optimizing oncologic and functional outcomes.

It is our hope that the book will provide a comprehensive resource for the multidisciplinary care of patients with laryngeal cancer, and a reflection of the expertise and the passion of those who care for them.

Rogério A. Dedivitis, MD, PhD, FACS
Giorgio Peretti, MD, PhD
Ehab Hanna, MD, FACS
Claudio R. Cernea, MD

About the Editors

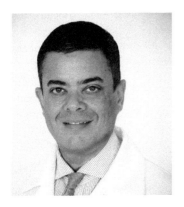

Rogério A. Dedivitis is Full Professor at University of São Paulo School of Medicine and Assistant Surgeon of the Head and Neck Service, Hospital das Clínicas, University of São Paulo School of Medicine, São Paulo, Brazil. He is the Chair of the Department of Head and Neck Surgery, Irmandade da Santa Casa da Misericórdia de Santos and Hospital Ana Costa, Santos, Brazil. He is the Chair Full Professor, Department of Surgery, Centro Universitário Lusíada, Santos, and Chair Professor, Department of Otorhinolaryngology–Head and Neck Surgery, Universidade Metropolitana de Santos, Brazil. He is Past President of the Brazilian Society of Head and Neck Surgery and Latin American Federation of Societies of Head and Neck Surgery.

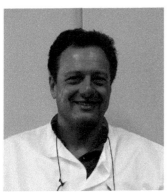

Giorgio Peretti is Full Professor and Chief of the Department of Otorhinolaryngology–Head and Neck Surgery, University of Genoa, Italy, and Past President of the European Laryngological Society.

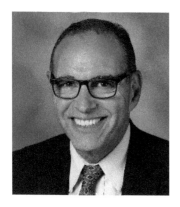

Ehab Hanna is currently Professor and Vice Chair of the Department of Head and Neck Surgery, with a joint appointment in the Department of Neurosurgery, MD Anderson Cancer Center. He also serves as an Adjunct Professor of Otolaryngology and Head and Neck Surgery at Baylor College of Medicine. He is an internationally recognized head and neck surgeon and expert in the treatment of patients with skull base tumors and head and neck cancer. He is the Medical Director of the Multidisciplinary Head and Neck Center and Co-director of the Skull Base Tumor program. For the last 15 years, Dr. Hanna has consistently been named one of America's Best Doctors and Top Doctors in Cancer. He authored over 350 publications. He co-edited two major textbooks, *Cancer of the Head and Neck* and *Comprehensive Management of Skull Base Tumors*. He is the Editor-in-Chief of the journal *Head & Neck*, which is the official journal of the International Federation of Head and Neck Societies. Dr. Hanna served as the President of the North American Skull Base Society (2014) and the President of the American Head and Neck Society (2018).

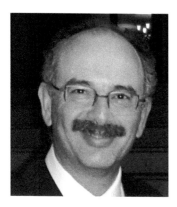

Claudio R. Cernea is Associate Professor and Chairman at the Department of Head and Neck Surgery and also, Chief of the Head and Neck Service at Hospital das Clínicas, University of São Paulo School of Medicine, São Paulo, Brazil. He is Past President of the Brazilian Society of Head and Neck Surgery and Director of the International Federation of Head and Neck Oncological Societies.

Contributors

Sundeep Alapati, DO
Head and Neck Surgery Clinical Fellow
Memorial Sloan Kettering Cancer Center
New York, New York

Helio R. Nogueira Alves, MD, PhD
Staff Surgeon
Department of Plastic Surgery
University of São Paulo Medical School;
Attending Surgeon
Instituto do Câncer do Estado de
    São Paulo (ICESP)
University of São Paulo Medical School
São Paulo, Brazil

Petra Ambrosch, MD
Professor and Chairman
Department of Otorhinolaryngology–Head and
    Neck Surgery, UKSH, Campus Kiel
University of Kiel
Kiel, Germany

Robert J. Amdur, MD
Professor
Department of Radiation Oncology
University of Florida
Gainesville, Florida

Mohssen Ansarin, MD
Chairman
Department of Otolaryngology–Head and Neck
    Surgery
European Institute of Oncology IRCCS
Milan, Italy

Houda Bahig, MD, PhD
Fellow in Radiation Oncology
Department of Radiation Oncology
The University of Texas MD Anderson
    Cancer Center
Houston, Texas;
Centre Hospitalier de l'Université de Montréal
Montreal, Canada

Antonio Augusto T. Bertelli, MD, MS
Professor of Surgery
Head and Neck Surgery Division
Department of Surgery
Santa Casa de São Paulo Medical School
São Paulo, Brazil

Arnaud F. Bewley, MD, FACS
Assistant Professor
Department of Otolaryngology–Head and Neck
    Surgery
University of California, Davis
Sacramento, California

Carol R. Bradford, MD, FACS
Executive Vice Dean for Academic Affairs
Professor, Department of Otolaryngology–Head
    and Neck Surgery
University of Michigan Medical School
Ann Arbor, Michigan

Michiel W.M. van den Brekel, MD, PhD
Professor
Department of Head and Neck Surgery and
    Oncology
Netherlands Cancer Institute/
    Antoni van Leeuwenhoek Hospital;
Academic Medical Center Amsterdam
Institute of Phonetic Sciences ACLC
University of Amsterdam
Amsterdam, The Netherlands

Filippo Carta, MD
Assistant Professor
Unit of Otorhinolaryngology
Department of Surgery
Azienda Ospedaliero-Universitaria
    di Cagliari
University of Cagliari
Cagliari, Italy

Genival B. de Carvalho, MD, MS
Attending Surgeon
Department of Otorhinolaryngology–Head and
  Neck Surgery
A.C. Camargo Cancer Center
São Paulo, Brazil

Marcos B. de Carvalho, MD, PhD
Medicine and Oncologic Doctor
Department of Head and Neck Surgery
Molecular Biology Laboratório
Heliópolis Hospital
São Paulo, Brazil

Mario Augusto F. Castro, PhD
Assistant Surgeon
Department of Surgery
University of Sao Paulo School of Medicine;
Departments of Head and Neck Surgery
Irmandade da Santa Casa da Misericordia de San-
  tos and Hospital Ana Costa
Santos, Brazil

Augusto Cattaneo, MD
Head and Neck Surgeon
Department of Otolaryngology–Head and Neck
  Surgery
European Institute of Oncology IRCCS
Milan, Italy

Claudio R. Cernea, MD, PhD
Associate Professor and Chairman
Department of Head and Neck Surgery
University of São Paulo School of Medicine
São Paulo, Brazil

Pankaj Chaturvedi, MS, FACS
Professor and Surgeon
Department of Head and Neck
  Surgery;
Deputy Director
Centre for Cancer Epidemiology
Tata Memorial Centre
Mumbai, India;
Secretary General
International Federation of Head and
  Neck Oncologic Societies

Francesco Chu, MD
Head and Neck Surgeon
Department of Otolaryngology–Head and Neck
  Surgery
European Institute of Oncology IRCCS
Milan, Italy

Erika Crosetti, MD, PhD
Senior Consultant of Otolaryngology
Head and Neck Oncology Service
Candiolo Cancer Institute - FPO IRCCS
Candiolo,Turin, Italy

Gustavo Cunha, MD
Postgraduate Program
Department of Otolaryngology–Head and Neck
  Surgery
Federal University of São Paulo
São Paulo, Brazil

Otavio Curioni, PhD, Full Professor
Medicine Doctor
Otolaryngology–Head and Neck Surgery
Molecular Biology Laboratório, Heliópolis Hospital
São Paulo, Brazil

Rogério A. Dedivitis, MD, PhD, FACS
Professor
Department of Head and Neck Surgery
University of São Paulo
  School of Medicine
São Paulo, Brazil

Pierre R. Delaere, MD, PhD
Professor of Otorhinolaryngology
Department of Head and Neck Surgery
University Hospitals Leuven;
Department of Immunology and Transplantation
KU Leuven
Leuven, Belgium

Gilles Delahaut, MD
Resident
Department of Otolaryngology–Head and Neck
  Surgery
CHU UCL Namur
Yvoir, Belgium

Fernando L. Dias, MD, PhD, FACS
Chief
Head and Neck Surgery Service
Brazilian National Cancer Hospital 1 Institute–INCA;
Chairman
Department of Head and Neck Surgery
Post Graduate School of Medicine
Catholic University of Rio de Janeiro
Rio de Janeiro, Brazil

Umamaheswar Duvvuri, MD, PhD
Assistant Professor
Department of Otolaryngology
University of Pittsburgh
Pittsburgh, Pennsylvania

Alessia Farneti, MD
Clinical Radiation Oncologist
Department of Radiation Oncology
IRCCS Regina Elena National Cancer Institute
Rome, Italy

D. Gregory Farwell, MD, FACS
Professor and Chair
Department of Otolaryngology–Head and Neck
  Surgery
University of California, Davis
Sacramento, California

Fabio Ferreli, MD
Consultant
Department of Otolaryngology–Head and Neck
  Surgery
Humanitas University
Milan, Italy

Arlene A. Forastiere, MD
Professor
Department of Oncology
Johns Hopkins University
Baltimore, Maryland

Emilson Q. Freitas, MD
Attending Surgeon
Head and Neck Surgery Service Cancer Hospital 1
Brazilian National Cancer Institute–INCA
Rio de Janeiro, Brazil

Antonio J. Gonçalves, MD, PhD
Full Professor, Head
Head and Neck Surgery Division
Department of Surgery
Santa Casa de São Paulo Medical School
São Paulo, Brazil

Christine G. Gourin, MD, MPH, FACS
Professor
Department of Otolaryngology–Head and Neck
  Surgery
Head and Neck Surgical Oncology
Johns Hopkins University
Baltimore, Maryland

Roberta Granata, MD
Clinical Fellow
Medical Oncology Unit 3 Fondazione
IRCCS Istituto Tumori Milano
University of Milano
Milan, Italy

André V. Guimarães, MD, PhD
Full Professor
Department of Head Neck Surgery
Hospital das Clinicas
University of São Paulo;
Chairman, Department of ENT and Head
  and Neck
Department of Universidade Metropolitana de
  Santos (UNIMES)
São Paulo, Brazil

G. Brandon Gunn, MD
Associate Professor
Department of Radiation Oncology
The University of Texas MD Anderson
  Cancer Center
Houston, Texas

Leonardo Haddad, PhD
Associate Professor
Department of Otolaryngology–Head and Neck
  Surgery
Federal University of São Paulo
São Paulo, Brazil

Ehab Hanna, MD, FACS
Professor and Vice Chairman
Department of Head and Neck Surgery
The University of Texas MD Anderson Cancer
    Center
Houston, Texas

Fabiola Incandela, MD
Consultant
Department of Otorhinolaryngology,
    Maxillofacial and Thyroid Surgery
Fondazione IRCCS
National Cancer Institute of Milan
University of Milan
Milan, Italy

Ana Ponce Kiess, MD
Assistant Professor
Department of Radiation Oncology
Johns Hopkins University
Baltimore, Maryland

Se-Heon Kim, MD, PhD
Professor
Department of Otorhinolaryngology
Yonsei Univesity College of Medicine
Seoul, Korea

Luiz P. Kowalski, MD, PhD
Director
Department of Otorhinolaryngology–Head and
    Neck Surgery
A.C. Camargo Cancer Center
São Paulo, Brazil

Marco A.V. Kulcsar, MD, PhD
Coordinator
Department of Head and Neck Surgery
Cancer Institute of the São Paulo
    State (ICESP) – FMUSP
São Paulo, Brazil

Georges Lawson, MD
Professor
Department of Otolaryngology–Head and Neck
    Surgery
CHU UCL Namur
Yvoir, Belgium

Nancy Y. Lee, MD, FASTRO
Vice Chair, Department of Radiation Oncology
Chief, Experimental Therapeutics
Director, Head and Neck Radiation Oncology
Memorial Sloan Kettering Cancer Center
New York, New York

C. René Leemans, MD, PhD
Professor and Chair
Department of Otolaryngology–Head and Neck
    Surgery
Amsterdam University Medical Centers
VU University Medical Center/Cancer
    Center Amsterdam
Amsterdam, The Netherlands

Carlos N. Lehn, MD
Director
Department of Head and Neck Surgery
Hospital do Servidor Público Estadual
    de Sao Paulo – FMO/IAMSPE
São Paulo, Brazil

Lisa Licitra, MD
Associate Professor
Medical Oncology Unit 3 Fondazione
IRCCS Istituto Tumori Milano
University of Milano
Milan, Italy

Roberto A. Lima, MD, PhD
Director, Cancer Hospital 1
Head and Neck Surgeon
Brazilian National Cancer Institute–INCA
Rio de Janeiro, Brazil

Manish Mair, MS, MCh
Assistant Professor
Department of Head and Neck Surgery
Tata Memorial Hospital
Mumbai, India

Laura Marucci, MD
Senior Radiation Oncologist
Department of Radiation Oncology
IRCCS Regina Elena National Cancer Institute
Rome, Italy

Leandro L. de Matos, MD, PhD
Assistant Professor
Department of Head and Neck Surgery
University of São Paulo Medical School;
Attending Surgeon
Instituto do Câncer do Estado de São Paulo (ICESP)
University of São Paulo Medical School;
Researcher
University of São Paulo Medical School
São Paulo, Brazil

Abie Mendelsohn, MD
Assistant Professor
Department of Head and Neck Surgery
David Geffen School of Medicine at UCLA
Los Angeles, California

William M. Mendenhall, MD
Professor
Department of Radiation Oncology
University of Florida
Gainesville, Florida

Catherine E. Mercado, MD
Chief Resident
Department of Radiation Oncology
University of Florida
Gainesville, Florida

Giuseppe Mercante, MD
Consultant
Department of Otolaryngology–Head and Neck
  Surgery
National Cancer Institute Regina Elena
Rome, Italy

Francesco Missale, MD
Resident
Department of Otorhinolaryngology–Head and
  Neck Surgery
University of Genoa
Genoa, Italy

Alberto Paderno, MD
Consultant
Department of Otolaryngology–Head and Neck
  Surgery
University of Brescia
Brescia, Italy

Young Min Park, MD, PhD
Assistant Professor
Department of Otorhinolaryngology
Yonsei University College of Medicine
  Seoul, Korea

Giorgio Peretti, MD
Professor and Chief
Department of Otorhinolaryngology–Head and
  Neck Surgery
University of Genoa
Genoa, Italy

Marije J.F. Petersen, MD
PhD Student
Department of Head and Neck Surgery and
  Oncology
Netherlands Cancer Institute/
  Antoni van Leeuwenhoek Hospital
Amsterdam, The Netherlands

Cesare Piazza, MD
Associate Professor and Head
Department of Otorhinolaryngology,
  Maxillofacial and Thyroid Surgery
Fondazione IRCCS
National Cancer Institute of Milan
University of Milan
Milan, Italy

Vincent Vander Poorten, MD, PhD, MSc
Professor
Department of Otorhinolaryngology–Head and
  Neck Surgery
University Hospitals Leuven;
Department of Oncology, Head and Neck
  Oncology Section
KU Leuven
Leuven, Belgium

Roberto Puxeddu, MD, FRCS
Professor
Unit of Otorhinolaryngology
Department of Surgery
Azienda Ospedaliero-Universitaria di Cagliari
University of Cagliari
Cagliari, Italy

Abrão Rapoport, PhD
Assistant Professor
Department of Otorhinolaryngology–Head and
    Neck Surgery
Hospital Heliópolis
São Paulo, Brazil

Marc Remacle, MD, PhD
Professor
Department of Otolaryngology–Head and Neck
    Surgery
CHU UCL Namur
Yvoir, Belgium

Giuseppe Sanguineti, MD
Director
Department of Radiation Oncology
IRCCS Regina Elena National Cancer Institute
Rome, Italy

Claudia Schmalz, MD
Radiation Oncologist
Department of Radiation Oncology,
    Karl-Lennert-Krebscentrum, UKSH, Campus Kiel
University of Kiel
Kiel, Germany

Jatin P. Shah, MD, PhD, DSc, FACS, FRCSE,
    FDSRCS, FRCSDS, FRCSI, FRACS
Professor of Surgery
E.W. Strong Chair in Head and Neck Oncology
Memorial Sloan Kettering Cancer Center
New York, New York

Matthew E. Spector, MD, FACS
Assistant Professor
Co-Director, Head and Neck Oncology Program
Department of Otolaryngology–Head and Neck
    Surgery
Michigan Medicine
Ann Arbor, Michigan

Giuseppe Spriano, MD
Professor and Chairman
Department of Otolaryngology–Head and Neck
    Surgery
Humanitas University
Milan, Italy

Shaum S. Sridharan, MD
Clinical Instructor
Department of Otolaryngology
University of Pittsburgh Medical Center
Pittsburgh, Pennsylvania

Jayne R. Stevens, MD
Major, Medical Corps, US Army
Clinical Lecturer
Department of Otolaryngology–Head and Neck
    Surgery
Michigan Medicine
Ann Arbor, Michigan

Sandro J. Stoeckli, MD
Professor
Department Otorhinolaryngology–Head and Neck
    Surgery
Kantonsspital St. Gallen
St. Gallen, Switzerland

Giovanni Succo, MD
Associate Professor of
    Otolaryngology
Department of Oncology
University of Turin;
Head and Neck Oncology Service
Candiolo Cancer Institute - FPO IRCCS
Turin, Italy

José G. Vartanian, MD, PhD
Attending Surgeon
Department of Otorhinolaryngology–Head and
    Neck Surgery
A.C. Camargo Cancer Center
São Paulo, Brazil

Sebastien Van der Vorst, MD, PhD
Assistant Professor
Head and Neck Surgeon
Department of Otolaryngology–Head and Neck
    Surgery
Amsterdam University
    Medical Centers
VU University Medical Center
Amsterdam, The Netherlands

Fernando Walder, MD
Full Professor Assistant
Department of ENT and Head and Neck Surgery
Federal University of São Paulo
São Paulo, Brazil

S. van Weert, MD
Head and Neck Surgeon
Department of Otolaryngology and Head and
  Neck Surgery
Amsterdam University Medical Centers
Amsterdam, The Netherlands

Yao Yu, MD
Assistant Attending L1
Department of Radiation Oncology
Memorial Sloan Kettering Cancer Center
New York, New York

Dan P. Zandberg, MD
Associate Professor of Medicine
Director, Head and Neck Cancer and
  Thyroid Cancer Disease Sections
Division of Hematology/Oncology
UPMC Hillman Cancer Center
Pittsburgh, Pennsylvania

1 T1a Glottic Carcinoma Undergoing Transoral Laser Surgery

Leonardo Haddad, Gustavo Cunha

Abstract

In this chapter we discuss the case of a T1a squamous cell carcinoma of the glottis treated with transoral laser microsurgery with complete removal of the cancer that showed no signs of recurrence for 3 years of follow-up. The first symptom of cancer of the glottis is usually hoarseness, and early diagnosis is extremely important. Laryngoscopy is the most important examination for diagnosing and staging of the disease; however, in cases which may not be possible to identify all the limits of the lesion during laryngoscopy, an imaging examination (CT or MRI) must be performed, which may help evaluate the tumor extension. Treatment goals are cure of the cancer and preservation of laryngeal function, such as voice and swallowing. Some of the most suitable treatment options are transoral laser microsurgery, radiotherapy, and open partial laryngectomy. The transoral laser microsurgery approach has been associated with good oncological and functional results, low complication rates and less severe complications when compared to the other techniques, including cases involving the anterior commissure. This technique also results in lower management costs and reduced hospitalization time. Patient selection, laryngeal exposure, and type of cordectomy are major points of surgical success, and there is still much controversy about free margins as a predictor of recurrence. While using CO_2 laser, potentially dangerous complications of the procedure must be avoided with appropriate protection of the endotracheal tube and the patient's eyes and face while using a CO_2 laser.

Keywords: laryngeal neoplasms, laryngeal cancer, glottic cancer, CO_2 laser, cordectomy, surgical treatment, transoral laser microsurgery

1.1 Case Report

A 58-year-old female physician, was admitted to our service complaining of progressive dysphonia that had developed in the past 3 months. She denied dyspnea, dysphagia, and dyspeptic symptoms. She admitted to cigarette smoking, (40 pack-years) and alcohol consumption socially. No comorbidities were identified and family history was negative for cancer.

Her voice was moderately rough and the videolaryngoscopy revealed extensive leukoplakia affecting the entire anteroposterior extension of the right vocal fold, without involvement of the anterior commissure (▶ Fig. 1.1). The neck was clinically negative.

After treatment options were discussed with the patient a transoral laser microsurgery technique was performed, with complete excision of the lesion. Intraoperative frozen section biopsy revealed a high-grade intraepithelial lesion without evidence of infiltration of the basement membrane (carcinoma in situ). A type II cordectomy with complete removal of the tumor was performed (▶ Fig. 1.2). Pathological examination revealed a superficially invasive, moderately differentiated squamous cell carcinoma (SCC) of the right vocal fold, with free margins.

This patient has been followed up regularly for 3 years, with no signs of recurrence. Laryngoscopy showed complete glottic closure. Voice quality was good and the patient was satisfied with it.

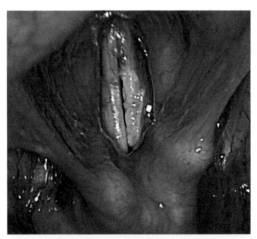

Fig. 1.1 Laryngoscopic view of the leukoplakia affecting the right vocal fold.

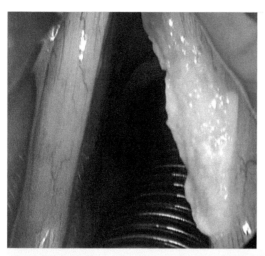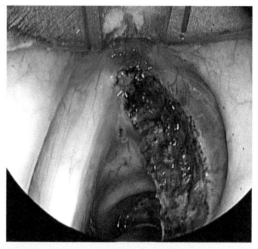

Fig. 1.2 Transoral laser microsurgery. View of the lesion (left) and final result after complete removal of the tumor (right).

1.2 Discussion

Cancer of the larynx accounts for 2 to 4.5% of all malignant neoplasms and 25% of the head and neck tumors, with 50% of these cancers involving the vocal folds. In males, the incidence is highest in Southern Europe, some countries of Central and Eastern Europe and of South America, and in the African-American population of the United States. In these populations, standardized incidence was 10/100.000. In females, the highest rate is found in the African American population, at around 3/100.000.[1]

Early cancer of the glottis refers to a cancer that has not spread to adjacent spaces of the larynx and corresponds to the stages Tis, T1, and T2 (AJCC/UICC TNM, 8th edition).[2] The first symptom of cancer of glottis is usually hoarseness and the early diagnosis is quite relevant, since advanced lesions require more aggressive treatment modalities. The use of imaging examinations, such as computed tomography (CT) and magnetic resonance imaging (MRI), may help evaluate the extent of the neoplasm particularly in cases in which all limits cannot be determined with direct laryngoscopy. However, laryngoscopy is the most important examination for diagnosing and staging of early cancer of the glottis.

Treatment goals are cure of the cancer and preservation of laryngeal function, such, as voice and swallowing, and minimizing the risk of serious complications. Different types of procedures can be used, such as transoral laser microsurgery (TLM), radiotherapy (RT), or open partial laryngectomy (OPL). Since the survival rates are almost equivalent, treatment choice is usually decided based on voice outcomes, treatment duration, and the patients' condition and preference.[3,4]

Recent studies about cost-effectiveness compared the main treatment modalities of early glottic cancer and revealed best results with TLM because of its low management costs, reduced hospitalization time, and good oncological and functional results, with low complication rates and less severe complications when compared to the other techniques.[5,6] The OPL is associated with longer hospitalization time, higher rate of complications (postoperative pain, edema, emphysema, and the required tracheotomy), high costs, and worse functional results, although it allows obtaining larger free margins and the possibility of treating the neck when required.[7] On the other hand, RT offers good oncological and voice outcomes, but higher costs, prolonged time of treatment, mucosal damage, and long-term side effects such as xerostomia.[8]

Although there is no current consensus, recent meta-analysis showed no significant difference in voice quality comparing laser cordectomy and RT in the treatment of T1 glottic carcinoma.[9] Longitudinal voice evaluation of patients treated with CO_2 laser cordectomy revealed immediate worsening of voice quality (< 3 months), followed by recovery and stabilization (> 6 months), and results comparable to preoperative patterns, especially in cases related to less extensive cordectomy, unilateral and without anterior commissure involvement.[10,11,12]

Despite the good oncologic and functional results of TLM in early cancer of the glottis, there has been ongoing debate regarding its application in patients with involvement of the anterior commissure. Although primary RT has been considered as an effective and voice-preserving treatment modality for cancer of the glottis, it has demonstrated worse results in cases involving the anterior commissure, but there is still no consensus regarding this matter. Some authors have advocated OPL due to the achievement of better local control (86–91%) compared to those treated with RT (56–76%).[13,14] However, considering the duration and possible complications of RT and open surgery, TLM may be the preferred treatment modality with shorter hospitalization, minimal morbidity, and comparable local control (79–92.8%).[15,16]

Surgical margins are also a major concern. Some authors have considered positive margins as a factor of bad prognosis.[16,17] However, others did not demonstrate the association of the margin status and patient's outcomes.[15,18] A resection margin of 2 mm is often considered as sufficient in cancer of the glottis, as opposed to other sites in the head and neck.[19] With resection artifacts and specimen shrinkage and carbonization around this tiny margin, pathological assessment could be hampered leading to false interpretation of tumor edges. Therefore, results of positive margins do not necessarily represent inadequate tumor removal.[17] Furthermore, the recent introduction of new endoscopic devices, namely, the use of narrow band imaging (NBI) has demonstrated enormous value in defining superficial extension of the cancer and delineating its margins of resection. This "biologic endoscopy" concept revealed a great reduction of superficial positive margins from 23.7 to 3.6%.[20]

Even though frozen section is reliable in laser-assisted cordectomies,[21] this procedure seems difficult to implement in a regular basis given that it is time-consuming and requires an available and experienced pathology team. On the other hand, biopsy of the tissue remaining in and around the tumor removal ground has been recommended.[17]

Besides, in an attempt to improve local control, some authors also suggest a routine second-look laryngoscopy to detect residual glottic cancers. However, while the identification of residual tumor may be beneficial for oncologic control, the routine practice second-look laryngoscopy is of questionable value due to the low rate of findings and high cost.[21,22]

1.3 Tips

- *Patient selection:* Adequate case selection regarding size, location, and extent of the cancer, surgical exposure of the larynx, and comorbidities are critical factors for successful treatment.
- *Suspension microlaryngoscopy:* One of the major points of transoral laser surgery is performing a good suspension microlaryngoscopy that provides the surgeon with the greatest exposure of the entire larynx. For the success of the surgery, it is important that all limits of the lesion can be determined for complete removal, and it is especially relevant when the anterior commissure is involved. Therefore, it is recommended that different kinds and sizes of laryngoscopes be available to achieve a complete view of the cancer.
- *Type of cordectomy:* The type of cordectomy will vary depending on the extension and degree of infiltration of the lesion. The major point to focus on is the complete removal of the cancer. If you are treating a case of leukoplakia and/or erythroplakia, we recommend a frozen section evaluation. If there is any degree of dysplasia, at least a type II cordectomy instead of a traditional type I cordectomy should be performed, in order to prevent further recurrences, as voice quality is not significantly different.
- *Margins:* Although we believe complete excision of the cancer is staisfactory for treatment, we also recommend collecting fragments from the margins after removing the cancer and considering an early second-look surgery if there is any positive margin.

1.4 Traps

- *Limits of the cancer.* If it is not possible to identify all the limits of the tumor during diagnostic laryngoscopy, an imaging examination (CT or MRI) may help to evaluate the extent of the cancer and to decide if it can be treated transorally. Remember that a T1 carcinoma involving the anterior commissure may actually be a T3 if it invades the thyroid cartilage.
- *Protection of the endotracheal.* Laser-induced endotracheal fire is the most feared complication

in these surgeries. The surgeon must be careful with the endotracheal tube and protect it from the laser beams in order to prevent the risks of fire hazards. The use of laser-safe tubes is recommended whenever possible and we also suggest filling the first cuff with saline, so it will help you detect laser damage to the cuff. It is also recommended to perform a burn test before the procedure to verify the beams' alignment and discuss with the anesthesia team the best anesthetic technique. Total intravenous anesthesia with low (< 40%) fraction of inspired oxygen (FiO_2) is preferred.

- *Eye and skin hazards.* The CO_2 laser beams have the potential to damage the eyes and skin of the patient and operating room personnel. Therefore, appropriate spectacles must be used in order to reduce the risk of ocular damage, and it is mandatory to protect the patient's eyes and face using a damp towel as a drape.

References

[1] Schultz P. Vocal fold cancer. Eur Ann Otorhinolaryngol Head Neck Dis. 2011; 128(6):301–308

[2] Amin MB, Sullivan DC, Jessup JM, et al, eds. American Joint Committee on Cancer Staging Manual. 8th ed. New York, NY: Springer; 2017

[3] Bertino G, Degiorgi G, Tinelli C, Cacciola S, Occhini A, Benazzo M. CO_2 laser cordectomy for T1–T2 glottic cancer: oncological and functional long-term results. Eur Arch Otorhinolaryngol. 2015; 272(9):2389–2395

[4] Mendenhall WM, Werning JW, Hinerman RW, Amdur RJ, Villaret DB. Management of T1–T2 glottic carcinomas. Cancer. 2004; 100(9):1786–1792

[5] Goor KM, Peeters AJ, Mahieu HF, et al. Cordectomy by CO_2 laser or radiotherapy for small T1a glottic carcinomas: costs, local control, survival, quality of life, and voice quality. Head Neck. 2007; 29(2):128–136

[6] Diaz-de-Cerio P, Preciado J, Santaolalla F, Sanchez-Del-Rey A. Cost-minimisation and cost-effectiveness analysis comparing transoral CO_2 laser cordectomy, laryngofissure cordectomy and radiotherapy for the treatment of T1–T2, N0, M0 glottic carcinoma. Eur Arch Otorhinolaryngol. 2013; 270(4):1181–1188

[7] Succo G, Crosetti E, Bertolin A, et al. Benefits and drawbacks of open partial horizontal laryngectomies, part A: early- to intermediate-stage glottic carcinoma. Head Neck. 2016; 38(s)(uppl 1):E333–E340

[8] Mendenhall WM, Amdur RJ, Morris CG, Hinerman RW. T1–T2N0 squamous cell carcinoma of the glottic larynx treated with radiation therapy. J Clin Oncol. 2001; 19(20):4029–4036

[9] Greulich MT, Parker NP, Lee P, Merati AL, Misono S. Voice outcomes following radiation versus laser microsurgery for T1 glottic carcinoma: systematic review and meta-analysis. Otolaryngol Head Neck Surg. 2015; 152(5):811–819

[10] Lee HS, Kim JS, Kim SW, et al. Voice outcome according to surgical extent of transoral laser microsurgery for T1 glottic carcinoma. Laryngoscope. 2016; 126(9):2051–2056

[11] Chu PY, Hsu YB, Lee TL, Fu S, Wang LM, Kao YC. Longitudinal analysis of voice quality in patients with early glottic cancer after transoral laser microsurgery. Head Neck. 2012; 34(9):1294–1298

[12] Mendelsohn AH, Matar N, Bachy V, Lawson G, Remacle M. Longitudinal voice outcomes following advanced CO_2 laser cordectomy for glottic cancer. J Voice. 2015; 29(6):772–775

[13] Rucci L, Gallo O, Fini-Storchi O. Glottic cancer involving anterior commissure: surgery vs radiotherapy. Head Neck. 1991; 13(5):403–410

[14] Zohar Y, Rahima M, Shvili Y, Talmi YP, Lurie H. The controversial treatment of anterior commissure carcinoma of the larynx. Laryngoscope. 1992; 102(1):69–72

[15] Lee HS, Chun BG, Kim SW, et al. Transoral laser microsurgery for early glottic cancer as one-stage single-modality therapy. Laryngoscope. 2013; 123(11):2670–2674

[16] Peretti G, Piazza C, Cocco D, et al. Transoral CO(2) laser treatment for T(is)-T(3) glottic cancer: the University of Brescia experience on 595 patients. Head Neck. 2010; 32(8):977–983

[17] Charbonnier Q, Thisse AS, Sleghem L, et al. Oncologic outcomes of patients with positive margins after laser cordectomy for T1 and T2 glottic squamous cell carcinoma. Head Neck. 2016; 38(12):1804–1809

[18] Michel J, Fakhry N, Duflo S, et al. Prognostic value of the status of resection margins after endoscopic laser cordectomy for T1a glottic carcinoma. Eur Ann Otorhinolaryngol Head Neck Dis. 2011; 128(6):297–300

[19] Hartl DM, Brasnu DF. Contemporary surgical management of early glottic cancer. Otolaryngol Clin North Am. 2015; 48(4):611–625

[20] Garofolo S, Piazza C, Del Bon F, et al. Intraoperative narrow band imaging better delineates superficial resection margins during transoral laser microsurgery for early glottic cancer. Ann Otol Rhinol Laryngol. 2015; 124(4):294–298

[21] Remacle M, Matar N, Delos M, Nollevaux MC, Jamart J, Lawson G. Is frozen section reliable in transoral CO(2) laser-assisted cordectomies? Eur Arch Otorhinolaryngol. 2010; 267(3):397–400

[22] Fang TJ, Courey MS, Liao CT, Yen TC, Li HY. Frozen margin analysis as a prognosis predictor in early glottic cancer by laser cordectomy. Laryngoscope. 2013; 123(6):1490–1495

2 Radiotherapy for T1a Glottic Cancer

Catherine E. Mercado, Robert J. Amdur, William M. Mendenhall

Abstracts

Primary radiotherapy (RT) for T1a cancer of the glottis is a highly effective treatment resulting in excellent outcomes. Treatment with primary RT for early-stage vocal cord cancer allows for voice preservation with a tolerable toxicity profile. For T1a cancer of the glottis, the recommended RT dose schedule is 63 Gy at 2.25 Gy per fraction once daily using a three-field technique.

Keywords: radiation therapy, early-stage glottic cancer, vocal cord cancer, T1 cancer of the glottis, clinical outcomes

2.1 Case Presentation

A 68-year-old male with a 40 pack-year history of smoking cigarettes presented for medical attention for persistent hoarseness lasting 5 months. After a course of oral antibiotics did not improve symptoms, he was referred to an otolaryngologist. On physical examination, there was no cervical adenopathy on palpation and examination of the oral cavity did not reveal any abnormal lesions. Flexible laryngoscopy demonstrated a white nodular lesion on the anterior one-third of the right true vocal cord (TVC). The left TVC was mildly edematous but without visible tumor. The TVCs had normal mobility (▶Fig. 2.1).

An axial computed tomography (CT) scan, with contrast of the larynx demonstrated an infiltrating mass involving the anterior one-half of the right TVC without extension to the midline at the anterior commissure (▶Fig. 2.2). There was no invasion of the thyroid cartilage and no extension into the subglottic region. No abnormal cervical or supraclavicular adenopathy was present and CT imaging of the chest was negative for pulmonary metastasis. Direct micro laryngoscopy under general anesthesia confirmed the absence of subglottic extension.

A biopsy of the right TVC was performed and the pathology report revealed a moderately differentiated squamous cell carcinoma. As per the eighth edition of the American Joint Committee on Cancer (AJCC) staging system, the disease was staged as a clinical T1a N0 M0 squamous cell carcinoma of the right TVC.

Treatment with primary external-beam radiotherapy (EBRT) was recommended. The patient received a total dose of 63 Gy at 2.25 Gy per fraction once daily. A three-field technique with 6-MV photons was used to deliver approximately 95% of the dose through opposed lateral wedged fields weighted to the side of the lesion; the remaining dose was delivered by an anterior field shifted

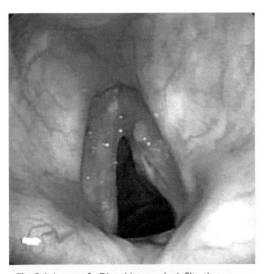

Fig. 2.1 Image of a T1a white papular infiltrating squamous cell carcinoma involving the anterior one-half of the right true vocal cord taken using a flexible fiberoptic endoscope.

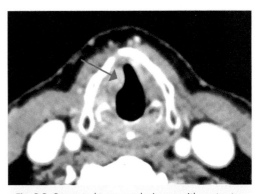

Fig. 2.2 Computed tomography image with contrast enhancement illustrating a cross section of the larynx at the level of the vocal cords. The *red arrow* highlights an infiltrating mass involving the anterior one-half of the right true vocal cord.

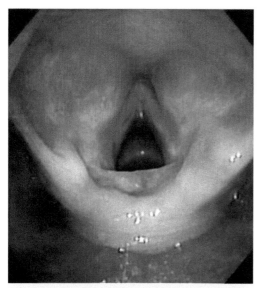

Fig. 2.3 Image of normal true vocal cords 1-year after primary radiotherapy for a T1 glottic cancer.

0.5 cm toward the side of the lesion. The tumor dose was specified to the 95% normalized isodose line (▶Fig. 2.3).

At the time of follow-up 1 year after treatment, examination using the flexible laryngoscope demonstrated bilateral TVCs without edema, lesions, or asymmetry. Bilateral vocal cord mobility was normal. The patient's voice had returned to normal. There were no late treatment toxicites.

2.2 Discussion

2.2.1 Clinical Presentation, Staging, and Diagnostic Evaluation

Most lesions of the TVC begin on the free margin and superior surface of the vocal cord. When diagnosed, about two-thirds are confined to the cords, typically one cord. Per the eighth edition of the AJCC staging system for primary laryngeal cancer, T1 glottic cancer is defined as a cancer limited to the vocal cord(s) (that may involve the anterior or posterior commissure) with normal mobility. T1 cancers are stratified into those involving one vocal cord (T1a) and those involving both vocal cords (T1b).[1]

Cancer arising on the TVC most commonly produces hoarseness at an early stage. Odynophagia, otalgia, pain localized to the thyroid cartilage, and airway obstruction are all features of advanced lesions. Diagnostic evaluation includes the following: a physical examination of the head and neck region, flexible fiberoptic endoscopy to best visualize the larynx, a CT scan with contrast enhancement of the larynx and neck, and a direct laryngoscopy with biopsy performed with the patient under general anesthesia.

2.2.2 Treatment Options

In treating cancer of the vocal cord, the goal is cure with the best functional result and the smallest risk of a serious complication. Patients who have early stage cancer, including those with T1a cancer, should receive larynx-preserving treatment,[2] which includes primary RT or surgery by transoral laser microsurgery (TLM) or transoral robotic surgery (TORS).[3]

At many treatment centers, RT is the initial treatment prescribed for T1 cancer of the glottis, with surgery reserved for salvage if there is a local recurrence occurs.[4,5,6] The major advantage of RT compared with partial laryngectomy is a better quality of voice preservation. However, it is important to note that primary surgery with TLM and TORS has shown comparable cure rates when compared to primary RT.[5,7,8] The advantages of surgery include avoidance of RT, a single treatment, and potential cost-effectiveness.

Most recurrences appear in the first 2 years after treatment, but late recurrences may appear even after 5 years. However, the latter instance may actually be a second primary cancer. If a patient recurs locally after primary RT, they may be salvaged by cordectomy, hemilaryngectomy, supracricoid partial laryngectomy, or total laryngectomy. Open partial laryngectomy and total laryngectomy are the most commonly used surgical salvage procedures.

If a patient recurs after primary surgery, salvage with RT may be possible. If a patient recurs after a combination of RT and partial laryngectomy, total laryngectomy may still be a successful option for salvage.

2.2.3 Radiation Therapy Dose and Technique

Many institutions use a dose-fractionation schedule of 66 Gy for T1 lesions given in 2-Gy fractions. However, there is evidence that increasing the dose per fraction and shortening the overall treatment time may improve local tumor control.[9,10,11,12,13]

Yamazaki et al reported a prospective trial in which a series of patients with T1 N0 squamous cell cancer of the glottic larynx were randomized to definitive RT at 2.0 or 2.25 Gy per fraction.[14] The 5-year local control rates were 77% after 2.0 Gy per fraction and 92% after 2.25 Gy per fraction (p = 0.004); there was no difference in either acute or late toxicity. At the University of Florida, patients with T1 vocal cord are treated with radiation to a total dose of 63 Gy in 2.25-Gy fractions once daily for a total of 28 fractions.

Primary RT for T1 cancer of the glottis consists of EBRT delivered by small treatment fields only covering the primary lesion in the larynx, and without including the cervical lymph nodes.[6] A three-field technique, using 4- or 6-MV X-rays, is used to deliver approximately 95% of the dose through opposed lateral wedged fields weighted to the side of the lesion; the remaining dose is delivered by an anterior field shifted 0.5 cm toward the side of the lesion.[15] RT treatment fields extend from the thyroid notch superiorly to the inferior border of the cricoid and fall off anteriorly. The posterior border depends on the posterior extension of the cancer. Field borders for a patient with T1 N0 cancer are depicted in ▶ Fig. 2.4. The field size ranges

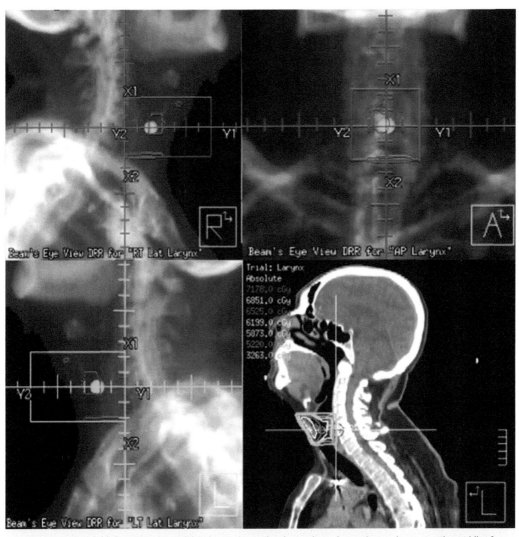

Fig. 2.4 Treatment fields for early cancer of the glottis. The top border is adjusted according to the cancer. The middle of the thyroid notch is the landmark for very early cancers. The posterior border is 1 cm posterior to the posterior edge of the thyroid cartilage if the cancer is confined to the anterior two-thirds of the vocal cord; if the posterior one-third of the vocal cord is involved, the posterior border is placed 1.0 to 1.5 cm behind the cartilage. The inferior border is placed at the inferior aspect of the cricoid cartilage if there is no subglottic extension.

from 4 × 4 to 5 × 5 cm (plus an additional anterior 1.0 cm of "flash"). Larger treatment fields could increase the risk of edema without improving the cure rate. The tumor dose is usually specified at the 95% normalized isodose line.

Intensity-modulated RT may be considered for T1–T2 glottic cancers to reduce the dose to carotid arteries.[6] The potential advantages of this technique must be weighed against the potential increased likelihood of a marginal miss.

2.2.4 Treatment Results from Primary Radiotherapy

The reported outcomes after primary RT of T1 cancer of the glottis are excellent, with a local control rate of over 90% at 5 years after treatment (►Table 2.1). Reported surgical outcomes have illustrated comparable cancer control rates to that of primary RT for T1 glottic cancer in multiple published series.[16,17,18]

2.2.5 Follow-up after Treatment

Post-RT follow-up of patients with early stage cancer is planned for every 4 to 8 weeks for 2 years, every 3 months for the third year, every 6 months until the fifth year, and then annually for life.

Follow-up of patients with cancer of the vocal cord lesions treated by RT or conservative surgery is essential since early detection of a recurrence usually results in salvage that may include cure with preservation of the voice. If a recurrence is suspected but the biopsy is negative, patients are re-examined at 2- to 4-week intervals until the issue is settled.

2.2.6 Radiation Therapy Sequelae

The acute toxicities from primary RT for early cancer of the vocal cord are relatively mild. During the first 2 to 3 weeks, the voice may improve as the cancer regresses. The voice typically becomes hoarse again because of RT-induced changes, even though the cancer continues to regress. A mild self-limiting sore throat commonly begins to develop at the end of the second week of RT. The voice begins to improve approximately 3 weeks after completing treatment, usually reaching a plateau in 2 to 3 months. Patients with T1a cancer of the vocal cord often recover a normal voice.

Edema of the larynx is the most common sequela after RT for cancer of the glottis. The rate of clearance of the edema is related to the RT dose, volume of tissue irradiated, continued use of alcohol and tobacco, and size and extent of the original lesion. Soft-tissue necrosis leading to chondritis occurs in less than 1% of patients, usually in those who continue to smoke cigarettes. Soft-tissue and cartilage necrosis mimics recurrence, with hoarseness, pain, and edema; a laryngectomy may be recommended as a last resort for fear of recurrent cancer, even though biopsy specimens may only reveal tissue necrosis.

Corticosteroids, such as dexamethasone (Decadron), have been used to reduce RT-induced edema after recurrence has been ruled out by biopsy. If ulceration and pain occur, administration of antibiotics may help. Of 519 patients with T1 N0 or T2 N0 cancer of the vocal cancer treated at the University of Florida, 5 (1%) experienced severe complications,[4] including total laryngectomy for a suspected local recurrence (1 patient), permanent tracheostomy for edema (3 patients), and a pharyngocutaneous fistula after a salvage total laryngectomy (1 patient).

Table 2.1 Local control after primary radiotherapy

Institution	Follow-up	No. of patients	Stage	Local control (interval) (%)
University of Florida[4]	Minimum, 2 y Median, 9.9 y	230	T1a	94 (5 y)
		61	T1b	93 (5 y)
Massachusetts General Hospital[19]	Not stated	665	T1	93 (5 y)
University of California, San Francisco[20]	Median, 9.7 y	315	T1	85 (5 y)
Princess Margaret Hospital[21]	Median, 6.8 y	403	T1a	91 (5 y)
		46	T1b	82 (5 y)

References

[1] Amin MB, Sullivan DC, Jessup JM, Brierley JD, Gaspar LE. Laryngeal cancer. AJCC Cancer Staging Manual. 8th ed. New York, NY: Springer; 2017

[2] Network NCC. NCCN Guidelines v.1 Head Neck. 2018

[3] Dziegielewski PT, Kang SY, Ozer E. Transoral robotic surgery (TORS) for laryngeal and hypopharyngeal cancers. J Surg Oncol. 2015; 112(7):702–706

[4] Mendenhall WM, Amdur RJ, Morris CG, Hinerman RW. T1–T2N0 squamous cell carcinoma of the glottic larynx treated with radiation therapy. J Clin Oncol. 2001; 19(20):4029–4036

[5] Mendenhall WM, Werning JW, Hinerman RW, Amdur RJ, Villaret DB. Management of T1–T2 glottic carcinomas. Cancer. 2004; 100(9):1786–1792

[6] Chera BS, Amdur RJ, Morris CG, Kirwan JM, Mendenhall WM. T1N0 to T2N0 squamous cell carcinoma of the glottic larynx treated with definitive radiotherapy. Int J Radiat Oncol Biol Phys. 2010; 78(2):461–466

[7] Day AT, Sinha P, Nussenbaum B, Kallogjeri D, Haughey BH. Management of primary T1–T4 glottic squamous cell carcinoma by transoral laser microsurgery. Laryngoscope. 2017; 127(3):597–604

[8] O'Sullivan B, Mackillop W, Gilbert R, et al. Controversies in the management of laryngeal cancer: results of an international survey of patterns of care. Radiother Oncol. 1994; 31(1):23–32

[9] Harwood AR, Beale FA, Cummings BJ, Keane TJ, Payne D, Rider WD. T4N0M0 glottic cancer: an analysis of dose-time volume factors. Int J Radiat Oncol Biol Phys. 1981; 7(11):1507–1512

[10] Kim RY, Marks ME, Salter MM. Early-stage glottic cancer: importance of dose fractionation in radiation therapy. Radiology. 1992; 182(1):273–275

[11] Schwaibold F, Scariato A, Nunno M, et al. The effect of fraction size on control of early glottic cancer. Int J Radiat Oncol Biol Phys. 1988; 14(3):451–454

[12] Woodhouse RJ, Quivey JM, Fu KK, Sien PS, Dedo HH, Phillips TL. Treatment of carcinoma of the vocal cord. A review of 20 years experience. Laryngoscope. 1981; 91(7):1155–1162

[13] Mendenhall WM, Riggs CE, Cassisi NJ. Treatment of head and neck cancers. In: DeVita VT, ed. DeVita Hellman, and Rosenberg's Cancer: Principles and Practice of Oncology. Philadelphia, PA: Lippincott Williams & Wilkins; 2008:809–814

[14] Yamazaki H, Nishiyama K, Tanaka E, Koizumi M, Chatani M. Radiotherapy for early glottic carcinoma (T1N0M0): results of prospective randomized study of radiation fraction size and overall treatment time. Int J Radiat Oncol Biol Phys. 2006; 64(1):77–82

[15] Million RR, Cassisi NJ, Mancuso AA. Larynx. In: Million RR, Cassisi NJ, eds. Management of Head and Neck Cancer: Multidisciplinary Approach. Philadelphia, PA: JB Lippincott; 1994:431–497

[16] Spector JG, Sessions DG, Chao KS, et al. Stage I (T1 N0 M0) squamous cell carcinoma of the laryngeal glottis: therapeutic results and voice preservation. Head Neck. 1999; 21(8):707–717

[17] Steiner W. Results of curative laser microsurgery of laryngeal carcinomas. Am J Otolaryngol. 1993; 14(2):116–121

[18] Gallo A, de Vincentiis M, Manciocco V, Simonelli M, Fiorella ML, Shah JP. CO_2 laser cordectomy for early-stage glottic carcinoma: a long-term follow-up of 156 cases. Laryngoscope. 2002; 112(2):370–374

[19] Wang CC. Carcinoma of the larynx. In: Wang CC, ed. Radiation Therapy for Head and Neck Neoplasms. New York, NY: Wiley-Liss; 1997:221–255

[20] Le QT, Fu KK, Kroll S, et al. Influence of fraction size, total dose, and overall time on local control of T1–T2 glottic carcinoma. Int J Radiat Oncol Biol Phys. 1997; 39(1):115–126

[21] Warde P, O'Sullivan B, Bristow RG, et al. T1/T2 glottic cancer managed by external beam radiotherapy: the influence of pretreatment hemoglobin on local control. Int J Radiat Oncol Biol Phys. 1998; 41(2):347–353

3 Robotic Surgery for Early-Stage Laryngeal Cancer

Umamaheswar Duvvuri, Shaum S. Sridharan

Abstract

Surgical management of early-stage laryngeal cancer has evolved in the recent past. Minimally invasive surgical strategies and techniques have gained increasing importance and are now used more frequently. While transoral laser surgery is the most commonly employed technique, robotic surgery is gaining traction. The da Vinci surgical robot is the most established and frequently used surgical robot. However, the size of this system makes access to the larynx/supraglottis challenging. Recently, the Flex system has been approved for transoral surgery. This chapter describes the role of robotic surgery in the management of early-stage laryngeal cancer. We describe a case of an early laryngeal tumor that was treated with transoral robotic resection using the Flex robotic system. We detail the considerations in patient management. The criteria for patient selection, both functional and anatomic, are discussed. We also discuss the important considerations to ensure adequate exposure of the tumor for transoral surgery. The postoperative management of patients treated with robotic surgery is described, along with tips and pitfalls. We also contrast the role of radiation therapy to robotic surgery for the management of this disease.

Keywords: laryngeal cancer, early-stage, robotic surgery, transoral

3.1 Case Report

A 54-year-old Caucasian female patient presented with progressive throat pain that had started 4 months previously, followed by episodes of choking on liquids. She admitted to tobacco use, with a 45 pack-year smoking history, and social alcohol use. The patient was otherwise healthy without significant comorbidities of dyspnea or pulmonary disease.

At the time of the consultation, the patient was healthy and presented some mild hoarseness. There was no lymphadenopathy. A direct laryngoscopy revealed an ulcer-infiltrative lesion in the right aryepiglottic fold, without extension to the anterior commissure or the glottis. The mobility of both vocal folds was normal. The lesion did not extend to the infraglottis, ventricle, or ipsilateral arytenoid.

For a better deeper evaluation of the extension of the lesion, and to assess the nodal disease burden, a CT scan with contrast, using fine cuts through the larynx, was performed. There were no signs of extension to the glottis or the paraglottic space (▶Fig. 3.1).

The ease of exposure of the tumor was confirmed with an operative endoscopy. The anatomopathological result showed a moderately differentiated squamous cell carcinoma. In order to facilitate control of the airway and improve surgical access, a tracheotomy was performed. Exposure of the lesion was obtained using a Flex retractor. The tumor was localized to the aryepiglottic region, without extension to the piriform sinuses or the postcricoid area (▶Fig. 3.2).

The patient then underwent a transoral robotic resection of the lesion using the Medrobotics Flex surgical robot. The surgical margins of resection required excision of the aryepiglottic fold, portion of the epiglottis, and mucosal resection for the interarytenoid area. Both arytenoids were preserved. The Flex robot was placed into the mouth and the tumor was exposed and prepared for resection.

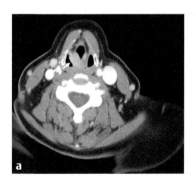
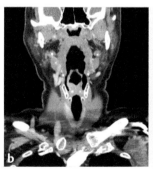

Fig. 3.1 MRI scan, in transversal and coronal scan, evidencing a lesion at the left vocal fold and partial invasion of the paraglottic space.

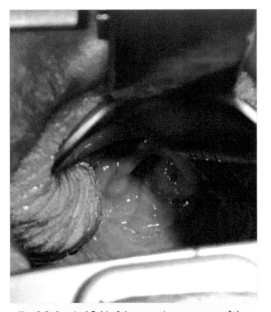

Fig. 3.2 Surgical field of the resection: exposure of the tumor using a Flex retractor. The extent of the tumor is easily seen, allowing for the verification of the tumor at direct view.

For the performance of the surgery, the tumor was exposed using the Flex retractor. This afforded excellent visualization of the tumor and surrounding anatomy. The resection was commenced by identifying the margins of the tumor. These extended anteriorly/medially to involve the hemiepiglottis, laterally to the pharyngoepiglottic fold, and posteriorly to the arytenoid. The dissection was initiated by transecting the epiglottis. The dissection was then carried laterally by incising into the mucosa in the vallecula. This allowed for dissection in the lateral aspect of the tumor. The pharyngoepiglottic fold was then transected. In this area, we encountered the arterial supply to the larynx, the superior laryngeal artery. This vessel was controlled using bipolar cautery and hemostatic clips. The remainder of the dissection is continued posteriorly. The arytenoid mucosa was preserved, but the aryepiglottic fold was completely resected to ensure adequacy of resection. The medial limit of the dissection is the interarytenoid space, which is preserved to avoid posterior glottic stenosis. It is important to note that the deep margin of resection must be assessed intraoperatively, by paying careful attention to the depth of resection. Additionally, the surgical assistant can use suction cannula to palpate the tissues, to ensure adequate resection margins.

Intraoperative pathologic consultation is used to ensure that the surgical margins are free of malignant disease. This is accomplished by submitted representative margins from the main resection specimen (▶ Fig. 3.3).

After finishing tumor resection, hemostasis is obtained in the surgical field using vasoconstrictive agents (such as dilute epinephrine or oxymetazoline) in combination with bipolar cautery. The tracheostomy is maintained until the lymphadenectomy is completed. The patient was returned to the operating theater 1 week later. At this time, bilateral neck dissections, levels 2 to 4, were performed.

The histopathological report showed well-differentiated squamous cell carcinoma adjacent to the thyroid cartilage, but with no invasion (▶ Fig. 3.4).

The patient progressed satisfactorily; the tracheotomy was occluded and the patient was discharged. The nasoenteral tube was retained for a total of 5 days. The tracheostomy tube was removed after the postoperative visit on postoperative day 10.

3.2 Discussion

In recent years, despite the new radiotherapy techniques and chemotherapy, surgery still offers excellent oncological results for patients with early-stage laryngeal cancer.[1,2,3,4] Radiotherapy, laser endoscopic excision, transoral robotic resection, and vertical partial laryngectomies in selected cases have been successfully used in the treatment of early-stage carcinomas.[1,2,3,4]

The decision between surgery and nonsurgical treatment in laryngeal cancer is a complex one. The treating physician must consider the patient's clinical condition (specifically the condition/function of the larynx), the patient's ability to tolerate and comply with 6 to 8 weeks of radiation/chemoradiotherapy, and their acceptance of a temporary tracheostomy. Most importantly, there must be shared decision-making so that the patient feels empowered in the decision-making process.

Arshad et al reported on data from the Surveillance, Epidemiology and End Results Program (SEER) database showing that conservation surgery with neck dissection yields improved oncologic outcomes when compared to radiation only for patients with early-stage/low-volume disease.[5] A recent meta-analysis suggested that surgical therapy for T1–T2 disease resulted in excellent control rates, although a definitive comparison to

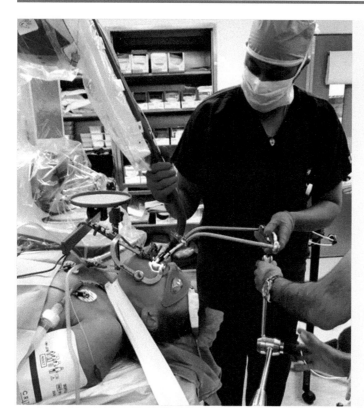

Fig. 3.3 Docking of the surgical robot. The Flex surgical robot is brought into the field and the robotic arm is introduced into the mouth. This allows for visualization of the tumor and dissection using the manually operated instruments.

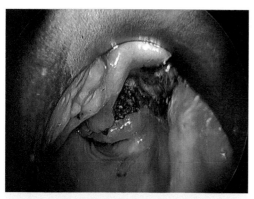

Fig. 3.4 Postresection view of the operative field. The postresection view demonstrates adequate resection of the lesion while preserving the integrity of the true vocal folds and the piriform sinuses.

intensity-modulated radiation therapy (IMRT) was limited by a lack of data.[6]

In the author's opinion, surgical treatment options should be offered to patients with low-volume disease who are at a high likelihood of avoiding adjuvant therapy. Adjuvant therapy after partial laryngeal surgery is often associated with

increased rates of dysphagia and possibly aspiration. The decision to subject the patient to adjuvant therapy is frequently driven by the nodal status (multiple positive nodes, and extranodal extension). Therefore, we prefer to limit surgical therapy to patients with T1–2 N0–1 disease.

In recent years, there has been a shift from performing open supraglottic laryngectomy to minimally invasive techniques such as transoral laser or transoral robotic resections. Transoral surgeries are associated with reduced rates of tracheotomy and quicker decannulation, if tracheotomy is performed.[7,8]

Supraglottic cancers have a high propensity for nodal metastases. Therefore, elective nodal dissection is recommended for these patients. If open partial surgery is performed, nodal dissection can be accomplished at the same time. When transoral surgery is performed, the decision can be made about whether to perform nodal dissection simultaneously or to stage the procedure. Each approach has advantages and disadvantages.

The main advantage of simultaneous dissection is that the operation can be performed at a single stage, eliminating the need for another operation. If availability of the surgical robot is limited, it may be advantageous to perform the nodal dissection at another time, so as to increase the utilization of the surgical robotic system. Another advantage with staging of neck dissections is to allow for clearance of surgical margins at the time of nodal dissection, particularly if the primary tumor resection results in a close or positive surgical margin.

Once the decision has been made to undertake a transoral resection, especially using a robotic system, the patient should be evaluated for candidacy. One of the key elements in facilitating surgical resection is exposure of the tumor. The patient should be evaluated for adequacy of exposure. This can be accomplished by performing an operative endoscopy prior to scheduling the extirpative procedure. After significant experience is obtained, the surgeon will be able to determine if a particular patient is a good candidate for transoral resection based on in-office consultation.

Some key cephalometric parameters can be useful in assessing adequacy of exposure. The patient should be able to extend the neck, and open the mouth. A high-arched palate, short thyromental distance, and narrow mandible are associated with increased difficulty of exposure.

One of the main advantages of transoral resection for laryngeal cancer is the ability to minimize tissue trauma by avoiding transcervical dissection. This potentially facilitates enhanced recovery. Transoral approaches facilitate a direct approach to the tumor, thereby obviating the need for reconstruction. The resection bed is often left to heal by intention and therefore does not routinely require reconstruction. Of course, in the case of large defects or if there is concern for communication into the fascial planes/spaces of the cervical region, a reconstructive option should be considered.

3.3 Tips

- Discuss at length with the patient the expectations for swallowing results, and options for other types of treatment, including radiotherapy.
- The ability to expose the lesion should be assessed, ideally in the operating room using a variety of retractors.
- Tumor extension and structures that need to be resected to ensure negative margins should be carefully assessed and mapping biopsies should be performed as indicated. We prefer to use mapping biopsies if an operative endoscopy is performed prior to resection.
- A protective tracheotomy should be considered in patients with difficult exposure, or those that

will require resection/dissection of the interarytenoid area.
- Partial laryngeal surgery will cause temporary dysphagia. A nasogastric feeding should be inserted to facilitate alimentation.

3.4 Traps

- Be careful with the staging! A T1b tumor that infiltrates the thyroid cartilage becomes a T4a tumor. Thus, it is important to perform a complementary image examination (CT or MRI).
- Inadequate exposure will compromise the quality of the resection. The ability to adequately expose the tumor must be carefully considered.
- Be careful with elderly patients and those with obstructive chronic pulmonary diseases.
- Invasion of the paraglottic and/or pre-epiglottic space will change the stage of the tumor to T3 and therefore the indication to perform conservation laryngeal surgery.

References

[1] Bhattacharyya T, Kainickal CT. Current status of organ preservation in carcinoma larynx. World J Oncol. 2018; 9(2):39–45
[2] Gorphe P. A contemporary review of evidence for transoral robotic surgery in laryngeal cancer. Front Oncol. 2018; 8:121
[3] Guimarães AV, Dedivitis RA, Matos LL, Aires FT, Cernea CR. Comparison between transoral laser surgery and radiotherapy in the treatment of early glottic cancer: a systematic review and meta-analysis. Sci Rep. 2018; 8(1):11900
[4] Pedregal-Mallo D, Sánchez Canteli M, López F, Álvarez-Marcos C, Llorente JL, Rodrigo JP. Oncological and functional outcomes of transoral laser surgery for laryngeal carcinoma. Eur Arch Otorhinolaryngol. 2018; 275(8):2071–2077
[5] Arshad H, Jayaprakash V, Gupta V, et al. Survival differences between organ preservation surgery and definitive radiotherapy in early supraglottic squamous cell carcinoma. Otolaryngol Head Neck Surg. 2014; 150(2):237–244
[6] Swanson MS, Low G, Sinha UK, Kokot N. Transoral surgery vs intensity-modulated radiotherapy for early supraglottic cancer: a systematic review. Curr Opin Otolaryngol Head Neck Surg. 2017; 25(2):133–141
[7] Ansarin M, Cattaneo A, De Benedetto L, et al. Retrospective analysis of factors influencing oncologic outcome in 590 patients with early-intermediate glottic cancer treated by transoral laser microsurgery. Head Neck. 2017; 39(1):71–81
[8] Ansarin M, Zabrodsky M, Bianchi L, et al. Endoscopic CO_2 laser surgery for early glottic cancer in patients who are candidates for radiotherapy: results of a prospective non-randomized study. Head Neck. 2006; 28(2):121–125

4 T1b Glottic Cancer Treated with Transoral Laser Surgery

Filippo Carta, Roberto Puxeddu

Abstract

T1b squamous cell carcinoma (SCC) of the glottis can be treated with radiotherapy or transoral laser surgery. Radiotherapy is usually advocated since voice results are considered better compared to transoral laser surgery; nevertheless, the transoral approach is also frequently performed for T1b at the request of the patients. In such cases, special care is needed to avoid unexpected scar. This chapter reports the typical case of a T1b SCC of the glottis with involvement of the anterior commissure observed in a 69-year-old male with a clinical history of daily cigarette smoking for 20 years, and progressive hoarseness lasting for 1 year, who underwent en bloc bilateral subligamental type II cordectomy. The patient, after 3 years of follow-up, is free of cancer. The endoscopic treatment in the form of type II cordectomy was chosen for the following reasons: (1) the surgical strategy has the advantages of a histologically proven resection without residual cancer and, in case of recurrence a further surgical treatment (including transoral surgery) and also radiotherapy are still available; (2) early cancer of the glottis is associated with a low incidence of occult metastasis and there is no indication for the neck dissection in cN0 patients; (3) the transoral approach allows for treatment of the cancer with minimal complications, low trauma to healthy tissue, and without the need for tracheostomy and/or nasogastric feeding tube; (4) the patient requested to be treated quickly in one stage. In our opinion, transoral CO_2 laser microsurgery is an important treatment option in T1b cancer of glottis.

Keywords: T1b glottic carcinoma, CO_2 laser, laryngeal microsurgery

4.1 Clinical Case

The eighth edition of the American Joint Committee on Cancer (AJCC) – TNM classification of laryngeal malignancies defines T1 cancer of the glottis as a cancer limited to the vocal cord(s) that may involve the anterior or posterior commissure with normal mobility; the cancer is classified as T1b when it involves both vocal cords.[1]

The role of open partial horizontal laryngectomy (OPHL) for the management of laryngeal squamous cell carcinoma (SCC) has decreased considerably in the last 15 years owing to the development of transoral laser microsurgery and with advances in radiation therapy.[2]

Although voice outcomes after transoral laser surgery for T1a cancer have been reported to be extremely favorable with type I to III cordectomies, results after endoscopic treatment for T1b can be worse, especially if the anterior commissure is involved and the resection is performed in one stage.

We report a typical case of a T1b SCC of the glottis with anterior commissure involvement observed in a 69-year-old male.

The patient reported a clinical history of daily cigarette smoking for 20 years, no alcohol intake, and progressive hoarseness during the past year.

Flexible laryngoscope examination of the larynx revealed a mildly vegetating leukoerythroplastic lesion of the glottis with superficial involvement of the anterior commissure and without impairment of the vocal cord mobility.

Voice analysis showed a voice handicap index (VHI) of, the grade, roughness, breathiness, asthenia, and strain (GRBAS) scale showed the following scores: 3, 3, 1, 1, and 2.

During preoperative counseling, the patient expressed his wish to be treated in one stage in the form of an excisional biopsy.

The day of surgery, the patient received ceftriaxone (1,000 mg IV) as antibiotic prophylaxis. The patient was evaluated under general anaesthesia using an endotracheal Mallinckrodt tube (internal diameter of 5.0–7.0 mm; Athlone, Ireland), and using white light and image-enhanced system (▶ Fig. 4.1), in order to assess the precise superficial extension of the lesion, to search for synchronous primary cancers, and to identify other precancerous lesions. The endoscopic evaluation was also associated with a contact endoscope performing an image-enhanced contact endoscopy (Image-ECE) that revealed a vascular pattern grade 4 according

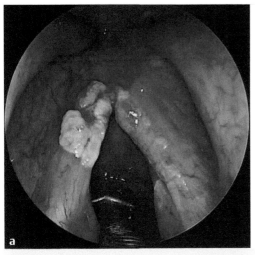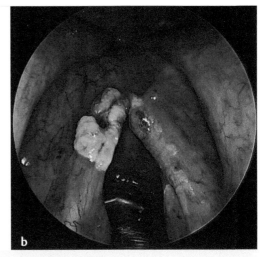

Fig. 4.1 Endoscopic view with Image1 S: white light **(a)** and Spectra A **(b)** modalities.

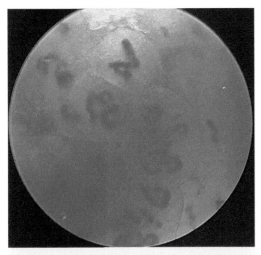

Fig. 4.2 Image-enhanced contact endoscopy ×60 of the cancer seen with Clara + Chroma modality, showing a vascular pattern IV suspicious for squamous cell carcinoma, according to the classification of Puxeddu et al.[3]

to the classification of Puxeddu et al[3] (▶Fig. 4.2), highly suspicious for SCC.

Palpation of the lesion showed adherence to the vocal ligament that was confirmed at hydrodissection.

After the intraoperative evaluation, the patient underwent en bloc bilateral subligamental type II cordectomy (▶Fig. 4.3 and ▶Fig. 4.4), according to the classification of the European Laryngological Society,[4,5] in macroscopically healthy tissue. The procedure was performed using Zeiss S21 (Jena, Germany) with 400-mm focal lens coupled with a AcuPulse (Tel Aviv, Israel) CO_2 laser with an AcuBlade (Tel Aviv, Israel) focusing system, with which it was possible to obtain a 150 µm spot. The superpulsed mode was used at 10 W in continuous wave. This technique allowed a precise dissection with minimal charring with the complete preservation of the vocalis muscle.

The postoperative course was uneventful, and the patient was discharged from the hospital after 2 days. On the 6th and 14th day after surgery, he underwent flexible scope examination under local anaesthesia with removal of the fibrin from the glottis.

Definitive histologic examination revealed a pT1b SCC according to the AJCC–TNM classification[1] resected in free margins of more than 0.5 mm.

The patient, after 3 years of follow-up, is free of cancer (▶Fig. 4.5). The last voice analysis performed 3 years after surgery showed a VHI of 20, the GRBAS scale showed the following scores: 2, 2, 0, 1, and 1.

4.2 Discussion

Most of the studies in the literature analyzed patients with T1a and T1b cancer together who are often considered as affected by T1N0 glottic SCC. Disease-free survival rate for T1b glottic SCC is reported to be slightly lower (85 vs. 88%);

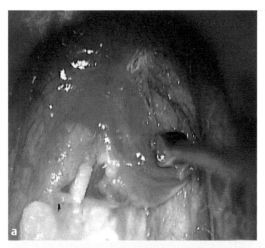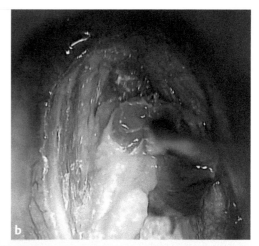

Fig. 4.3 Intraoperative view of the progressive dissection of the anterior commissure.

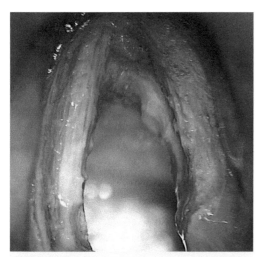

Fig. 4.4 Endoscopic view of the surgical field after type II bilateral cordectomy.

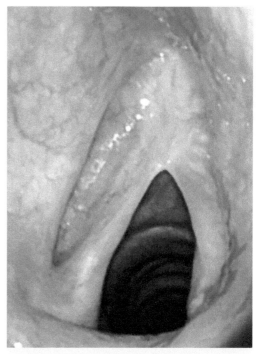

Fig. 4.5 Fibrolaryngoscopic view 3 years after surgery demonstrating an anterior commissure web but no cancer.

conversely, only a minimal difference was observed in disease-specific survival rates for T1b in comparison to T1a patients (respectively, 96 vs. 97%).[6]

Bilateral lesions can be treated endoscopically with good oncologic results, but voice outcomes can be poor as the result of the bilateral impairment of the mucosal wave and scar. The anterior commissure has been identified in several studies as a laryngeal subsite at risk for local treatment failure, especially when the vertical plane of the anterior commissure is involved,[7,8,9] and some investigators believe that anterior commissure involvement should be a contraindication to endoscopic laser surgery.[10] Avoiding the long discussion about the negative impact of the anterior commissure involvement on local control, the most evident complication after the removal of T1b with anterior commissure involvement in en bloc procedure is an anterior commissure web with mild to severe stenosis.

4.2.1 Different Approaches

Radiotherapy offers good voice and oncologic outcomes in patients with early glottic SCC, but it is a time-consuming and expensive procedure; no statistically significant alteration of the fundamental frequency was found in T1 patients who underwent radiotherapy and those who underwent endoscopic surgery; neither treatment can be considered superior from the patients' point of view.[11]

Sjögren et al studied a series of 36 patients who had involvement of the anterior commissure who had radiotherapy as their primary treatment. Their 5-year local control and laryngeal preservation rates were 88 and 91%, respectively.[12]

OPHLs still play an important role in contemporary conservative management of laryngeal cancer. Mendenhall et al, in 2004, compared the results of several studies dealing with the management of T1–T2 cancer. Local control rates after laser excision ranged from 80 to 90% for T1 cancer, and OPHL showed local control ranges from 90 to 95%.[13] However, in recent years, traditional OPHLs have been largely replaced by transoral laser microsurgery for most T1 and some T2 lesions of the larynx, since it results in less morbidity.[14,15]

In reviewing the first major series of supracricoid laryngectomy, the majority of the cases were T1b with or without anterior commissure involvement; currently laser surgery has dramatically reduced the need for open partial laryngectomy, which is the great advantage of the transoral approach for the trauma to healthy tissue, while conventional open surgery requires dissection through the skin and disrupts the integrity of the cartilage to gain best exposure to the tumor site.[16]

Different authors reported good oncologic outcomes after endoscopic surgery for glottic lesions with or without anterior commissure involvement: Rödel et al studied 89 T1 glottic cancer patients and reported 21 local recurrences; their 5-year local control, laryngeal preservation rate, ultimate local control, and overall survival were 71, 95, 98, and 88%, respectively[17]; Motta et al evaluated 169 patients, and their 5-year ultimate local control and overall survival rates were 83 and 84%, respectively[18]; Gallo et al studied 22 patients, and their local control and overall survival were 91 and 95%, respectively[18]; Peretti et al in a retrospective analysis of 595 patients with Tis–T3 glottic cancer reported an overall 5-year organ-preservation rate of 97.1% (98.5% for Tis, 98.1% for T1, 95% for T2, and 72% for T3).[8]

4.2.2 Rationale for Considering the Therapeutic Decision

The optimal treatment of laryngeal cancer should be individualized according to the size and extent of the cancer, the age, and physical condition of the patient and his needs; the skill and experience of the surgeon also play an important role, but the center should offer all the possible options for the best oncological results while preserving laryngeal functions.

The endoscopic treatment in the form of type II cordectomy was chosen on the basis of the following considerations:
- Compared to primary radiotherapy, surgical approach has the advantages of a histologically proven resection without residual cancer, and, in case of recurrences, a further surgical treatment (including transoral surgery) and radiotherapy are still available.[17]
- Early cancer of the glottis is associated with a low incidence of occult metastasis[20] and there is no indication for the surgical treatment of the neck in cN0 patients.
- Although the endoscopic CO_2 laser treatment and OPHL yield similar local control and survival rates, the transoral approach allows treatment of the cancer with minimal complications, minimal trauma to healthy tissue, and the convenience of sparing a tracheostomy and nasogastric feeding tube.[17]
- Last but not least, the choice of the patient to treat the cancer in the most expedited manner.

4.3 Tips

Laryngeal exposure is one of the most limiting factors in transoral CO_2 laser microsurgery. A complete and proper endoscopic exposure of the anterior commissure, may be difficult in some instances for the narrow-angle and V-shaped configuration of the thyroid cartilage; as a consequence, a complete set of laryngoscopes is mandatory, and for difficult exposures, smaller laryngoscopes of different shapes are required. A wide resection of the vocal false cord and good external counterpressure during surgery can also be useful.[9] The lack of dentures in this particular case allowed for an easy approach.

In the case of bilateral glottic carcinoma of the anterior third of the vocal cords with healthy mucosa at the anterior commissure, a two-step procedure can be accomplished in selected cases, with the most prominent lesion excised first and the contralateral lesion excised 3 to 4 weeks later, to reduce the risk of anterior web formation.

The anterior commissure can be treated by a wide subperichondrial resection, by dissecting the inner aspect of the cartilage that attaches to Broyles' ligament and removing the dense fibroelastic tissue of this area,[21] or by a superficial dissection in the form of type I or II cordectomies if the lesion is in situ or microinvasive as evaluated by hydrodissection. The CO_2 laser with new-generation micromanipulators offers a very gentle tool to perform a precise resection.

Since the infiltration of the vocalis muscle occurs in only 2.6 to 5.5% of patients affected by T1 glottic carcinoma,[21,22] lesions limited to one vocal cord with slight impairments of laryngostroboscopic findings would benefit oncologically from a type II resection, while more extended cordectomies (types III–V) should be reserved for cases of invasive SCC involving the vocalis muscle. In the cases of previous vocal cord "stripping," type II cordectomy is usually mandatory.

The intraoperative evaluation allows not only for a "biologic" endoscopy but also for the precise staging and recording of the lesion. Biologic endoscopy in this case was accurate in predicting the histology.

4.4 Traps

While subperichondrial resection for more locally advanced T1b (major anterior commissure involvement) appears to be burdened by less *webbing*, the superficial en bloc resection of a T1b lesion is usually followed by major scar on the glottic plane and this has to be considered for patients who need their voice. In these cases, radiotherapy should be considered; the removal of fibrin to reduce the entity of the web may be also used.

References

[1] Amin MB, Greene FL, Edge SB, et al. The eighth edition AJCC Cancer Staging Manual: continuing to build a bridge from a population-based to a more "personalized" approach to cancer staging CA Cancer J Clin. 2017; 67:93–99

[2] Marcotullio D, de Vincentiis M, Iannella G, Bigelli C, Magliulo G. Surgical treatment of T1b glottic tumor, 10-years follow-up. Eur Rev Med Pharmacol Sci. 2014; 18(8):1212–1217

[3] Puxeddu R, Sionis S, Gerosa C, Carta F. Enhanced contact endoscopy for the detection of neoangiogenesis in tumors of the larynx and hypopharynx. Laryngoscope. 2015; 125(7):1600–1606

[4] Remacle M, Eckel HE, Antonelli A, et al. Endoscopic cordectomy. A proposal for a classification by the Working Committee, European Laryngological Society. Eur Arch Otorhinolaryngol. 2000; 257(4):227–231

[5] Remacle M, Van Haverbeke C, Eckel H, et al. Proposal for revision of the European Laryngological Society classification of endoscopic cordectomies. [Erratum]. Eur Arch Otorhinolaryngol. 2007; 264(5):499–504

[6] Gioacchini FM, Tulli M, Kaleci S, Bondi S, Bussi M, Re M. Therapeutic modalities and oncologic outcomes in the treatment of T1b glottic squamous cell carcinoma: a systematic review. Eur Arch Otorhinolaryngol. 2017; 274(12):4091–4102

[7] O'Hara J, Markey A, Homer JJ. Transoral laser surgery versus radiotherapy for tumour stage 1a or 1b glottic squamous cell carcinoma: systematic review of local control outcomes. J Laryngol Otol. 2013; 127(8):732–738

[8] Peretti G, Piazza C, Cocco D, et al. Transoral CO(2) laser treatment for T(is)-T(3) glottic cancer: the University of Brescia experience on 595 patients. Head Neck. 2010; 32(8):977–983

[9] Carta F, Bandino F, Olla AM, Chuchueva N, Gerosa C, Puxeddu R. Prognostic value of age, subglottic, and anterior commissure involvement for early glottic carcinoma treated with CO_2 laser transoral microsurgery: a retrospective, single-center cohort study of 261 patients. Eur Arch Otorhinolaryngol. 2018; 275(5):1199–1210

[10] Mortuaire G, Francois J, Wiel E, Chevalier D. Local recurrence after CO_2 laser cordectomy for early glottic carcinoma. Laryngoscope. 2006; 116(1):101–105

[11] Lombardo N, Aragona T, Alsayyad S, Pelaia G, Terracciano R, Savino R. Objective and self-evaluation voice analysis after transoral laser cordectomy and radiotherapy in T1a-T1b glottic cancer. Lasers Med Sci. 2018; 33(1):141–147

[12] Sjögren EV, Langeveld TP, Baatenburg de Jong RJ. Clinical outcome of T1 glottic carcinoma since the introduction of endoscopic CO_2 laser surgery as treatment option. Head Neck. 2008; 30(9):1167–1174

[13] Mendenhall WM, Werning JW, Hinerman RW, Amdur RJ, Villaret DB. Management of T1-T2 glottic carcinomas. Cancer. 2004; 100(9):1786–1792

[14] Succo G, Peretti G, Piazza C, et al. Open partial horizontal laryngectomies: a proposal for classification by the working committee on nomenclature of the European Laryngological Society. Eur Arch Otorhinolaryngol. 2014; 271(9):2489–2496

[15] Succo G, Crosetti E, Bertolin A, et al. Benefits and drawbacks of open partial horizontal laryngectomies, part A: early- to intermediate-stage glottic carcinoma. Head Neck. 2016; 38(suppl 1):E333–E340

[16] Weiss BG, Ihler F, Pilavakis Y, et al. Transoral laser microsurgery for T1b glottic cancer: review of 51 cases. Eur Arch Otorhinolaryngol. 2017; 274(4):1997–2004

[17] Rödel RM, Steiner W, Müller RM, Kron M, Matthias C. Endoscopic laser surgery of early glottic cancer: involvement of the anterior commissure. Head Neck. 2009; 31(5):583–592

[18] Motta G, Esposito E, Motta S, Tartaro G, Testa D. CO_2 laser surgery in the treatment of glottic cancer. Head Neck. 2005; 27(7):566-573

[19] Gallo A, de Vincentiis M, Manciocco V, Simonelli M, Fiorella ML, Shah JP. CO_2 laser cordectomy for early-stage glottic carcinoma: a long-term follow-up of 156 cases. Laryngoscope. 2002; 112(2):370–374

[20] Ansarin M, Cattaneo A, De Benedetto L, et al. Retrospective analysis of factors influencing oncologic outcome in 590 patients with early-intermediate glottic cancer treated by transoral laser microsurgery. Head Neck. 2017; 39(1):71–81

[21] Peretti G, Nicolai P, Piazza C, Redaelli de Zinis LO, Valentini S, Antonelli AR. Oncological results of endoscopic resections of Tis and T1 glottic carcinomas by carbon dioxide laser. Ann Otol Rhinol Laryngol. 2001; 110(9):820–826

[22] Pittore B, Ismail-Koch H, Davis A, et al. Thyroarytenoid muscle invasion in T1 glottic carcinoma. Eur Arch Otorhinolaryngol. 2009; 266(11):1787–1791

5 T1b Glottic Cancer

Yao Yu, Nancy Y. Lee

Abstract

Early-stage squamous cell carcinomas of the glottic larynx can be treated with either larynx-preserving surgery or definitive radiotherapy with high rates of cure and excellent voice preservation. T1b cancers involving both vocal folds represent a unique cohort deserving of special anatomic and staging considerations. In this chapter, we discuss strategies for patient selection, with particular attention to the significance of anterior commissure involvement and depth of invasion. Practical guidelines for radiation simulation, field design, and dose fractionation are reviewed, along with common clinical pitfalls. Investigational strategies, including intensity-modulated radiotherapy, are also explored.

Keywords: glottic cancer, anterior commissure, larynx preservation, cordectomy, intensity-modulated radiotherapy, accelerated fractionation

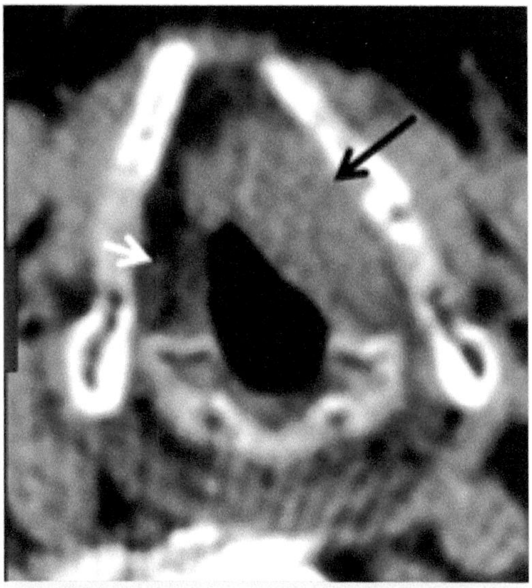

Fig. 5.1 Thin-cut CT can reveal paraglottic extension and anterior extension that is not appreciated on clinical examination.

5.1 Introduction

Patients with Tis-T2 cancer of the glottis can be treated with larynx-preserving strategies such as radiotherapy, transoral laser microsurgery (TLM), or open partial laryngectomy. Within this group, patients with T1b disease represent a unique subset requiring special consideration and careful attention to the anatomic extent of disease, resectability, and voice quality.

5.2 Evaluation

A complete history, including current or former tobacco use, changes in voice quality, and history of rigorous voice use, is important for discussion of treatment options.

Careful evaluation of the larynx using indirect laryngoscopy, video stroboscopy, and direct laryngoscopy is essential for pretreatment staging and decision-making. Evaluation should include an assessment of anterior commissure (AC) involvement, extent and location of mucosal disease, supra- or infraglottic extension, and impairment of vocal fold mobility. On direct laryngoscopy and biopsy, the depth of invasion may have prognostic implications for voice quality following TLM.

For patients with a bulky cancer or cancer involving the AC, thin-cut CT of the neck or MRI may be useful for identifying early cartilage invasion or paraglottic extension that is not appreciated on clinical examination alone (▶Fig. 5.1). Imaging may also be useful in cases with submucosal cancer, where clinical examination can underestimate the true extent of the cancer.

5.3 Selection of Treatment Modality

TLM and hemilaryngectomy are the primary alternatives to radiotherapy. TLM is minimally invasive and can achieve high rates of local control, although repeated applications are sometimes required. There are no randomized trials powered to assess the differences in oncologic outcomes between TLM and radiotherapy.[1,2,3,4,5] Depending on the extent of disease and treatment modality, excellent oncologic and voice outcomes can be achieved with both radiotherapy and TLM.[6,7,8] Compared with radiotherapy and TLM, hemilaryngectomy is associated with increased morbidity and is therefore reserved for bulky disease or as salvage.[9]

The selection of a definitive treatment modality is highly dependent upon the availability of technical expertise and referral patterns.

In practice, superficial lesions and lesions involving the posterior portions of the cord are often amenable to TLM with very limited morbidity. Lesions that are more deeply invasive, requiring European Laryngological Society (ELS) type III to VI resections, may be associated with poorer voice outcomes, and these cases are often referred for radiotherapy. Similarly, some authors routinely refer patients with AC involvement for radiotherapy due to concerns regarding operative exposure, difficulty achieving clear margins, and the potential for impaired vocal outcomes with extensive anterior commissure involvement.[10,11,12] Finally, many patients are referred for refractory disease despite multiple surgical attempts.

5.3.1 Anterior Commissure Involvement

Historically, AC involvement has been a negative prognostic factor for patients treated with either radiotherapy or TLM.[13]

Tumors involving the AC can be difficult to expose completely for resection, and it can be difficult to achieve negative margins at this location.[11,12,13,14,15] Hoffmann and colleagues showed that AC was associated with a disease-free survival of 54.6%, compared with 79.8% for cancers without AC involvement, and that a greater number of these patients required other modalities for salvage, including total laryngectomy.[11] Similarly, Rödel and colleagues found that AC involvement was associated with lower rates of local control with surgery (5-year local control 73 vs. 89% for T1a, 68 vs. 86% for T1b).[15] Other authors have reported higher rates of local control, albeit with a smaller number of patients.[12] Following resection, patients may be at risk for development of an anterior laryngeal web, which can negatively influence voice quality.

The prognostic importance of AC involvement on outcomes following radiotherapy is more controversial. Much of the clinical data supporting these findings come from an era predating the routine use of CT or MRI imaging and modern dosimetry, potentially resulting in cancers that were understaged or even missed. Additionally, many treatment series span decades and include patients treated with significant variability and technique and dosimetric precision. In a small series, Nozaki and colleagues[16] found AC involvement was associated with worse 5-year local control (58 vs. 89%) and potentially attributable to underdosage anteriorly. Chen and colleagues showed that the impact of AC involvement could be overcome by using higher doses per fraction.[17] In more contemporary series using accelerated fractionation and 3D dosimetry, the effect of AC involvement appears to be attenuated. Le and colleagues identified a difference of borderline statistical significance (80 vs. 91%) for patients with T1 lesions.[18] Chera and colleagues reported on a series of 585 patients with T1–T2 glottic larynx cancer treated with definitive radiation, including 369 patients with AC involvement. Patients with T1a and T1b disease achieved 10-year local control of 93 and 91%, and AC involvement was not associated with adverse outcomes.[19]

5.4 Voice Quality

Voice quality preservation is similar using both TLM and radiation. Aaltonen and colleagues conducted a randomized trial of TLM versus radiation for T1a cancers of the glottic larynx, using multimodal assessments of voice quality as the primary endpoint. Patients were assessed 6 and 24 months after treatment using expert-rated voice quality videolaryngostroboscopic findings, and self-rated voice quality. In this study, TLM was associated with a more breathy voice and a wider glottal gap. At 2 years, patients treated with radiation had less hoarseness-related inconvenience.[6] More recently, Ma and colleagues conducted a retrospective review of long-term voice quality for patients treated with TLM or radiotherapy for Tis-T2 cancer of the glottic larynx, to address the possibility that radiotherapy could result in long-term voice impairment. The authors report that TLM was associated with better expert-rated quality and objective voice measures, but this difference did not translate into a different patient-reported voice quality. Importantly, 76% of patients in this study were treated with type I and II cordectomies. The authors hypothesized that radiotherapy-associated voice changes may take longer to occur than postsurgical changes.[7] In contrast, Watson and colleagues followed patients for a mean of 11 years after radiotherapy and showed only slight deterioration in voice quality beyond 1 year of follow-up.[20]

5.4.1 Superficial versus Deeply Invasive Tumors

Tumors that are deeply invasive require more extensive surgery, which are in turn associated with worse voice outcomes. Lee and colleagues conducted a longitudinal study of voice quality before and after TLM for T1 glottic tumors. They demonstrated that patients who underwent type I or II cordectomies had improvement in their perceptual voice and voice handicap index (VHI) compared with pretreatment baseline, whereas those undergoing type III to V cordectomies did not. Patients who had T1b cancer or AC involvement experienced deterioration in their voice quality.[8] Similarly, Núñez Batalla and colleagues found that radiotherapy resulted in better voice outcomes compared with a group of TLM patients who were treated with transmuscular cordectomies.[21]

In our practice, patients with deep tissue extension requiring type III or greater cordectomies are referred for radiotherapy consultation.

5.5 Simulation and Planning

The traditional beam arrangements for early cancer of the glottis entail a pair of 5 × 5 cm opposed lateral beams centered on the vocal cords (▶ Fig. 5.2). The collimator is rotated to match the angle of the vertebrae. The borders are set as follows: anterior—1 cm anterior to the skin; posterior—anterior border of the vertebral body; superior—thyroid notch; and inferior—caudal to the cricoid cartilage.

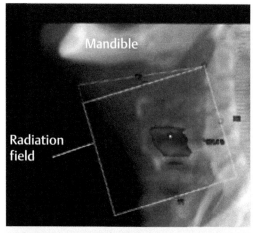

Fig. 5.2 A standard 5 × 5 cm field centered on the vocal cord with 1 cm anterior flash.

Wedges can be used to reduce anterior inhomogeneity with this approach; however, overwedging may result in a cold spot anteriorly, increasing the risk for local failure. Hot spots should be avoided. Attention to wedging is particularly important for patients with T1b disease who often have tumor near the anterior larynx or involving the AC. Thin patients and those patients with an angulated thyroid cartilage may require 0.5 to 1 cm of bolus anterior to the thyroid cartilage to ensure adequate buildup and coverage of the anterior cord. The plan should be adjusted until uniform coverage of the true cords, false cords, and the upper subglottis (▶ Fig. 5.3).

Patients with a short neck present a challenge for setup because the shoulders interrupt the path of the beam. For borderline cases, the arms and shoulders can be stretched inferiorly. Patients may be treated with a couch kick, at the cost of increased lung dose. At the Memorial Sloan Kettering Cancer Center (MSKCC), intensity-modulated radiotherapy is being for these patients.

Intensity-modulated radiotherapy is being investigated for early stage cancers of the larynx. This technique may improve sparing of adjacent normal tissues in the neck, including the carotid arteries, potentially mitigating long-term carotid artery stenosis.[22,23] This is of particular concern for patients with early larynx cancers because the majority of patients are cured with therapy and life expectancy is long (▶ Fig. 5.4).

5.6 Fractionation

Accelerated hypofractionated radiotherapy, 63 Gy in 28 fractions at 2.25 Gy per fraction, is our standard dose for T1 cancers of the larynx. The importance of fraction size was demonstrated in a randomized trial comparing hypofractionated radiotherapy (63 Gy/28 fractions) to standard fractionation (66 Gy/33 fractions). At 5 years, local control favored the hypofractionated arm (92 vs. 77%; $p = 0.004$), and there was no difference in acute or late toxicities. Cause-specific survival was high regardless of treatment arm due to the success of salvage surgery.[24] The Danish Head and Neck Cancer Group (DAHANCA) group randomized patients with nonmetastatic glottic cancers to five or six fractions per week, which was associated with lower local failures rates (13.7 vs. 22.0% at 10 years) and fewer disease-specific deaths for T1–T2 tumors.[25] Registry studies have shown improvement in local control over several decades,

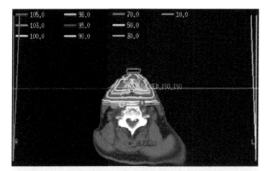

Fig. 5.3 A 2 × 2 cm slab of 0.5- to 1-cm-thick bolus can be used to improve coverage anteriorly.

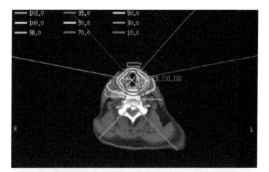

Fig. 5.4 Intensity-modulated radiotherapy is currently being studied to reduce the risk of carotid-sparing radiotherapy.

potentially attributable to increased use of altered fractionation, technical advances in radiotherapy, and reduced rates of smoking.[26]

5.7 Long-term Considerations and Secondary Malignancy

Long-term toxicities from radiation and concern regarding secondary malignancies are often cited as the primary reasons for withholding radiation, especially among younger patients. Among all patients with cancer of the head and neck treated with radiotherapy, the risk of a subsequent malignancy is approximately 25%; however, only 20% of these will occur in the head and neck.[26,27,28] These tumors are largely due to the field cancerization effects from known head and neck risk factors such as smoking and alcohol, rather than direct carcinogenic effects from radiotherapy.[29]

5.8 Smoking Cessation

Patients should be counseled on smoking cessation before initiation of treatment. Continued tobacco use is associated with worse local control, higher rates of secondary malignancy, and lower overall survival.[30]

References

[1] Sjögren EV. Transoral laser microsurgery in early glottic lesions. Curr Otorhinolaryngol Rep. 2017; 5(1):56–68

[2] Yoo J, Lacchetti C, Hammond JA, Gilbert RW; Head and Neck Cancer Disease Site Group. Role of endolaryngeal surgery (with or without laser) versus radiotherapy in the management of early (T1) glottic cancer: a systematic review Head Neck. 2014; 36:1807–1819

[3] Warner L, Chudasama J, Kelly CG, et al. Radiotherapy versus open surgery versus endolaryngeal surgery (with or without laser) for early laryngeal squamous cell cancer Cochrane Database Syst Rev. 2014; 3:CD002027

[4] Mendenhall WM, Werning JW, Hinerman RW, Amdur RJ, Villaret DB. Management of T1–T2 glottic carcinomas. Cancer. 2004; 100(9):1786–1792

[5] Higgins KM, Shah MD, Ogaick MJ, Enepekides D. Treatment of early-stage glottic cancer: meta-analysis comparison of laser excision versus radiotherapy. J Otolaryngol Head Neck Surg. 2009; 38(6):603–612

[6] Aaltonen L-M, Rautiainen N, Sellman J, et al. Voice quality after treatment of early vocal cord cancer: a randomized trial comparing laser surgery with radiation therapy. Int J Radiat Oncol Biol Phys. 2014; 90(2):255–260

[7] Ma Y, Green R, McCabe D, Goldberg L, Woo P. Long-term voice outcome following radiation versus laser microsurgery in early glottic cancer. J Voice. 2017: S0892–1997(17)30326–0

[8] Lee HS, Kim JS, Kim SW, et al. Voice outcome according to surgical extent of transoral laser microsurgery for T1 glottic carcinoma. Laryngoscope. 2016; 126(9):2051–2056

[9] Rosier JF, Grégoire V, Counoy H, et al. Comparison of external radiotherapy, laser microsurgery and partial laryngectomy for the treatment of T1N0M0 glottic carcinomas: a retrospective evaluation. Radiother Oncol. 1998; 48(2):175–183

[10] Hoffmann C, Cornu N, Hans S, Sadoughi B, Badoual C, Brasnu D. Early glottic cancer involving the anterior commissure treated by transoral laser cordectomy. Laryngoscope. 2016; 126(8):1817–1822

[11] Hoffmann C, Hans S, Sadoughi B, Brasnu D. Identifying outcome predictors of transoral laser cordectomy for early glottic cancer. Head Neck. 2016; 38(suppl 1):E406–E411

[12] Mendelsohn AH, Kiagiadaki D, Lawson G, Remacle M. CO_2 laser cordectomy for glottic squamous cell carcinoma involving the anterior commissure: voice and oncologic outcomes. Eur Arch Otorhinolaryngol. 2015; 272(2):413–418

[13] Bradley PJ, Rinaldo A, Suárez C, et al. Primary treatment of the anterior vocal commissure squamous carcinoma. Eur Arch Otorhinolaryngol. 2006; 263(10):879–888

[14] Chone CT, Yonehara E, Martins JEF, Altemani A, Crespo AN. Importance of anterior commissure in recurrence of early glottic cancer after laser endoscopic resection. Arch Otolaryngol Head Neck Surg. 2007; 133(9):882–887

[15] Rödel RMW, Steiner W, Müller RM, Kron M, Matthias C. Endoscopic laser surgery of early glottic cancer: involvement of the anterior commissure. Head Neck. 2009; 31(5):583–592

[16] Nozaki M, Furuta M, Murakami Y, et al. Radiation therapy for T1 glottic cancer: involvement of the anterior commissure. Anticancer Res. 2000; 20(2B):1121–1124

[17] Chen M-F, Chang JT-C, Tsang N-M, Liao CT, Chen WC. Radiotherapy of early-stage glottic cancer: analysis of factors affecting prognosis. Ann Otol Rhinol Laryngol. 2003; 112(10):904–911

[18] Le QT, Fu KK, Kroll S, et al. Influence of fraction size, total dose, and overall time on local control of T1–T2 glottic carcinoma. Int J Radiat Oncol Biol Phys. 1997; 39(1):115–126

[19] Chera BS, Amdur RJ, Morris CG, Kirwan JM, Mendenhall WM. T1N0 to T2N0 squamous cell carcinoma of the glottic larynx treated with definitive radiotherapy. Int J Radiat Oncol Biol Phys. 2010; 78(2):461–466

[20] Watson M, Drosdowsky A, Frowen J, Corry J. Voice outcomes after radiotherapy treatment for early glottic cancer: long-term follow-up. J Voice. 2017:S0892–1997(17)30264–3

[21] Núñez Batalla F, Caminero Cueva MJ, Señaris González B, et al. Voice quality after endoscopic laser surgery and radiotherapy for early glottic cancer: objective measurements emphasizing the Voice Handicap Index. Eur Arch Otorhinolaryngol. 2008; 265(5):543–548

[22] Gomez D, Cahlon O, Mechalakos J, Lee N. An investigation of intensity-modulated radiation therapy versus conventional two-dimensional and 3D-conformal radiation therapy for early stage larynx cancer. Radiat Oncol. 2010; 5:74

[23] Zumsteg ZS, Riaz N, Jaffery S, et al. Carotid sparing intensity-modulated radiation therapy achieves comparable locoregional control to conventional radiotherapy in T1–2N0 laryngeal carcinoma. Oral Oncol. 2015; 51(7):716–723

[24] Yamazaki H, Nishiyama K, Tanaka E, Koizumi M, Chatani M. Radiotherapy for early glottic carcinoma (T1N0M0): results of prospective randomized study of radiation fraction size and overall treatment time. Int J Radiat Oncol Biol Phys. 2006; 64(1):77–82

[25] Lyhne NM, Primdahl H, Kristensen CA, et al. The DAHANCA 6 randomized trial: Effect of 6 vs 5 weekly fractions of radiotherapy in patients with glottic squamous cell carcinoma. Radiother Oncol. 2015; 117(1):91–98

[26] Lyhne NM, Johansen J, Kristensen CA, et al. Pattern of failure in 5001 patients treated for glottic squamous cell carcinoma with curative intent: a population based study from the DAHANCA group. Radiother Oncol. 2016; 118(2):257–266

[27] McDonald S, Haie C, Rubin P, Nelson D, Divers LD. Second malignant tumors in patients with laryngeal carcinoma: diagnosis, treatment, and prevention. Int J Radiat Oncol Biol Phys. 1989; 17(3):457–465

[28] Cooper JS, Pajak TF, Rubin P, et al. Second malignancies in patients who have head and neck cancer: incidence, effect on survival and implications based on the RTOG experience. Int J Radiat Oncol Biol Phys. 1989; 17(3):449–456

[29] Berrington de Gonzalez A, Curtis RE, Kry SF, et al. Proportion of second cancers attributable to radiotherapy treatment in adults: a cohort study in the US SEER cancer registries. Lancet Oncol. 2011; 12(4):353–360

[30] Al-Mamgani A, van Rooij PH, Mehilal R, Verduijn GM, Tans L, Kwa SL. Radiotherapy for T1a glottic cancer: the influence of smoking cessation and fractionation schedule of radiotherapy. Eur Arch Otorhinolaryngol. 2014; 271(1):125–132

6 T1b Glottic Cancer, Vertical Partial Laryngectomy

André V. Guimarães, Marco A.V. Kulcsar

Abstract

T1b glottic cancer is a cancer that has more than one kind of treatment and the results are approximately the same. In some developed countries, the first treatment is radiotherapy and in others, transoral laryngectomies with or without laser. However, both treatments are expensive and need special materials. Despite the popularization of these techniques, vertical partial laryngectomy yields the same results, provides good voice rehabilitation, and does not need special materials. In this chapter, frontolateral (vertical) partial laryngectomy is described step by step, from diagnosis to surgery, with its tips and traps.

Keywords: laryngeal neoplasms, laryngectomy, glottic cancer, organ preservation, early laryngeal cancer

6.1 Case Report

A 45-year-old Caucasian male, laborer, presented to our clinic with a history of progressive dysphonia that had started 3 months previously, followed by dyspnea. He stated that he smoked one pack of cigarettes per day for 28 years as well as drinking 700 mL of draft beer during the weekend for the last 5 years. There were no comorbidities.

In the first evaluation, the patient presented a good general clinical condition and a 100% Karnofsky performance scale and complained of a 4-month dysphonia. He presented with hoarseness with little vocal range. No abnormalities were noticed during oroscopy and cervical palpation. Laryngoscopy revealed a vegetative mass occupying the entire right vocal fold (VF), up to the anterior commissure (AC). The left VF appeared normal. Both VFs presented normal mobility. The lesion did not extend to the infraglottis, ventricle or ipsilateral arytenoid (▶Fig. 6.1). He underwent a nasofibrolaryngoscopy and biopsy which revealed a squamous cell carcinoma.

For more detailed evaluation of the extension of the lesion, a CT scan was performed which demonstrated an irregular lesion on the right VF, with heterogeneous contrast enhancement, and no invasion of the paraglottic space or the AC, and, the ipsilateral arytenoid was preserved.

There were no signs of extension to the left VF. The patient underwent a frontolateral laryngectomy (FLL), under general anesthesia. Perioperative prophylactic antibiotics were administered. A tracheostomy was performed through a separate incision above the third tracheal ring. A second horizontal incision was made at approximately the level of the thyroid notch (▶Fig. 6.2a). Skin flaps were elevated above the hyoid and below the cricoid cartilage. The strap muscles were then elevated, exposing the thyroid lamina and external perichondrium. The thyroid cartilage was incised at the midline and a posteriorly based perichondrial flaps were elevated bilaterally (▶Fig. 6.2b). The extent of the elevation reflected the intended thyroid cartilage resection.

Vertical parallel thyroid cartilage cuts were made approximately 5 mm from each other including the notch (▶Fig. 6.2c).

A wide cricothyrotomy allowed access to the subglottis. The tumor occupied the right VF. The thyrotomy was performed extensively on both sides. The left VF was then incised 2 mm laterally from the AC, through the cricothyrotomy. A dissection was made on the right side from the thyroid cartilage and an incision above and below the fold was performed, with the tumor under direct visualization, with approximately 3 mm of margin up to the vocal process of the right arytenoid (▶Fig. 6.3 and ▶Fig. 6.4).

New margins from both sides of the VF were submitted to frozen section assessment and were free of tumor invasion. The left VF was fixed anteriorly to the residual thyroid cartilage and epiglottic residual petiole with a Vicryl suture. Reconstruction of the VF was done with a mucosal flap from

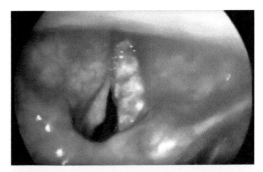

Fig. 6.1 Telelaryngoscopy with the tumor on the right vocal fold.

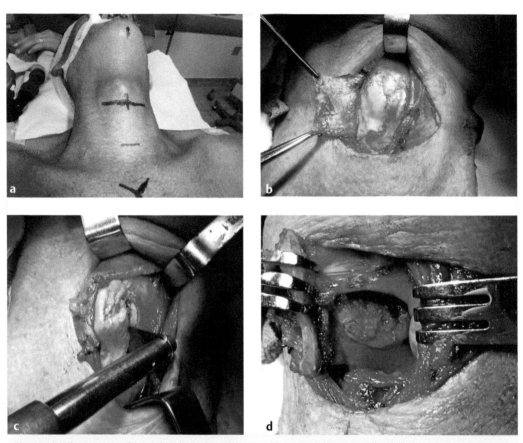

Fig. 6.2 (a) Skin incisions. (b) Perichondrium flap of the thyroid cartilage. (c) Cutting the thyroid cartilage. (d) Right vocal fold with the tumor.

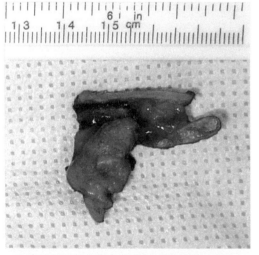

Fig. 6.3 Tumor specimen with the thyroid cartilage wedge.

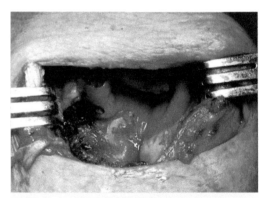

Fig. 6.4 View of the larynx without the right vocal fold.

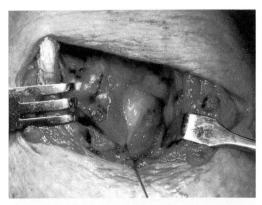

Fig. 6.5 Flap for reconstruction and fixation to the left vocal fold.

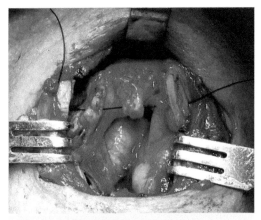

Fig. 6.6 Closure of the thyroid cartilage with the fixation of the epiglottis.

the ventricular fold (▸Fig. 6.5 and ▸Fig. 6.6). The thyroid cartilage was approximated in the midline with nylon suture and the strap muscles were approximated as a second layer. A Penrose drain was then inserted. The skin was reapproximated in layers and a cuffed tracheostomy tube was introduced.

The patient made satisfactory progress and was discharged on the third postoperative day; the tracheostomy was occluded on the seventh day and the cannula was removed 7 days later. The patient was found to be eupneic and the voice was rough. A laryngoscopy 3 months after the surgery showed edema on the right side of the larynx; on the left side, the VF was mobile. A histopathological specimen showed the tumor adjacent to AC cartilage (▸Fig. 6.7).

Fig. 6.7 Histopathological aspect, showing the tumor adjacent to anterior commissure cartilage (high magnification [HE], ×100x).

6.2 Discussion

T1b glottic carcinoma involves both VFs.[1] The goal of larynx-preservation therapy is to offer improved function and quality of life for patients with laryngeal cancer, without compromising survival.

The FLL technique for treating early-stage glottic carcinomas was first defined by Leroux-Robert in 1956.[2] FLL is applied for glottic cancers having a VF involvement, reaching the AC, the anterior are third of the opposite VF, and the overlying medial thyroid cartilage, but without impaired VC movement.[3] However, FLL should not be performed when there is extension to the ventricle and paraglottic space; or for infraglottic extension up to 2 to 3 mm. This procedure can achieve free margins with a reasonable limit, considering that a positive margin is a prognostic factor for local recurrence.[4,5] Previous biopsy is recommended in order to avoid

confusion with granulomatosis diseases (blastomycosis and tuberculosis). Tuberculosis and squamous cell carcinoma may also occur together.

The AC is a well-studied interface between soft tissues (Broyles' ligament) and cartilage that allows the spread of cancer due to the proximity of the thyroid cartilage to mucosa, absence of inner perichondrium, and the early ossification of the cartilage at this level. When a glottic cancer invades the supraglottic AC, the risk of cartilage invasion is higher.[6] Cartilage invasion may not affect VC mobility, increasing the risk of understaging. Consequently, a carcinoma with AC involvement requires more aggressive procedures, especially in the case of focal infiltration of the inner thyroid cartilage upstaging the cancer to T4a. FLL is not recommended for T4a stage; however, another laryngeal-preserving modality could be.

Radiotherapy sounds less aggressive for patients as a treatment option for larynx neoplasms, and for this purpose we observed an increase in indication for this nonsurgical approach due to patient preference. Radiotherapy is acceptable for cases without AC invasion; involvement is a predictor of poor response to radiotherapy.[7] In spite of this tendency, there is a selection treatment bias when comparing outcomes between surgery and radiotherapy groups. This bias is inherent in retrospective studies. We have observed in the literature the decrease in the vertical open partial laryngectomy approach, which was replaced by the endolaryngeal microscopic laser surgery technique, as it may avoid a tracheostomy with adequate oncological outcome, although it is possible to perform FLL without tracheostomy.[8] There is no doubt that endoscopic surgery is of great value, but underdeveloped countries may have few medical centers with appropriate expert surgeons and equipment for endolaryngeal oncological laser surgery. Nevertheless, there is no reason for shifting surgery indication to radiotherapy. In addition, in case of radiotherapy failure, salvage total laryngectomy was more than 13 times more common in patients treated with radiotherapy ($p = 0.002$) when compared to those who underwent surgery. Nevertheless, mortality due to recurrence did not differ between surgery and radiotherapy groups.[9] The prognostic significance of AC involvement in glottic cancer remains controversial. For instance, if there is any doubt as to AC invasion, it would be better to remove the AC and part of one or both VFs in a single unit, together with the cartilaginous framework at the cost of poorer functional outcome.[10]

FLL reconstruction of the endolarynx results in a neoglottic coaptation, thus raising maximum phonation time and avoiding aspiration. There are several techniques which can be used, such as bipedicled strap muscle transposition, epiglottic cartilage rotation, and ventricular band flap.

Inadequate endolaryngeal exposure is an anatomical factor that would shift endolaryngeal surgery to a transcervical approach.[11] This adequacy of endolaryngeal exposure may be evaluated by a laryngoscopy as a preoperative clinical predictor.[12]

There is no reason to compare voice outcome between FLL and endoscopic surgery. The evaluation of acoustic voice quality after FLL reconstructed with the bipedicled sternohyoid muscle flap showed an important increase in the fundamental frequency, and the values of all parameters were changed regardless of the AC synechia findings.[13] In our series, the voice was still rougher, but intelligible and swallowing was not a problem.

In conclusion, FLL is an effective option for T1b glottic tumor with voice preservation, without dysphasia and rare stenosis in need of definitive tracheostomy. Moreover, FLL allows for a supracricoid horizontal partial laryngectomy as a salvage surgery.

6.3 Tips

- FLL is recommended for T1b cancers with or without extension to the AC and up to the vocal process of one arytenoid.
- The infraglottic anterior extension up to 2 to 3 mm permits the procedure with free margins.
- One VF and up to one-thirds of the opposite vocal fold can be removed.
- After sawing the cartilage notch between two parallel lines, open the cricothyroid membrane and start incising the VF contralateral to the cancer.
- Remove part of the epiglottic petiole near the AC.
- When closing the larynx with three separate sutures, do not forget to fix the VF to the remaining epiglottic petiole, forming a neocommissure.
- Replace VF with a reconstructive technique suturing inside the larynx.
- No feeding tube is necessary.
- Inform the patient that every partial laryngectomy can shift to total in the same intraoperative stage.
- Discuss at length with the patient the expectations for vocal results, considering the other types of treatment, including radiotherapy.

6.4 Traps

- Check tumor stage (spread) under general anaesthesia (rigid laryngoscopy with Hopkins 30-degree optics). Ventricular, infraglottic, or posterior to arytenoid process disease may surprise you.
- Perform a complementary CT scan because a T1b tumor that infiltrates the thyroid cartilage becomes a T4a.
- Invasion of the pre-epiglottic or paraglottic spaces are contraindications.
- Thyroid cartilage may fracture with forceful closure.
- When closing the larynx, perforate the cartilage, then put the sutures through it.

- Be cautious when operating on elderly patients and those with chronic obstructive pulmonary diseases.
- Subcutaneous emphysema due to early tracheostomy closure or skin sutures placed too closely.
- If the tracheostomy remains in place more than 14 days. Evaluate for stenosis.

References

[1] Byrd DR, Greene FL. The eighth edition of TNM: implications for the surgical oncologist. Ann Surg Oncol. 2018; 25(1):10–12

[2] Leroux-Robert J. Conservative surgery in cancer of larynx Boll Soc Med Chir Cremona. 1956; 10(4):68–76

[3] Fiorella R, Di Nicola V, Mangiatordi F, Fiorella ML. Indications for frontolateral laryngectomy and prognostic factors of failure. Eur Arch Otorhinolaryngol. 1999; 256(8):423–425

[4] Dedivitis RA, de Andrade-Sobrinho J, de Castro MA. Prognostic factors and comorbidity impact upon the frontolateral laryngectomy Rev Col Bras Cir. 2009; 36(5):392–397

[5] Peretti G, Piazza C, Bolzoni A, et al. Analysis of recurrences in 322 Tis, T1, or T2 glottic carcinomas treated by carbon dioxide laser. Ann Otol Rhinol Laryngol. 2004; 113(11):853–858

[6] Ulusan M, Unsaler S, Basaran B, Yılmazbayhan D, Aslan I. The incidence of thyroid cartilage invasion through the anterior commissure in clinically early-staged laryngeal cancer. Eur Arch Otorhinolaryngol. 2016; 273(2):447–453

[7] Maheshwar AA, Gaffney CC. Radiotherapy for T1 glottic carcinoma: impact of anterior commissure involvement. J Laryngol Otol. 2001; 115(4):298–301

[8] Brumund KT, Gutierrez-Fonseca R, Garcia D, Babin E, Hans S, Laccourreye O. Frontolateral vertical partial laryngectomy without tracheotomy for invasive squamous cell carcinoma of the true vocal cord: a 25-year experience. Ann Otol Rhinol Laryngol. 2005; 114(4):314–322

[9] Mahler V, Boysen M, Brøndbo K. Radiotherapy or CO(2) laser surgery as treatment of T(1a) glottic carcinoma? Eur Arch Otorhinolaryngol. 2010; 267(5):743–750

[10] Laccourreye O, Muscatello L, Laccourreye L, Naudo P, Brasnu D, Weinstein G. Supracricoid partial laryngectomy with cricohyoidoepiglottopexy for "early" glottic carcinoma classified as T1–T2N0 invading the anterior commissure. Am J Otolaryngol. 1997; 18(6):385–390

[11] Milovanovic J, Jotic A, Djukic V, et al. Oncological and functional outcome after surgical treatment of early glottic carcinoma without anterior commissure involvement. BioMed Res Int. 2014; 2014:464781

[12] Piazza C, Mangili S, Bon FD, et al. Preoperative clinical predictors of difficult laryngeal exposure for microlaryngoscopy: Laryngoscope. 2014; 124(11):2561–2567

[13] Pfuetzenreiter EG, Jr, Dedivitis RA, Queija DS, Bohn NP, Barros AP. The relationship between the glottic configuration after frontolateral laryngectomy and the acoustic voice analysis. J Voice. 2010; 24(4):499–502

7 Transoral Laser Microsurgery for Intermediate Supraglottic Cancer

Alberto Paderno, Fabiola Incandela, Cesare Piazza

Abstract

Locally intermediate supraglottic squamous cell carcinoma (SCCs) may be managed by a variety of surgical and nonsurgical approaches. First, when planning transoral laser microsurgery (TLM), the surgeon should fully delineate superficial and deep tumor infiltration. This may be done by careful endoscopic examination (using both white light and narrowband imaging) and cross-sectional imaging (CT and/or MR). Furthermore, nodal involvement should be routinely assessed (ideally by ultrasonography) in order to get a comprehensive view of the extension of the disease. TLM resection of each supraglottic subsite is characterized by different outcomes in terms of survival and function. While the quality of the voice is usually not influenced, a varied degree of swallowing impairment and aspiration should be expected temporarily. In general, patient evaluation has a crucial role in determining the optimal treatment and should be aimed at balancing oncologic and functional outcomes. For this reason, when assessing the "ideal" treatment for a given clinical scenario, it is mandatory to tailor the therapeutic choice in consideration of both patient- and tumor-related factors. The main limiting factors influencing the treatment choice when considering TLM in locally intermediate supraglottic carcinomas will be presented and discussed in the text, with particular emphasis on preoperative evaluation and planning.

Keywords: laryngeal cancer, supraglottic carcinoma, transoral laser microsurgery, supraglottic laryngectomy, survival, functional outcomes

7.1 Case Report

A 67-year-old male, with a long history of cigarette smoking, presented to our office complaining of progressive dysphagia, hoarseness, and loss of appetite lasting 2 months. In this period, he noticed some difficulties in swallowing solid foods that progressively worsened. He did not report any chronic comorbidities.

A transnasal videoendoscopic evaluation of the upper aerodigestive tract (UADT) was performed. This procedure was carried out in the office under topical anesthesia using a flexible ENF-V2 videoendoscope connected to an EvisExera II CLV-180B light source (Visera Elite OTV-S190, Olympus Medical Systems Corporation, Tokyo, Japan), integrated with a high-definition television (HDTV) and narrowband imaging (NBI) column. Videolaryngoscopic examination showed an exophytic lesion on the laryngeal aspect of the epiglottis at the junction between the suprahyoid and infrahyoid epiglottis. The lesion was irregular, ulcerated, and bled easily touched, characterized by an abnormal vascular pattern suspicious for malignancy at the HDTV-NBI examination (▶Fig. 7.1).[1] Physical examination

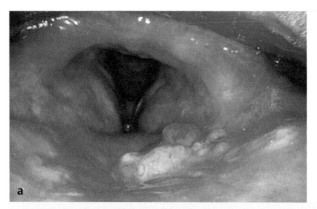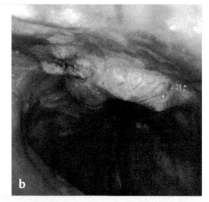

Fig. 7.1 Preoperative videoendoscopy of the supraglottic cancer under **(a)** high-definition television (HDTV) white light and **(b)** HDTV-NBI (narrowband imaging).

did not reveal any suspicious lymph nodes in the neck.

Contrast-enhanced computed tomography (CT) confirmed the presence of an exophytic lesion of the epiglottis without invasion of the pre-epiglottic space (PES) fat pad or extension in other adjacent laryngeal subsites (▶ Fig. 7.2). No suspicious lateral neck lymph nodes were detected by imaging. Clinical staging was therefore confirmed to be supraglottic cT2N0.

The case was discussed at the Multidisciplinary Tumor Board and transoral laser microsurgery (TLM) was proposed as the treatment of choice.

The patient was intubated transorally with a laser-safe endotracheal tube (Mallinckrodt Laser Oral Tracheal Tube, Codivien, Mansfield, Ireland). Adequate laryngeal exposure was obtained by a "vallecular laryngoscope" (Microfrance Laryngoscope 124, Medtronic ENT, Jacksonville, FL), allowing visualization of the entire epiglottis and valleculae. The diagnostic evaluation was integrated by an intraoperative rigid endoscopy by 0- and 70-degree telescopes (Olympus 5-mm telescopes, Hamburg, Germany) to get a more precise three-dimensional assessment of the boundaries of the cancer. Before starting resection of the cancer, a biopsy was carried out for histopathological confirmation.

TLM was accomplished with a carbon dioxide laser (Ultrapulse Laser CO_2, Lumenis, Yokneam, Israel), set on an ultrapulse mode, at 3 W of delivered power and at 400 mm of working distance.

Resection of the cancer was performed with a "multibloc technique" (i.e., progressively disassembling the lesion in an ordinated fashion without any attempt to perform an "en bloc" procedure), performing a transoral supraglottic laryngectomy (type IIb according to the European Laryngological Society classification).[2] The resection included the entire epiglottis, and the anterior line of resection went through the PES fat pad to provide complete tumor resection with free surgical margins. Vascular clips were applied on the superior laryngeal pedicles bilaterally, at the level of the pharyngoepiglottic folds. Frozen sections were performed to check the lateral, cranial, and distal (mucosal) margins of resection. No tracheostomy was carried out. A nasogastric feeding tube was positioned at the end of the surgical procedure. The patient was extubated at the end of surgery and sent to the Department of Head and Neck Surgery. Prophylactic antibiotic therapy (sulbactam and penicillin 1.5 g twice a day) was started at the end of surgery and prolonged for 10 days. Nonopioid analgesics were also prescribed.

On the first postoperative day (POD), videoendoscopy did not evidence any local edema and/or bleeding. On the third POD, videoendoscopic swallowing examination was performed, confirming the absence of dysphagia and/or aspiration. The nasogastric feeding tube was therefore removed and the patient gradually resumed oral feeding without significant issues. He was discharged on the fourth POD without complications.

Clinical evaluation of swallowing and EAT-10 score[3] was normal and the patient received a score of 1 on the penetration–aspiration scale.[4] During follow-up, the patient gradually developed a supraglottic circular synechia with no sign of dyspnea (▶ Fig. 7.3).

The histopathologic report confirmed the lesion to be a moderately differentiated (G2) squamous cell carcinoma (SCC) of the epiglottis. No signs of

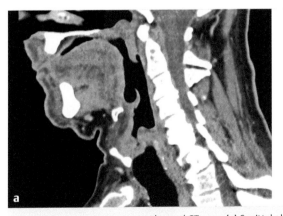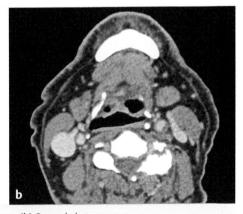

Fig. 7.2 Preoperative contrast enhanced CT scan. (a) Sagittal plane. (b) Coronal plane.

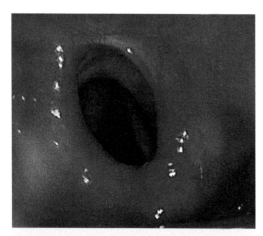

Fig. 7.3 Videoendoscopic examination, 28 months after surgery, showing no signs of recurrent disease.

perineural and/or lymphovascular invasion were found. No involvement of the PES fat pad was detected. All superficial and deep resection margins were confirmed to be negative. Pathological staging was therefore defined as pT2NxG2R0. The patient had no indication for adjuvant treatments after discussion at the Multidisciplinary Tumor Board. Follow-up was performed by periodic transnasal flexible videoendoscopic examination in the office every 2 months and imaging (CT every year and neck ultrasonography every 4 months in the first year and every 6 months in the second). The patient is without evidence of locoregional or distant disease at 28 months after surgery.

7.2 Discussion

Locally intermediate supraglottic SCCs are a relatively infrequent disease presentation that may be managed by a variety of surgical and nonsurgical approaches. For this reason, comprehensive characterization of both the cancer and patient features is essential in guiding the most appropriate therapeutic choice.

First, preoperative evaluation should be focused on determining superficial and deep extension of the cancer: this may be obtained by combining endoscopic evaluation (i.e., flexible videoendoscopy with and without HDTV-NBI) and cross-sectional imaging (i.e., MR and/or CT). Second, given the non-negligible rate of lateral neck metastases even in locally intermediate tumors, complete evaluation of all potentially involved levels in the neck should always be performed (by ultrasonography

or CT/MR). Suspicious lymph nodes should be further evaluated by fine-needle aspiration cytology to direct the therapeutic approach.

When planning TLM, the surgeon should fully delineate superficial extension of the cancer under general anesthesia by performing a comprehensive examination of the larynx using rigid telescopes, in order to confirm the surgical indication and to precisely tailor the excision in each individual patient.

In particular, a subtle extension to the glottic plane should be carefully evaluated as it leads to significant changes in the surgical approach, with possible inferior extension of the transoral resection to the anterior commissure and adjacent anterior thirds of the vocal folds. Similarly, superficial extension from the aryepiglottic fold may easily lead to involvement of the glottic plane through the arytenoid and should be thoroughly evaluated. A similar approach should be employed to exclude or better evaluate unexpected superficial extensions to other nearby subsites, such as the base of the tongue and hypopharynx.

Once major superficial and/or multifocal extensions outside the supraglottis have been excluded, a further step is to assess the deep tumor infiltration toward laryngeal visceral spaces (in particular the PES). Partial invasion of the PES fat pad is not a contraindication for TLM. However, attention must be paid to evaluate possible tumor diffusion from the PES laterally into the upper paraglottic space, since no strong anatomical barrier prevents local spread. Moreover, encroachment of the cancer into the PES up to the thyrohyoid membrane, hyoid bone, and upper third of the thyroid cartilage may not allow us to obtain reliable surgical margins due to an unfavorable line of sight and incomplete visualization of the deepest extension of the lesion. In addition, apart from related technical difficulties, the biological behavior of such a lesion becomes unpredictable and hardly manageable by a transoral approach. In fact, neoplastic medullary spread within the thyroid cartilage is not amenable to intraoperative visualization and/ or histopathological confirmation. According to our experience, cancers retaining a cuff of healthy adipose tissue between the deep front of invasion and the thyrohyoid membrane can still be safely resected by a TLM approach.[5] However, when this prerequisite is not met (massive T3), our policy is to shift to an open partial horizontal laryngectomy (OPHL type I according to the European Laryngological Society classification),[6] in order to obtain more adequate cancer-free surgical margins.

TLM resection of each supraglottic subsite is characterized by different outcomes in terms of survival and function. While the quality of voice is generally not influenced, a varied degree of swallowing impairment and aspiration should be expected. In particular, this may be more severe when resection is extended to the aryepiglottic fold and/or one arytenoid.[7]

Regarding the treatment policy of the neck, T2 supraglottic SCCs clinically N0 after neck ultrasound can be treated by elective neck dissection simultaneously to the TLM or 1 month later, unilaterally or bilaterally according to the tumor relationship with the midline and histopathologic evaluation of the specimen. We prefer the latter option since it gives the possibility to get more precise prognostic information on the tumor: close surgical margins, aggressive biological behavior, and presence of perineural and/or lymphovascular invasion may all prompt a 1-month-delayed neck dissection (and a second-look TLM), in order to treat occult metastases that are potentially present. By contrast, a wait-and-see policy for the neck can be chosen in selected frail patients with severe comorbidities and/or "small" T2 lesions (defined as lesions with a volume that would define them as T1 if not located at the junction between two supraglottic subsites; the present case was a typical example of "small" T2). Conversely, all patients who are clinically N+ should be treated with therapeutic unilateral or bilateral neck dissection performed simultaneously to the TLM.

In general, patient evaluation has a crucial role in determining the optimal treatment and should be aimed at balancing oncologic and functional outcomes. Some degree of aspiration should be expected after any form of surgical and nonsurgical conservative therapy: TLM, OPHL, radiotherapy (RT), or chemoradiotherapy (CRT). Patient's age and cardiopulmonary performance have a significant impact on postoperative rehabilitation and survival. The patient should be able to tolerate at least a chronic subclinical passage of liquids in the airways, which is sometimes only seen by objective (videoendoscopic and/or videofluoroscopic) evaluation of the swallowing. Notably, the most feared complication is aspiration pneumonia, which retains a non-negligible mortality rate especially in the early postoperative period and in fragile patients. On the other hand, its true impact in the long run and its role in determining late nontumor-related deaths are still to be precisely quantified. In the case of severe comorbidities and significant preoperative functional impairment, total laryngectomy should not be excluded even for intermediate cancers.

When considering locally intermediate cancer (T2 and T3), different authors have described optimal oncologic and functional outcomes that are at least comparable with those of OPHL and (chemo) radiotherapy (RT and CRT). However, there is no prospective randomized study comparing these different treatment options.

In a systematic review, of 232 patients with supraglottic T2 treated by TLM, local control ranged from 63 to 100% (weighted average, 83%).[8] When comparing it with the only intensity-modulated RT study, TLM had better local control rates (83 vs. 70%).

Consequently, data concerning supraglottic T3 treated by TLM are scarce and mainly originating from highly specialized institutions. Furthermore, the results are significantly influenced by the variability of selection criteria among different institutions. Five-year disease-free survival ranged from 67 to 76% in the three major retrospective series present in the literature to date.[5,9,10]

Finally, TLM offers better functional outcomes compared to those of OPHLs, which routinely require a tracheostomy, nasogastric feeding tube, and longer hospitalization time. Tracheostomy after TLM is seldom required since airway patency is usually not compromised. Swallowing rehabilitation is faster since the anatomical integrity of the laryngeal framework is preserved, as are most branches of the superior laryngeal nerve, as well as mucosa of the base of the tongue and musculature, pharyngeal constrictor muscles, hyoid bone, and strap muscles. This permits physiological laryngeal mobility and elevation during swallowing, provided that this organ maintains its anatomic position in the neck.

In conclusion, when considering the "ideal" treatment for a given clinical scenario, it is mandatory to tailor the therapeutic choice in consideration of both patient- and tumor-related factors. In this view, the main advantages of TLM are represented by the following:

- Oncologic outcomes comparable to those of OPHL and RT/CRT in selected locally intermediate supraglottic cancer.
- Optimal functional results and short hospital stay with favorable cost-effectiveness ratio.
- Repeatable treatment in case of positive surgical margins or recurrence of the disease.

7.3 Tips

- Extension of the cancer should be precisely determined in the preoperative phase. This can be done by employing different tools that allow us to precisely define the superficial and deep tumor extension. Laryngeal, hypopharyngeal, and oropharyngeal mucosa can be accurately examined by HDTV videolaryngoscopy with NBI. Deep extension of the cancer can be assessed by contrast-enhanced fine-cut CT or MR.
- Optimal laryngeal exposure can be obtained by using a large bore laryngoscope optimized for supraglottic exposure. This may be a fixed generic "vallecular" or a Lindholm laryngoscope. Distending bivalved laryngoscopes, such as the Hinni or the Steiner, may also offer some advantages.
- A multibloc resection is often necessary to adequately mobilize the bulky supraglottic structures and allow optimal visualization of the most critical anatomical sites (hyoid bone, thyroid cartilage, PES, upper paraglottic space, medial wall of the piriform sinus). The specimen should be carefully marked with ink and oriented to allow precise and reliable identification of the "true" surgical margins by the pathologist.

7.4 Traps

- Suboptimal exposure and incomplete tumor visualization (or manipulation) of the cancer can lead to higher rates of positive margins and inferior oncologic results after TLM. In these cases, it may be useful to consider shifting to an OPHL, especially when a concomitant neck dissection is needed.
- Extensive infiltration of the PES fat pad, with tumor encroachment at the level of the hyoid bone, thyrohyoid membrane, and upper half of the thyroid cartilage, cannot be safely managed through a TLM approach. In such a clinical situation, it is essential to consider other therapeutic approaches.

- The surgeon should expect poorer functional outcomes after type III and IV supraglottic resections, especially when extending to the aryepiglottic fold. In these cases, resumption of oral feeding can be delayed and swallowing rehabilitation should be particularly careful.

References

[1] Arens C, Piazza C, Andrea M, et al. Proposal for a descriptive guideline of vascular changes in lesions of the vocal folds by the committee on endoscopic laryngeal imaging of the European Laryngological Society. Eur Arch Otorhinolaryngol. 2016; 273(5):1207–1214

[2] Remacle M, Hantzakos A, Eckel H, et al. Endoscopic supraglottic laryngectomy: a proposal for a classification by the working committee on nomenclature, European Laryngological Society. Eur Arch Otorhinolaryngol. 2009; 266(7):993–998

[3] Belafsky PC, Mouadeb DA, Rees CJ, et al. Validity and reliability of the Eating Assessment Tool (EAT-10). Ann Otol Rhinol Laryngol. 2008; 117(12):919–924

[4] Robbins J, Coyle J, Rosenbek J, Roecker E, Wood J. Differentiation of normal and abnormal airway protection during swallowing using the penetration-aspiration scale. Dysphagia. 1999; 14(4):228–232

[5] Peretti G, Piazza C, Penco S, et al. Transoral laser microsurgery as primary treatment for selected T3 glottic and supraglottic cancers. Head Neck. 2016; 38(7):1107–1112

[6] Succo G, Peretti G, Piazza C, et al. Open partial horizontal laryngectomies: a proposal for classification by the working committee on nomenclature of the European Laryngological Society. Eur Arch Otorhinolaryngol. 2014; 271(9):2489–2496

[7] Piazza C, Barbieri D, Del Bon F, et al. Functional outcomes after different types of transoral supraglottic laryngectomy. Laryngoscope. 2016; 126(5):1131–1135

[8] Swanson MS, Low G, Sinha UK, Kokot N. Transoral surgery vs intensity-modulated radiotherapy for early supraglottic cancer: a systematic review. Curr Opin Otolaryngol Head Neck Surg. 2017; 25(2):133–141

[9] Canis M, Ihler F, Martin A, Wolff HA, Matthias C, Steiner W. Results of 226 patients with T3 laryngeal carcinoma after treatment with transoral laser microsurgery. Head Neck. 2014; 36(5):652–659

[10] Vilaseca I, Blanch JL, Berenguer J, et al. Transoral laser microsurgery for locally advanced (T3-T4a) supraglottic squamous cell carcinoma: sixteen years of experience. Head Neck. 2016; 38(7):1050–1057

8 The Role of Radiation Therapy in Early-Stage Supraglottic Cancer

Houda Bahig, G. Brandon Gunn

Abstract

Early-stage supraglottic squamous cell carcinoma (ES-SSCC) has access to a relatively rich lymphatic drainage and therefore associated with an elevated risk of occult cervical lymph node involvement, even in clinically node negative patients. ES-SSCC is typically managed with larynx-preserving strategies, which include transoral laser microsurgery/robotic surgery, radiotherapy ± chemotherapy, or open supraglottic or suprahyoid laryngectomy. With appropriate selection, these modalities yield similar outcomes, with reported local control between 70 and 100% for stage T1N0M0 and 60 and 90% for stage T2N0M0. In addition to cancer cure rate, the choice of treatment modality is also based on anticipated speech and swallowing function, airway protection, patient choice, and institutional expertise. Comprehensive pretreatment assessment by a multidisciplinary team including, at the minimum, head and neck surgery, radiation oncology, medical oncology, and speech language pathology is critical. In patients with larger or unfavorable cancers treated with radiotherapy alone, intensification with accelerated or hyperfractionated radiotherapy is recommended as these altered fractionation regimens have been associated with improved locoregional control. Speech and swallowing rehabilitation, nutritional follow-up, and referral to a smoking cessation program should be carried out for optimal functional and quality-of-life outcomes.

Keywords: supraglottic cancer, squamous cell carcinoma, early-stage, larynx preservation, radiotherapy, altered fractionation, transoral laser microsurgery, robotic surgery

8.1 Case Report

A 76-year-old Caucasian female, retired nurse aid, presented with a 3-month history of odynophagia and involuntary weight loss of 10 pounds. She was an active cigarette smoker, with a 30 pack-year history and drank alcohol socially. Her past medical history was relevant for chronic obstructive pulmonary disease (COPD), hypertension, osteoporosis, and previous hysterectomy for uterine fibroids. Her medications included an antihypertensive and vitamins.

On physical examination, she had an Eastern Cooperative Oncology Group (ECOG) performance status of 1 and no palpable cervical or supraclavicular adenopathy. Examination of the oral cavity and oropharynx was unremarkable. Fiberoptic nasopharyngolaryngoscopy demonstrated obvious thickening of the epiglottis, with a friable exophytic mass involving the supra- and infrahyoid epiglottis, with the epicenter at the left laryngeal surface of the epiglottis. The cancer involved and expanded the left aryepiglottic fold without definite involvement of the left arytenoid or pyriform sinus. The vocal cords were free of cancer and fully mobile. There was no involvement of the base of the tongue or pharyngeal walls (▶ Fig. 8.1).

The patient had a contrast-enhanced computed tomography (CT) of the neck, which revealed an enhancing mass at the epiglottis (maximal thickness of 7 mm) over a length of 3 cm craniocaudally, with extension to the left aryepiglottic fold, and

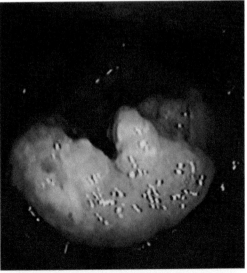

Fig. 8.1 Pretreatment image from fiberoptic videoendoscopy. Friable exophytic mass involving the supra- and infrahyoid epiglottis and thickened epiglottis with extension into left aryepiglottic fold.

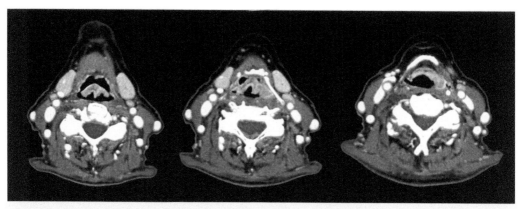

Fig. 8.2 Pretreatment CT neck. Axial images of pretreatment CT of the neck reveal an enhancing mass and thickened epiglottis with extension to the left aryepiglottic fold.

presence of nonspecific bilateral cervical lymph nodes (▸ Fig. 8.2). She underwent direct micro-suspension laryngoscopy with a biopsy of the supraglottic mass and rigid esophagoscopy. The biopsy revealed moderately to poorly differentiated invasive squamous carcinoma, p16 negative on immunohistochemistry. Fluorodeoxyglucose positron emission tomography (PET) /CT confirmed the primary extent and showed no hypermetabolic adenopathy. Chest images revealed findings consistent with COPD. There were no distant metastases. As the cancer involved more than one subsite of the supraglottis, had normal laryngeal/vocal fold mobility, and no signs of pre-epiglottic or extralaryngeal spread, final clinical stage was T2N0M0, American Joint Committee on Cancer (AJCC) group II (as per the eighth edition of the AJCC).[1] Upon interview, she reported mild dysphagia and odynophagia, but denied any signs or symptoms of aspiration. Evaluation with a speech-language pathologist and modified barium swallow showed mild dysphagia but no penetration or aspiration.

Following evaluation by head and neck surgery, and medical and radiation oncology, the patient's case was discussed at the multidisciplinary tumor board. Considering her good swallowing function and adequate airway protection, tumor location, extent, and stage as well as patient factors such as older age and history of COPD, definitive radiation therapy was recommended. Concurrent chemotherapy was considered, but given her age, final recommendations were for altered fractionation radiation therapy alone. In addition, the patient was referred to a smoking cessation program. At the time of radiotherapy simulation, the patient was positioned in a supine position, immobilized with a custom head, neck, and shoulder thermoplastic mask, to ensure reproducibility of the patient's position. CT images were obtained at 2-mm slice thickness for treatment planning purposes. To reduce internal cancer/laryngeal motion, the patient was given specific instruction for quiet respiration and not to swallow during simulation, image acquisition, or treatment delivery.

The radiation therapy target volumes were as follows: (1) a high-risk target volume encompassing the gross tumor volume (defined by combination of endoscopic and diagnostic imaging findings) plus an 8-mm margin as well as the adjacent larynx at risk in order to account for internal laryngeal motion (largely in the craniocaudal direction) and (2) a standard risk or elective target volume encompassing the bilateral cervical lymph nodes at risk for harboring microscopic regional disease, namely, lymph node levels II to IV bilaterally, the most cranial extent being the subdigastric nodes (▸ Fig. 8.3). A modified Danish Head and Neck Cancer Group (DAHANCA) fractionation schedule was administered, with a dose of 70 Gy to the high-risk target volume and 57 Gy to the standard-risk target volume, given in 35 fractions over 6 weeks, with 6 fractions per week (BID one day per week with ≥ 6 hours between fractions) for 5 of the 6 weeks. Treatment was planned and delivered using volumetric-modulated arc therapy (VMAT), with two full arcs, each with slight collimator rotation. The treatment plan was optimized to cover the aforementioned targets while respecting spinal cord tolerance and constraining as feasible the

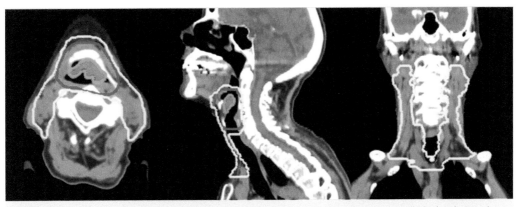

Fig. 8.3 Simulation CT and radiation therapy target volumes. (a) Gross tumor volume (*green*); (b) high-risk clinical target volume (*red*); and (c) standard risk clinical target volume (*yellow*).

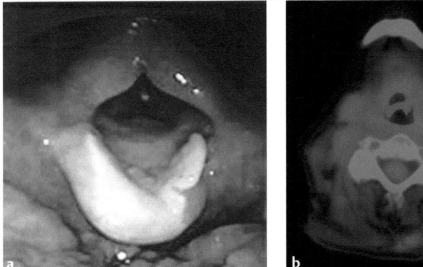
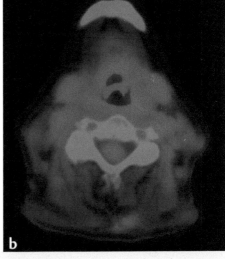

Fig. 8.4 Posttreatment assessments. **(a)** Image of fiberoptic videoendoscopy performed 2 months after radiation therapy completion. **(b)** Fluorodeoxyglucose (FDG)-PET/CT performed 3 months after radiation completion showing no residual avidity.

bilateral parotid glands, bilateral submandibular glands, oral cavity, lungs, shoulders, and cervical esophagus.

The patient tolerated the treatment well and completed it without interruption, hospitalization, or feeding tube placement. Acute toxicities included grade 2 dermatitis and grade 3 mucositis for which she required temporary use of narcotics. Contrast-enhanced CT of the neck and videoendoscopy 2 months after completion of radiation therapy showed resolution of the supraglottic cancer with treatment effects, namely, edema with anatomic distortion (▶ Fig. 8.4a). PET/CT carried out 3 months after the completion of treatment demonstrated no residual metabolic activity (▶ Fig. 8.4b). The patient remains disease free and able to eat a regular solid diet now 3 years after treatment.

8.2 Discussion

Early-stage supraglottic squamous cell carcinoma (ES-SSCC) generally includes stage I (T1N0M0) or stage II (T2N0M0) and perhaps those with N1 disease. While T1 cancers are limited to one subsite of the supraglottis with normal vocal cord mobility, T2 cancers invade the mucosa of more than one adjacent subsite of the supraglottis or have impaired vocal cord mobility, without laryngeal fixation or pre-epiglottic invasion. Due to the richness of draining lymphatics of the supraglottis, node-negative ES-SSCC may have up to a 40% risk microscopic nodal involvement.[2] Treatment strategies generally seek to address this risk for microscopic disease (e.g., elective nodal irradiation) and compared to the excellent outcomes of their early-stage glottic cancer counterpart, the 5-year overall survival for ES-SSCC is generally below 70%.[3] Treatment strategies for ES-SSCC are typically single modality, based on organ preservation and focus on maximizing disease control and survival while maintaining good laryngeal function (e.g., swallowing, airway protection, and vocal quality) and patient's quality of life.[4,5] Treatment options for ES-SSCC include (1) transoral laser microsurgery, transoral robotic surgery, or open supraglottic or suprahyoid laryngectomy (selected cases) ± neck dissection ± adjuvant radiotherapy[6,7,8,9] or (2) definitive radiotherapy alone, or in combination with systemic therapy for selected more unfavorable cancers with goals to improve local control and larynx preservation probability.[10,11,12] These treatment approaches yield local control between 70 and 100% for stage I and 60 and 90% for stage II.[9,10,12,13,14,15,16] ▶ Table 8.1 presents some published institutional outcomes for definitive radiotherapy in ES-SSCC. Retrospective studies, systematic reviews, and meta-analysis have compared outcomes of organ-preserving surgery versus radiotherapy, but conclusions have been inconsistent.[17,18,19,20] In the context of the inherent selection biases associated with retrospective comparisons and in the absence of randomized study, the optimal treatment strategy for ES-SSCC remains a subject of debate.

As per the most recent American Society of Clinical Oncology Clinical Practice Guidelines, both organ-preserving surgery and radiotherapy offer larynx preservation potential without compromising survival, and optimal management of ES-SSCC should be selected individually after careful consideration of patient and cancers characteristics, patient choice, and institutional expertise. Treatment decision should involve multidisciplinary evaluation and thorough physician-to-patient discussions eliciting personal preference, considering the potential advantages and trade-offs between approaches. As a general rule, most T1N0 tumors and nonbulky T2N0 cancers can be effectively managed with definitive radiotherapy as a single modality. Patient's characteristics, such as the presence of major medical problems precluding the use of general anesthesia, inadequate pulmonary reserve such as the presence of COPD, advanced age, or judged elevated risk of aspiration after supraglottic laryngectomy are factors in favor of a radiotherapy-based approach.[21] In addition, involvement of the vocal cords, anterior commissure, or bilateral arytenoids can preclude adequate organ-preserving surgery.[22] Organ-preserving surgery is generally favored for younger patients when feasible.[23] Indications for postoperative radiotherapy include close/positive margins, presence of perineural invasion or lymphovascular invasion,[24] or incidental upstaging features (e.g., multiple nodes, extranodal extension).

Table 8.1 Institutional local control (LC) outcomes following radical radiotherapy for early-stage supraglottic squamous cell carcinoma (ES-SSCC)

Author	Year	Institution	No. of patients	Dose	Outcomes
Hinerman et al[15]	2002	University of Florida	T1 = 18 T2 = 109	Not specified	*5-year LC* T1 = 100% T2 = 86%
Nakfoor et al[14]	1998	Massachusetts General Hospital	T1 = 21 T2 = 58	Hyperfractionation 67.2–72 Gy/1.6 Gy twice daily	*5-year LC* T1 = 96% T2 = 86%
Wendt et al[10]	1989	MD Anderson Cancer Center	T1 = 2 T2 = 23 T3 = 15	Hyperfractionation 72–79 Gy/1.2 Gy twice daily	*2-year LC* T1 = 100% T2–T3 = 87%

For patients with ES-SSCC with an unfavorable or bulky cancer to be treated with radiotherapy alone, treatment intensification through altered fractionation, namely, accelerated or hyperfractionated radiotherapy, is favored to improve local control.[25] Standard fractionation is defined as administration of approximately 2 Gy per daily fraction, 5 fractions per week, over 6.5 to 7 weeks, to a total dose of 66 to 70 Gy. Altered fractionation is accomplished by either shortening the overall treatment time, escalating the total dose, or sometimes both, and is generally achieved by delivering multiple smaller fractions per day for some of or the entire treatment course. Radiotherapy regimens vary between institutions; common altered fractionation schedules include the following:

- *Modified, moderately accelerated DAHANCA fractionation* of 66 to 70 Gy in 33 to 35 fractions of 2 Gy each delivered over 6 weeks; 6 fractions a week (twice a day once per week with ≥ 6 hours between fractions), delivered over a total of 6 weeks.
- *Accelerated fractionation using concomitant boost*, administering a total of 72 Gy in 42 fractions with an initial plan of 54 Gy in 30 fractions and a second plan focused on the high-risk volume of 18 Gy in 12 fractions of 1.5 Gy. The second plan is administered concurrently with the first plan over the last 12 days of treatment, given as a second daily fraction, with ≥6 hours between fractions.
- *Hyperfractionated regimen* of 76.8 to 79.2 Gy in 64 to 66 fractions of 1.2 Gy, administered twice a day with ≥ 6 hours between fractions.

A meta-analysis of 15 trials, involving 6,515 patients treated with head and neck radiotherapy, including 34% primary cancer of the larynx, revealed a 3.4 and 6.4% absolute benefit in 5-year overall survival and locoregional control, respectively, with altered fractionation versus standard fractionation.[25] The absolute overall survival benefit was found higher with hyperfractionation versus accelerated radiotherapy (8 vs. 2%). Additionally, when medically fit, patients with an unfavorable or deeply invasive T2N0 cancer are considered for concurrent platinum-based chemoradiation or sequential chemoradiation, in an attempt to further intensify treatment in patients felt to be at higher risk of poorer disease control.[12,26] When given concomitantly with chemotherapy, the standard radiotherapy fractionation schedule is generally used.

Intensity-modulated radiotherapy (IMRT) is the preferred technique for the delivery of locoregional radiotherapy to the head and neck. In fact, compared to 3D conformal radiotherapy, IMRT allows for relative sparing of many normal organs, particularly the parotid glands. In a randomized trial, IMRT was shown to reduce the rates of grade ≥ 2 xerostomia by 50% at 1-year postradiotherapy.[27] VMAT is a contemporary form of IMRT, where variable gantry speed, dose rate, and dynamic multileaf collimation are used, which significantly shorten radiation delivery time.[28] VMAT can therefore be specifically advantageous in the treatment of cancer of the larynx where swallowing motion is a concern. Likewise, intensity-modulated proton therapy is another advanced form of highly conformal radiotherapy with the potential to further improve patient outcomes through the elimination of unnecessary radiation to surrounding nontarget tissues.

For optimal functional and quality-of-life outcomes as well as for airway protection, assessment of speech, swallowing, and nutritional status should be carried out at baseline, during and after radiotherapy. Speech and swallowing rehabilitation, including early implementation of prophylactic exercises and swallowing maneuvers teaching (a.k.a. "eat and exercise"), is crucial for accelerated and full posttreatment recovery.[29,30] In addition, patients with supraglottic cancers receiving voice rehabilitation were shown to have improvements in voice outcomes after therapy.[31] An expert dietician should closely monitor the patient's body weight, nutritional needs, and hydration throughout treatment and after treatment to reduce the loss of weight and lean body mass, minimize treatment delays, and hospitalization rates, and to improve treatment outcomes.[32]

As per the National Comprehensive Cancer Network guidelines version 2.2017, surveillance after treatment completion should include history, physical examination, and fiberoptic nasopharyngolaryngoscopy every 1 to 3 months for the first year, every 2 to 6 months for the second year, every 6 months for the third to fifth year, and annually thereafter. A CT of the neck is typically obtained at 2 months after treatment, and further imaging as indicated in the presence of worrisome signs or symptoms, although ongoing surveillance neck imaging is routine at many centers. With rates of hypothyroidism after head and neck irradiation being around 30%,[33] routine thyroid-stimulating hormone levels should be obtained at every visit or at least every 6 months and thyroid hormone replacement should be prescribed for patients who are clinically hypothyroid. Chest imaging should be considered in patients with a significant history of smoking for detection of second primary cancers. Adequate speech and swallowing therapy and rehabilitation should be pursued during the follow-up period.

8.3 Tips

- Comprehensive pretreatment assessment is necessary for appropriate treatment selection. All patients should be evaluated by a head and neck surgeon, radiation oncologist, and medical oncologist, and should undergo a baseline assessment of voice and swallowing function by a speech-language pathologist. Appropriate counseling regarding the potential impact of radiation on swallowing function, voice, and quality of life should be carefully undertaken with the patient.
- Smoking cessation is important. Active smoking during radiotherapy has been associated with worse acute reactions and adverse survival and cancer control outcomes.[34] All patients should be encouraged to quit smoking and should be referred to smoking cessation programs, when appropriate.
- Interruption of radiotherapy has been associated with 1.6% absolute loss of local control with each missed treatment day.[35] In case of missed fraction, efforts to maintain the overall treatment time should be made. This can be achieved by either treating on weekends or by delivering two fractions on the same day, with ≥ 6 hour intervals between fractions.

8.4 Traps

- Underestimation of cancer extensions/staging could lead to geographic miss or undertreatment. It is important for the treating radiation oncologist to perform fiberscopic nasopharyngolaryngoscopy to carefully determine tumor extent in order to facilitate radiation therapy target volume design.
- Before starting radiotherapy, ensure that the patient is at minimal risk of respiratory compromise from radiation-induced laryngeal edema or development of aspiration. Likewise, airway safety should be closely monitored during radiotherapy through careful history and physical

examination. Fiberscopic nasopharyngolaryngoscopy is performed at many centers during radiotherapy to ensure a patent airway and to monitor treatment response.

- When selecting treatment modality, it is important to consider freedom from dysphagia, aspiration, voice quality, and airway protection as important functional endpoints in addition to disease control.

References

[1] American Joint Committee on Cancer. AJCC Staging Manual. 8th ed. New York, NY: Springer; 2017
[2] Lindberg R. Distribution of cervical lymph node metastases from squamous cell carcinoma of the upper respiratory and digestive tracts. Cancer. 1972; 29(6):1446–1449
[3] Piccirillo F. Cancer of the Larynx. In: SEER Survival Monograph: Cancer Survival Among Adults—U.S. SEER Program, 1988–2001. Patient and Tumor Characteristics. Bethesda, MD: National Cancer Institute; 2007
[4] Tufano RP Stafford EM. Organ preservation surgery for laryngeal cancer. Otolaryngol Clin North Am. 2008; 41(4):741–755, vi
[5] Moore BA, Holsinger FC, Diaz EM, Jr, Weber RS. Organ-preservation laryngeal surgery in the era of chemoradiation. Curr Probl Cancer. 2005; 29(4):169–179
[6] Thomas L, Drinnan M, Natesh B, Mehanna H, Jones T, Paleri V. Open conservation partial laryngectomy for laryngeal cancer: a systematic review of English language literature. Cancer Treat Rev. 2012; 38(3):203–211
[7] Ozer E, Alvarez B, Kakarala K, Durmus K, Teknos TN, Carrau RL. Clinical outcomes of transoral robotic supraglottic laryngectomy. Head Neck. 2013; 35(8):1158–1161
[8] Mendelsohn AH, Remacle M, Van Der Vorst S, Bachy V, Lawson G. Outcomes following transoral robotic surgery: supraglottic laryngectomy. Laryngoscope. 2013; 123(1):208–214
[9] Ambrosch P. The role of laser microsurgery in the treatment of laryngeal cancer. Curr Opin Otolaryngol Head Neck Surg. 2007; 15(2):82–88
[10] Wendt CD, Peters LJ, Ang KK, et al. Hyperfractionated radiotherapy in the treatment of squamous cell carcinomas of the supraglottic larynx. Int J Radiat Oncol Biol Phys. 1989; 17(5):1057–1062
[11] Sykes AJ, Slevin NJ, Gupta NK, Brewster AE. 331 cases of clinically node-negative supraglottic carcinoma of the larynx: a study of a modest size fixed field radiotherapy approach. Int J Radiat Oncol Biol Phys. 2000; 46(5):1109–1115
[12] Denaro N, Russi EG, Lefebvre JL, Merlano MC. A systematic review of current and emerging approaches in the field of larynx preservation. Radiother Oncol. 2014; 110(1):16–24
[13] Wang CC, Suit HD, Blitzer PH. Twice-a-day radiation therapy for supraglottic carcinoma. Int J Radiat Oncol Biol Phys. 1986; 12(1):3–7
[14] Nakfoor BM, Spiro IJ, Wang CC, Martins P, Montgomery W, Fabian R. Results of accelerated radiotherapy for supraglottic carcinoma: a Massachusetts General Hospital and Massachusetts Eye and Ear Infirmary experience. Head Neck. 1998; 20(5):379–384

[15] Hinerman RW, Mendenhall WM, Amdur RJ, Stringer SP, Villaret DB, Robbins KT. Carcinoma of the supraglottic larynx: treatment results with radiotherapy alone or with planned neck dissection. Head Neck. 2002; 24(5):456–467

[16] Wang CC, Montgomery WW. Deciding on optimal management of supraglottic carcinoma. Oncology (Williston Park). 1991; 5(4):41–46, discussion 46, 49, 53

[17] Arshad H, Jayaprakash V, Gupta V, et al. Survival differences between organ preservation surgery and definitive radiotherapy in early supraglottic squamous cell carcinoma. Otolaryngol Head Neck Surg. 2014; 150(2):237–244

[18] Sessions DG, Lenox J, Spector GJ. Supraglottic laryngeal cancer: analysis of treatment results. Laryngoscope. 2005; 115(8):1402–1410

[19] Goudakos JK, Markou K, Nikolaou A, Themelis C, Vital V. Management of the clinically negative neck (N0) of supraglottic laryngeal carcinoma: a systematic review. Eur J Surg Oncol. 2009; 35(3):223–229

[20] Patel KB, Nichols AC, Fung K, Yoo J, MacNeil SD. Treatment of early stage supraglottic squamous cell carcinoma: meta-analysis comparing primary surgery versus primary radiotherapy. J Otolaryngol Head Neck Surg. 2018; 47(1):19

[21] Parsons JT, Mendenhall WM, Stringer SP, Cassisi NJ, Million RR. Radiotherapy alone for moderately advanced laryngeal cancer (T2–T3). Semin Radiat Oncol. 1992; 2(3):158–162

[22] Jenckel F, Knecht R. State of the art in the treatment of laryngeal cancer. Anticancer Res. 2013; 33(11):4701–4710

[23] Suárez C, Rodrigo JP, Silver CE, et al. Laser surgery for early to moderately advanced glottic, supraglottic, and hypopharyngeal cancers. Head Neck. 2012; 34(7):1028–1035

[24] Bernier J, Cooper JS, Pajak TF, et al. Defining risk levels in locally advanced head and neck cancers: a comparative analysis of concurrent postoperative radiation plus chemotherapy trials of the EORTC (#22931) and RTOG (# 9501). Head Neck. 2005; 27(10):843–850

[25] Bourhis J, Overgaard J, Audry H, et al; Meta-Analysis of Radiotherapy in Carcinomas of Head and neck (MARCH) Collaborative Group. Hyperfractionated or accelerated radiotherapy in head and neck cancer: a meta-analysis. Lancet. 2006; 368(9538):843–854

[26] Forastiere AA, Ismaila N, Wolf GT. Use of larynx-preservation strategies in the treatment of laryngeal cancer: American Society of Clinical Oncology Clinical Practice Guideline Update Summary. J Oncol Pract. 2018; 14(2):123–128

[27] Nutting CM, Morden JP, Harrington KJ, et al; PARSPORT trial management group. Parotid-sparing intensity modulated versus conventional radiotherapy in head and neck cancer (PARSPORT): a phase 3 multicentre randomised controlled trial. Lancet Oncol. 2011; 12(2):127–136

[28] Verbakel WF, Cuijpers JP, Hoffmans D, Bieker M, Slotman BJ, Senan S. Volumetric intensity-modulated arc therapy vs. conventional IMRT in head-and-neck cancer: a comparative planning and dosimetric study. Int J Radiat Oncol Biol Phys. 2009; 74(1):252–259

[29] Hutcheson KA, Bhayani MK, Beadle BM, et al. Eat and exercise during radiotherapy or chemoradiotherapy for pharyngeal cancers: use it or lose it. JAMA Otolaryngol Head Neck Surg. 2013; 139(11):1127–1134

[30] Kotz T, Federman AD, Kao J, et al. Prophylactic swallowing exercises in patients with head and neck cancer undergoing chemoradiation: a randomized trial. Arch Otolaryngol Head Neck Surg. 2012; 138(4):376–382

[31] Jamal N, Ebersole B, Erman A, Chhetri D. Maximizing functional outcomes in head and neck cancer survivors: assessment and rehabilitation. Otolaryngol Clin North Am. 2017; 50(4):837–852

[32] Ackerman D, Laszlo M, Provisor A, Yu A. Nutrition management for the head and neck cancer patient. Cancer Treat Res. 2018; 174:187–208

[33] Tell R, Lundell G, Nilsson B, Sjödin H, Lewin F, Lewensohn R. Long-term incidence of hypothyroidism after radiotherapy in patients with head-and-neck cancer. Int J Radiat Oncol Biol Phys. 2004; 60(2):395–400

[34] Browman GP, Wong G, Hodson I, et al. Influence of cigarette smoking on the efficacy of radiation therapy in head and neck cancer. N Engl J Med. 1993; 328(3):159–163

[35] Hendry JH, Bentzen SM, Dale RG, et al. A modelled comparison of the effects of using different ways to compensate for missed treatment days in radiotherapy Clin Oncol (R Coll Radiol). 1996; 8(5):297–307

9 Early Supraglottic Cancer: Horizontal Supraglottic Laryngectomy

Otavio Curioni, Abrão Rapoport, Marcos B. de Carvalho

Abstract

There is no consensus about the best treatment for supraglottic squamous cell carcinoma because we do not have randomized controlled trials comparing the different treatments. Five accepted surgical and nonsurgical oncological treatments have been currently established: standard horizontal supraglottic laryngectomy, supraglottic microsurgery, transoral robotic surgery, radiotherapy alone, and radiotherapy in combination with chemotherapy. Current treatment guidelines indicate, for early cancer, a single modality of treatment either by radiotherapy or by conservative surgery. The decision between surgery and radiotherapy should consider the patient's choice (accept tracheostomy and feeding tube, even if temporarily), expectation regarding vocal outcome, and general clinical conditions. Based on a clinical case, this chapter discusses the rational decision-making process for an early primary supraglottic cancer, considering the clinical, radiological, and natural history of head and neck squamous cell carcinoma. In addition, we provide a step-by-step description of the horizontal standard supraglottic laryngectomy.

Keywords: squamous cell carcinoma, supraglottis, surgery, radiotherapy, horizontal partial laryngectomy

9.1 Case Report

A 49-year-old Caucasian male toolmaker presented with nonspecific sore throat and dysphagia for 3 months, not associated with comorbidities. His social history was positive for heavy alcohol drinking and smoking 64 packs of cigarettes per year.

The Eastern Cooperative Oncology Group (ECOG) performance status was zero or compared as a healthy person. A nasolaryngofibroscopic evaluation revealed an ulcerative lesion of the epiglottis with minimal extension to the vallecula and left aryepiglottic fold (the anatomical position of the epiglottis impaired the visualization of the lesion). The true vocal cords were mobile and mild edema is shown in ▶ Fig. 9.1.

Computed tomography (CT) scan revealed an irregular lesion of the epiglottis, left aryepiglottic fold, and vallecula without extra laryngeal extension and no enlarged cervical lymph nodes (▶ Fig. 9.2).

A biopsy using direct laryngoscopy (DL) confirmed the diagnosis of moderately differentiated squamous cell carcinoma, improving the evaluation of the extension of the lesion. The cancer was staged as cT2N0M0.

A supraglottic horizontal laryngectomy was carried out with resection of the epiglottis, vestibular and aryepiglottic folds, hyoid bone, superior portion of the thyroid cartilage, and pre-epiglottic space, in addition to with bilateral selective neck dissections.

An apron flap incision was made at the level of the thyroid cartilage extending to both sternocleidomastoid muscles (▶ Fig. 9.3).

The superior laryngeal nerves were identified and preserved at the midpoint between the superior corner of the hyoid bone and the thyroid cartilage, running along the superior laryngeal artery, a branch of the superior thyroid artery (▶ Fig. 9.4).

The infrahyoid musculature was skeletonized from the hyoid bone, followed by the transverse section of the thyroid cartilage (▶ Fig. 9.5).

The mucosa was opened at the level of the laryngeal ventricles. A transverse pharyngotomy, and section of the musculature of the base of the tongue

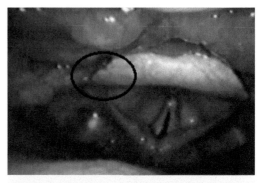

Fig. 9.1 Laryngoscopy revealed an irregular lesion in the epiglottis, vallecula, and left aryepiglottic fold (*circle*).

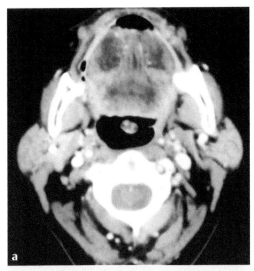
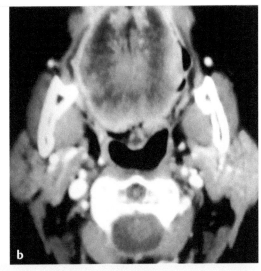

Fig. 9.2 (a, b) CT scan, demonstrating a lesion of the epiglottis, left aryepiglottic fold, and vallecula.

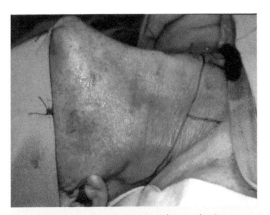

Fig. 9.3 Neck incision for horizontal supraglottic laryngectomy with bilateral neck dissections.

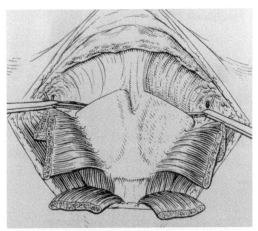

Fig. 9.4 The superior laryngeal nerves are identified and protected from injury during subsequent maneuvers. (Adapted from Barbosa.[1])

were performed. After the pharyngotomy, the cancer was resected with cancer free mucosal margins. Reconstruction was done by the mucosal suture of the pyriform sinus and three separate sites transferring the thyroid cartilage and base of the tongue.

A tracheostomy and a feeding tube were placed at the end of the procedure. The patient was decannulated on the twenty-fifth postoperative day and around same time started to receive an oral diet. Pathological examination revealed squamous cell carcinoma G3: pT2N1M0, R0, LVI0, PN0, and ECS0.

9.2 Discussion

Cancer of the larynx is the second most common malignancy of the head and neck region worldwide and squamous cell carcinoma accounts for more than 90% of all malignancies.[1]

The larynx is divided into three subsites anatomically and oncologically. Cancer arising in these subsites have their own individual oncologic behavior.

Supraglottic cancer tend to have more local regional advanced stages and present with nonspecific sore throat, dysphagia, and suspicious neck nodes at initial presentation.[2,3,4]

Supraglottic cancers can be treated effectively by radiotherapy, open surgery, or transoral laser microsurgery and robotic surgery. In the recent

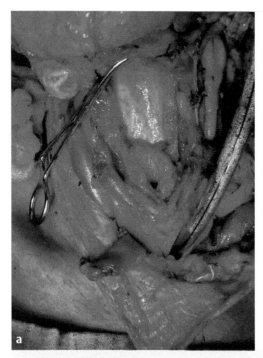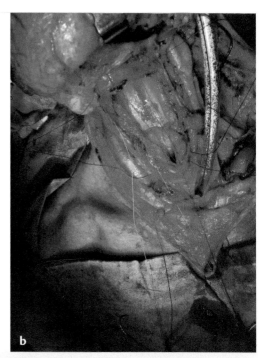

Fig. 9.5 **(a)** The thyroid cartilage was incised transversely and **(b)** the sutures were appropriately placed.

years, there has been an increasing trend of using organ preservation treatments, such as radiotherapy, with or without chemotherapy, in order to improve the patients' quality of life without decreasing oncological results. Either open conservative surgery or transoral microsurgery are mainly indicated for early cancer (T1–T2 tumors), and the goal is cure of the cancer with preservation of voice and deglutition.

There is no consensus on the best treatment for early supraglottic cancer because we do not have randomized controlled trials comparing the different treatments. Even today, physicians and patients rely on cohort studies and case series for decision-making.[5,6,7]

Current treatment guidelines indicate, for early cancer, a single modality of treatment either by radiotherapy or by conservative surgery.[8] The decision between surgery or radiotherapy should consider the patient's choice (accept tracheostomy and feeding tube, even if temporarily), expectation regarding vocal outcome, and general clinical conditions.

Finally, during treatment planning of head and neck cancer, especially in the larynx, the high incidence of metachronous cancer diagnosed after the control of the index cancer should also be considered.[9,10]

With surgery, treatment times are short, and a surgical specimen provides critical information about the primary cancer and, sometimes, about the regional lymph nodes, which provides important information for more accurate disease staging. Prognostic factors, such as positive margins, perineural spread, lymph node status, and the presence of extracapsular spread can be known only after surgery. This information can then be used to optimize the patient's treatment and the prognostic outcome. In addition, surgery leaves all other options for adjuvant or salvage treatment open. Radiotherapy can then be reserved for future treatment of recurrent or second primary cancers.[11,12]

The disadvantages of surgery stem from its possible complications, which include surgical site infection, bleeding, fistula formation, tracheostomy dependence, and chronic dysphagia. Transoral laser or robotic resection has been shown to reduce the incidence of major complications, such as permanent gastrostomy and tracheostomy, when compared with open surgery, without compromising survival outcomes.[13] However, it requires availability of modern technology, not always accessible in all centers.

One of the benefits of radiation over surgery is that it avoids general anesthesia. This is an important consideration for patients with underlying medical issues and other comorbidities. On the other hand, the volume seems to be more important than T-stage in predicting control in laryngeal squamous cell carcinoma patients in the planning of radiotherapy.

The present case was a cancer of the epiglottis with extension to the vallecula and aryepiglottic fold. Here, our option for conventional open surgery was the possibility of oncological control and the pathological study of the surgical specimen (primary cancer and neck lymph node) for better staging and prognosis. He was also a young patient with good performance profile and good pulmonary function, where possible adjuvant treatment could be better planned after the pathological information.

After a 30-month follow-up, the patient developed a second primary cancer in the pyriform sinuses and was treated with radiotherapy.

9.3 Tips

- Attention to the technical detail is required for safe supraglottic laryngectomy, which also depends on margin control and surgical technique.
- Neck metastasis is a serious problem with early supraglottic cancer, because both sides of the neck are at risk.
- Careful selection is the key to successful treatment.
- In the intraoperative stage, the supraglottic laryngectomy may be converted to a total laryngectomy.
- Depending on the expectations for vocal results, consider other types of treatment, including radiotherapy.

9.4 Traps

The T classification is an important prognostic marker; however, for predicting postoperative swallowing function, the radiological and endoscopic determination of the dimension of the cancer is very important.

Horizontal supraglottic laryngectomy can be a safe surgical option for elderly patients, but previous evaluation of the pulmonary function before surgery is mandatory because of an increased risk for aspiration pneumonia in patients with pulmonary problems.

References

[1] Barbosa JB, ed. Surgical treatment of head and neck. Ed. New York, NY: Grune & Stratton, 1974:178–184

[2] Peller M, Katalinic A, Wollenberg B, Teudt IU, Meyer JE. Epidemiology of laryngeal carcinoma in Germany, 1998–2011. Eur Arch Otorhinolaryngol. 2016; 273(6):1481–1487

[3] Curioni OA, Carvalho MB. A importância do diagnóstico clínico do carcinoma epidermoide de laringe em uma fase inicial da doença. Diagn Tratamento. 2001; 6:14–17

[4] Ganly I, Patel SG, Matsuo J, et al. Predictors of outcome for advanced-stage supraglottic laryngeal cancer. Head Neck. 2009; 31(11):1489–1495

[5] Mor N, Blitzer A. Functional anatomy and oncologic barriers of the larynx. Otolaryngol Clin North Am. 2015; 48(4):533–545

[6] DeSanto LW. Cancer of the supraglottic larynx: a review of 260 patients. Otolaryngol Head Neck Surg. 1985; 93(6):705–711

[7] Warner L, Chudasama J, Kelly CG, et al. Radiotherapy versus open surgery versus endolaryngeal surgery (with or without laser) for early laryngeal squamous cell cancer. Cochrane Database Syst Rev. 2014(12):CD002027

[8] Arshad H, Jayaprakash V, Gupta V, et al. Survival differences between organ preservation surgery and definitive radiotherapy in early supraglottic squamous cell carcinoma. Otolaryngol Head Neck Surg. 2014; 150(2):237–244

[9] Carlson RW, Larsen JK, McClure J, et al. International adaptations of NCCN Clinical Guidelines in Oncology. J Natl Compr Canc Netw. 2014; 12:643–648

[10] Bron LP, Pasche P, Monnier P, Schweizer V. Functional analysis after supracricoid partial laryngectomy with CHEP or CHP. Laryngoscope. 2002; 112:1289–1293

[11] León X, Martínez V, López M, et al. Second, third, and fourth head and neck tumors. A progressive decrease in survival. Head Neck. 2012; 34(12):1716–1719

[12] Freeman DE, Mancuso AA, Parsons JT, Mendenhall WM, Million RR. Irradiation alone for supraglottic larynx carcinoma: can CT findings predict treatment results? Int J Radiat Oncol Biol Phys. 1990; 19(2):485–490

[13] Rapoport A, Botelho RA, Souza RP, et al. The importance of pre-epiglottis space invasion in the treatment planning of larynx and hypopharynx cancer. Rev Bras Otorrinolaringol (Engl Ed). 2008; 74(1):74–78

10 Locally Intermediate Glottic Cancer: Transoral Laser Microsurgery

Giorgio Peretti, Fabiola Incandela, Francesco Missale

Abstract

Transoral laser microsurgery (TLM) is strongly recommended for early cancer of the glottis, since this technique is capable of achieving optimal outcomes in terms of recurrence-free survival and disease-specific survival provided by a minimally invasive approach with a low incidence of complications and very good functional results. The management of locally intermediate (T2–T3) glottic cancer is more challenging, because of a higher risk of recurrence, technical difficulty, and a wide range of other available treatment modalities such as TLM, open neck conservation surgery, and nonsurgical organ-preserving protocols. In this group of patients, the choice of treatment options is often guided by the technical facilities of the oncologic center. Some recommendations should be followed if TLM is the strategy chosen. We present the clinical case of a patient affected by a T3 glottic cancer treated by TLM in a highly specialized center as an example of the workflow that should guide the choice of such an approach.

Keywords: laryngeal cancer, laryngectomy, laser therapy, endoscopy, larynx, voice

10.1 Case Report

A 69-year-old male reported to our clinic with a history of progressive dysphonia for 4 months; he had never smoked and did not abuse alcohol. He had no chronic comorbidities and he had been treated 5 years earlier with radiotherapy for uveal melanoma of the left eye.

During outpatient consultation, transnasal videoendoscopic evaluation of the upper aerodigestive tract (UADT) was carried out using a flexible ENF-V2 videoendoscope connected to an EvisExera II CLV-180B light source (Visera Elite OTV-S190, Olympus Medical Systems Corporation, Tokyo, Japan), integrated with high-definition television and narrowband imaging (HDTV-NBI).

The examination revealed an exophytic lesion involving the entire true right vocal cord, which did not reach the arytenoid but extended to the anterior commissure, and toward the ipsilateral subglottis and supraglottis. The vocal cord was fixed, but arytenoid mobility was preserved. The lesion was characterized by atypical vascular changes suspicious for malignancy by HDTV-NBI examination (▶Fig. 10.1a, b).[1] The feasibility of a transoral approach was assessed in the preoperative setting considering a Laryngoscore of 4.[2]

To evaluate deep extension of the tumor and its relationship with the paraglottic space (PGS), pre-epiglottic space (PES), and cartilaginous framework, CT was performed, which revealed deep invasion of the lesion toward both the anterior PGS and subglottis without erosion of the thyroid cartilage. No suspicious cervical lymph nodes were detected (▶Fig. 10.1c). The clinical staging was a glottic tumor cT3N0M0 C2.

The patient was discussed by the multidisciplinary team and surgical treatment using transoral laser microsurgery (TLM) was proposed.

Laryngeal exposure, was obtained using a large bore laryngoscope (Microfrance Laryngoscopes 121, Medtronic ENT, Jacksonville, FL) which allowed visualization of the anterior commissure with external counter opressure on the neck. The diagnostic evaluation was integrated by intraoperative endoscopy with rigid endoscopes (0- and 70-degree angles). A superficial extension to the contralateral true vocal fold, ipsilateral supraglottis, and subglottis was confirmed (▶Fig. 10.1d). A biopsy with frozen sections confirmed the diagnoses of squamous cell carcinoma (SCC).

TLM was performed by CO_2 laser (Ultrapulse Laser CO_2, Lumenis, Yokneam, Israel), set on ultrapulse mode, which 3-W delivered power at 400-mm working distance.

The resection started with, exposing and removing the false vocal cords overlying the cancer. An endoscopic extended cordectomy, type Va–Vd according to European Laryngological Society (ELS) classification,[3] was performed with a "multiblock technique" to excise the entire tumor in five blocks (▶Fig. 10.2a, b). This technique allowed more precise and accurate assessment of the depth of the and comprehensive dissection of the PGS including the inner perichondrium of the thyroid cartilage. The resection was carried across the cricothyroid membrane as far as the first ring of the

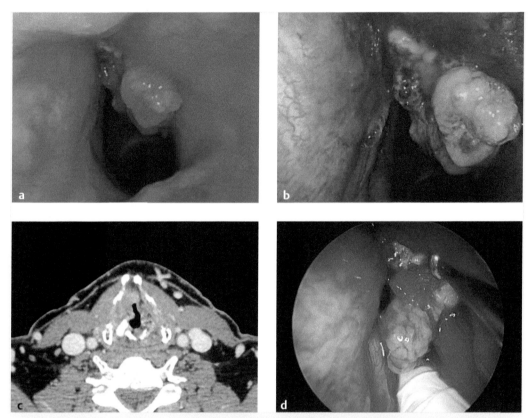

Fig. 10.1 Preoperative videoendoscopy of the tumor involving the entire right vocal cord with extension to the anterior commissure and subglottis and supraglottis in white light (a) narrowband imaging of the lesion (b). Preoperative CT of the neck which revealed invasion of the right anterior paraglottic space without signs of cartilage erosion (c). Intraoperative endoscopy with 0-degree endoscope demonstrating invasion of the floor of the right ventricle (d).

trachea. Care was taken not to penetrate the cricothyroid membrane or extend through the tracheal rings (▶ Fig. 10.2c).

On the first postoperative day, videoendoscopy was performed to evaluate laryngeal mobility. No edema or bleeding was present and after a swallowing examination that confirmed absence of dysphagia or aspiration, the patient started oral feeding without any problems. He was discharged the second day after surgery without the need for tracheostomy.

The histopathological report confirmed a moderately differentiated (G2) SCC of the right vocal cord, extending to the anterior commissure and to the subglottis with invasion of the vocal is muscle and paraglottic space. No evidence of perineural or lymphovascular invasion was found and all superficial and deep margins were negative; the pathologic staging was pT3G2R0 C3 cN0M0 C2.

The patient was scheduled for follow-up with imaging (CT and US of the neck) he 6 months and bimonthly endoscopic examinations for the first 2 years. The patient is currently free of 24 months after the surgery with good voice quality.

10.2 Discussion

Locally intermediate glottic cancer encompasses a heterogeneous variety of different lesions with distinct biological behavior and prognosis. Neoplastic pathways of diffusion toward visceral spaces (PGS and PES), invasion of the cartilaginous framework, and fixation of the vocal cord and/or the arytenoid represent critical issues that must be carefully considered during therapeutic planning.[4,5]

Such cancers are treatable by a wide range of different therapeutic strategies including TLM, open partial horizontal laryngectomy (OPHL), total

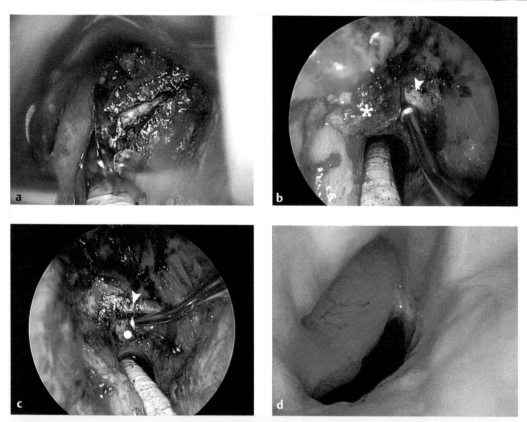

Fig. 10.2 **(a)** Intraoperative image of transtumoral resection using CO_2 laser across the middle third of the true vocal cord. **(b)** Endoscopic view after removal of the posterior portion of the cancer and dissection of the posterior paraglottic space (*star on the anterior aspect of the cancer and the arrowhead pointing to the thyroid cartilage*). **(c)** Final endoscopy at the end of surgery (*the arrowhead pointing to the thyroid cartilage and the circle the cricothyroid membrane*). **(d)** Videoendoscopy at 24 months revealing no recurrence of the cancer.

laryngectomy (TL), and nonsurgical organ-preserving protocols; the choice of treatment should be tailored, taking into account the highest cure rate with least morbidity, most favorable functional outcome, and costs.

In the last decades, increasing numbers of studies have confirmed that TLM has successfully expanded its indications, is reproducible in different oncologic centers, and is even suitable in combination with adjuvant therapy when necessary (▶ Table 10.1). However, evidence-based data of its utility in intermediate-advanced tumors are limited to case series performed by expert surgeons from a few institutions.[6,7,8,9,10,11,12] Therefore, its degree of recommendation remains limited. Moreover, several "weak points" of TLM such as inadequate exposure of the larynx, anterior commissure involvement in the craniocaudal direction,

infiltration of the PGS with arytenoid fixation, massive invasion of the PES, and erosion of the laryngeal framework are still under debate, thus restricting its application compared with more traditional surgical and nonsurgical options.[13]

For intermediate glottic SCC, functional outcomes in terms of voice, swallowing, and preservation of normal airway patency are also critical issues in the decision-making process. These factors may, in fact, dramatically impact the patient's emotional and physical life. The quality of the voice after TLM is related to the extent of resection and most authors have reported acceptable vocal outcomes, or at least comparable to those obtained after OPHL.[14,15]

Moreover, in contrast to the OPHL, TLM can better customize the mucosal and deep extension of the resection according to the size and location of

Table 10.1 Review of literature of oncological outcomes for intermediate-advanced glottic cancer treated by TLM

	N	T-stage	Treatment	5-y DFS (%)	5-y DSS (%)	5-y OS (%)
Mantsopoulos et al[6]	143	T2	TLM ± ND±RT	n/a	90.8	64.5
Peretti et al[7]	89	T2–T3	TLM ± RT	n/a	98.7	92.4
Caicedo-Granados et al[8]	32	T2–T3	TLM ± ND±RT	39.6	n/a	53.8
Canis et al[9]	142	T2a	TLM ± ND ± RT	76.4	93.2	72.2
Canis et al[9]	127	T2b	TLM ± ND ± RT	57.3	83.9	64.9
Canis et al[9]	122	T3	TLM ± ND ± RT	57.8	84.1	58.6
Pantazis et al[10]	19	T3	TLM ± RT	52.6	63.2	63.2
Peretti et al[11]	34	T3	TLM ± ND ± RT	72.9	87	65.2
Ansarin et al[12]	90	T2	TLM ± RT	75.3	n/a	n/a
Ansarin et al[12]	36	T3	TLM ± RT	68.6	n/a	n/a

Abbreviations: DFS, disease-free survival; DSS, disease-specific survival; n/a, not available; OS, overall survival; ND, neck dissection; RT, Radiotherapy; TLM, transoral laser microsurgery.

the cancer, thus minimizing the removal of uninvolved tissues resulting in preservation of healthy surrounding structures without modifying the physiologic laryngeal elevation. This is an essential aspect in adequate bolus progression, and thus greatly avoiding postoperative swallowing problems.

The negligible rate of aspiration following TLM represents an excellent result, especially when compared with the data reported after OPHL (temporary aspiration ranging from 32 to 89%) and chemoradiation (CRT; up to 84% of patients with temporary aspiration).[15,16,17,18] The same holds true for reduced perioperative and late morbidity, shorter hospitalization time, and fewer side effects. In particular, compared to OPHL and CRT, duration of hospitalization after TLM is significantly shorter (8.3 vs. 20–24 days, according to the specific protocol). Normal swallowing without permanent gastrostomy is achieved in 98% of cases and physiologic breathing without tracheostomy in 100% of patients.[16,19,20]

Another key strength of TLM is its feasibility in fragile elderly patients (older than 70 years) for whom open partial laryngectomies and nonsurgical organ preservation strategies are contraindicated due to associated comorbidities or age limits.[10]

A debated issue about management of laryngeal carcinomas is planning of follow-up. MR, in the hands of dedicated and experienced head and neck radiologists, has a higher diagnostic accuracy than CT in detecting recurrence of previously untreated intermediate glottic SCC and in all patients who underwent previous treatments. Therefore, this imaging technique should be always preferred, when available and feasible instead of CT.[21]

10.3 Tips

- Accurate and tailored patient selection, application of a multistep diagnostic evaluation based on pre- and intraoperative endoscopy, surgically oriented imaging assessment by dedicated head and neck radiologists, and use of a state-of-the-art laser technology are required to obtain outstanding and reproducible results.
- Adequate exposure of the larynx, particularly of the anterior commissure, allowing an accurate infrapetiolar exploration, is one of the main issues influencing the success of TLM; its prediction with objective assessment should be always considered in the preoperative counseling.[22,23]
- The use of high-frequency jet ventilation allows easier and safer management of lesions involving the posterior laryngeal compartment.[24]
- A "multiblock technique" of resection is strongly recommended in case of bulky lesions to optimize the three-dimensional view of the lesion and to assess the inferior and deep surgical margins.[25]
- The involvement of the posterior paraglottic space combined with the fixation of the cricoarytenoid joint represents the most controversial application for TLM affecting oncologic outcomes and determining higher recurrence rates than those obtained with open-neck procedures.[12,13]

10.4 Traps

- Given the wide range of technological tools and dedicated instrumentation currently available, even extended resection can be technically performed by TLM. However, when the surgeon is faced with unfavorable anatomy, inadequate exposure, and an unacceptably high risk of complications, the procedure should be changed without delay to an alternative external surgical approach or nonsurgical therapeutic options.
- In local intermediate lesions, recurrences tend to grow submucosally and are not visible by standard endoscopic examination until they reach a more advanced stage. Our data indicate that in such cancers the rate of submucosal persistence/recurrence increases to 43%, thereby augmenting the false-negative rate of postoperative endoscopic evaluation alone and highlighting the need for a customized follow-up policy with the combination of endoscopy and planned imaging.[21]

References

[1] Arens C, Piazza C, Andrea M, et al. Proposal for a descriptive guideline of vascular changes in lesions of the vocal folds by the committee on endoscopic laryngeal imaging of the European Laryngological Society. Eur Arch Otorhinolaryngol. 2016; 273(5):1207–1214

[2] Piazza C, Mangili S, Bon FD, et al. Preoperative clinical predictors of difficult laryngeal exposure for microlaryngoscopy: the Laryngoscore. Laryngoscope. 2014; 124(11):2561–2567

[3] Remacle M, Eckel HE, Antonelli A, et al. Endoscopic cordectomy. A proposal for a classification by the Working Committee, European Laryngological Society. Eur Arch Otorhinolaryngol. 2000; 257(4):227–231

[4] Canis M, Ihler F, Martin A, Wolff HA, Matthias C, Steiner W. Results of 226 patients with T3 laryngeal carcinoma after treatment with transoral laser microsurgery. Head Neck. 2014; 36(5):652–659

[5] Vilaseca I, Bernal-Sprekelsen M, Luis Blanch J. Transoral laser microsurgery for T3 laryngeal tumors: prognostic factors. Head Neck. 2010; 32(7):929–938

[6] Mantsopoulos K, Psychogios G, Koch M, Zenk J, Waldfahrer F, Iro H. Comparison of different surgical approaches in T2 glottic cancer. Head Neck. 2012; 34(1):73–77

[7] Peretti G, Piazza C, Del Bon F, et al. Function preservation using transoral laser surgery for T2-T3 glottic cancer: oncologic, vocal, and swallowing outcomes. Eur Arch Otorhinolaryngol. 2013; 270(8):2275–2281

[8] Caicedo-Granados E, Beswick DM, Christopoulos A, et al. Oncologic and functional outcomes of partial laryngeal surgery for intermediate-stage laryngeal cancer. Otolaryngol Head Neck Surg. 2013; 148(2):235–242

[9] Canis M, Martin A, Ihler F, et al. Transoral laser microsurgery in treatment of pT2 and pT3 glottic laryngeal squamous cell carcinoma - results of 391 patients. Head Neck. 2014; 36(6):859–866

[10] Pantazis D, Liapi G, Kostarelos D, Kyriazis G, Pantazis TL, Riga M. Glottic and supraglottic pT3 squamous cell carcinoma: outcomes with transoral laser microsurgery. Eur Arch Otorhinolaryngol. 2015; 272(8):1983–1990

[11] Peretti G, Piazza C, Penco S, et al. Transoral laser microsurgery as primary treatment for selected T3 glottic and supraglottic cancers. Head Neck. 2016; 38(7):1107–1112

[12] Ansarin M, Cattaneo A, De Benedetto L, et al. Retrospective analysis of factors influencing oncologic outcome in 590 patients with early-intermediate glottic cancer treated by transoral laser microsurgery. Head Neck. 2017; 39(1):71–81

[13] Peretti G, Piazza C, Mora F, Garofolo S, Guastini L. Reasonable limits for transoral laser microsurgery in laryngeal cancer. Curr Opin Otolaryngol Head Neck Surg. 2016; 24(2):135–139

[14] Roh JL, Kim DH, Park CI. Voice, swallowing and quality of life in patients after transoral laser surgery for supraglottic carcinoma. J Surg Oncol. 2008; 98(3):184–189

[15] Benito J, Holsinger FC, Pérez-Martín A, Garcia D, Weinstein GS, Laccourreye O. Aspiration after supracricoid partial laryngectomy: Incidence, risk factors, management, and outcomes. Head Neck. 2011; 33(5):679–685

[16] Hutcheson KA, Barringer DA, Rosenthal DI, May AH, Roberts DB, Lewin JS. Swallowing outcomes after radiotherapy for laryngeal carcinoma. Arch Otolaryngol Head Neck Surg. 2008; 134(2):178–183

[17] Bernal-Sprekelsen M, Vilaseca-González I, Blanch-Alejandro JL. Predictive values for aspiration after endoscopic laser resections of malignant tumors of the hypopharynx and larynx. Head Neck. 2004; 26(2):103–110

[18] Ellies M, Steiner W. Peri- and postoperative complications after laser surgery of tumors of the upper aerodigestive tract. Am J Otolaryngol. 2007; 28(3):168–172

[19] Alicandri-Ciufelli M, Piccinini A, Grammatica A, et al. Voice and swallowing after partial laryngectomy: factors influencing outcome. Head Neck. 2013; 35(2):214–219

[20] Pinar E, Imre A, Calli C, Oncel S, Katilmis H. Supracricoid partial laryngectomy: analyses of oncologic and functional outcomes. Otolaryngol Head Neck Surg. 2012; 147(6):1093–1098

[21] Marchi F, Piazza C, Ravanelli M, et al. Role of imaging in the follow-up of T2–T3 glottic cancer treated by transoral laser microsurgery. Eur Arch Otorhinolaryngol. 2017; 274(10):3679–3686

[22] Zeitels SM. Infrapetiole exploration of the supraglottis for exposure of the anterior glottal commissure. J Voice. 1998; 12(1):117–122

[23] Peretti G, Piazza C, Bolzoni A, et al. Analysis of recurrences in 322 Tis, T1, or T2 glottic carcinomas treated by carbon dioxide laser. Ann Otol Rhinol Laryngol. 2004; 113(11):853–858

[24] Mora F, Missale F, Incandela F, et al. High frequency jet ventilation during transoral laser microsurgery for Tis-T2 Laryngeal Cancer. Front Oncol. 2017; 7:282

[25] Hinni ML, Salassa JR, Grant DG, et al. Transoral laser microsurgery for advanced laryngeal cancer. Arch Otolaryngol Head Neck Surg. 2007; 133(12):1198–1204

11 Locally Intermediate Glottic Cancer: Chemoradiotherapy

Ana Ponce Kiess, Christine G. Gourin, Arlene A. Forastiere

Abstract

A case report of locally intermediate glottic cancer, cT3N0M0, stage III, is presented with discussion of the multidisciplinary evaluation, options for preserving the larynx, and the treatment course. Endoscopy revealed a left glottic mass extending to the left false cord, arytenoid, and aryepiglottic fold. The vocal fold was fixed. CT imaging demonstrated involvement of the left paraglottic space with no cervical lymphadenopathy. Swallowing function was normal with no penetration or aspiration, and vocal quality was hoarse with moderately reduced intensity. Concurrent chemoradiation was chosen by the patient whose employment entailed high occupational voice demands. The patient received a cumulative radiation dose of 7,000 cGy to gross disease, 6,125 cGy to the uninvolved larynx, and 5,600 cGy to bilateral cervical nodal levels II to IV that was planned and delivered using image-guided volumetric modulated arc therapy. Chemotherapy concurrent with radiation was seven weekly doses of cisplatin 40 mg/m^2 with hydration, antiemetics, and pain management. The patient required enteral nutritional support until 6 weeks following completion of treatment. PET/CT imaging at 12 weeks demonstrated non-fluorodeoxyglucose avid posttreatment changes indicative of a complete response. The surgical and nonsurgical larynx preservation treatment options, standard of care recommendations, expected outcomes, and supporting literature are discussed. Accurate staging and baseline assessment of swallowing and voice function are emphasized. Other factors to consider in the treatment decision are comorbidities, patient preference, and expectations for long-term voice quality.

Keywords: glottic cancer, larynx preservation, chemotherapy, radiotherapy, chemoradiotherapy, laryngectomy

11.1 Case Report

A 57-year-old Caucasian male presented with a 3 month history of progressive sore throat and hoarseness. He was an active smoker of one pack of cigarettes per day for 42 years and social use of alcohol. He also noted occasional shortness of breath at night when lying flat. He denied dysphagia or weight loss. He worked as a railroad manager with high occupational voice demands. His medical history was significant for hypertension treated with metoprolol and valsartan, and atrial fibrillation anticoagulated with rivaroxaban. He was referred to an Otolaryngologist, and flexible laryngoscopy revealed a left glottic mass extending to the left false cord, arytenoid, and aryepiglottic fold. The left vocal fold was fixed in the median position. CT of the neck with contrast showed an enhancing mass involving the left glottis and aryepiglottic fold with involvement of the left paraglottic space. There was no cervical lymphadenopathy on physical examination or CT of the neck. He underwent direct laryngoscopy with biopsy of the laryngeal mass. Pathology reported invasive squamous cell carcinoma. CT of the chest showed no suspicious pulmonary nodules, and the clinical staging by the seventh edition of AJCC was cT3N0M0 (stage III).

The patient was seen in a multidisciplinary head and neck clinic by an otolaryngologist, radiation oncologist, medical oncologist, and speech-language pathologist (SLP). Fiberoptic endoscopic evaluation of swallowing demonstrated normal baseline swallow function with no penetration or aspiration across all consistencies. The patient's vocal quality was moderately rough and hoarse with mildly reduced intensity. Surgical and nonsurgical treatment options were discussed with the patient, including total laryngectomy, partial laryngectomy, or definitive chemoradiation with weekly cisplatin.

Larynx-preserving surgery for this cancer would require a supracricoid laryngectomy, which includes removal of the true and, false vocal cords, supraglottis, and pre-epiglottic space, and may be extended to include one arytenoid or the epiglottis.[1] Anatomic contraindications to this procedure are bilateral arytenoid involvement, subglottic extension of the cancer more than 1 cm anteriorly and 0.5 cm posteriorly, cricoid cartilage involvement, base of tongue involvement, and extension into the hypopharynx or the pyriform apex. Functional considerations are aspiration and breathy voice resulting from surgery. Patients with pulmonary impairment are poor candidates for larynx-preserving surgery, because aspiration is common and the availability of speech-language pathology in rehabilitation is a critical component of surgical decision-making. Evaluation of pulmonary function is critical to successful surgery, with the ability to climb two flights of stairs without dyspnea an excellent indicator of the patient's ability to tolerate the functional sequelae of partial laryngectomy. Because surgery results in a U-shaped laryngeal inlet, dysphonia results with a voice that is breathy and of low volume.

The patient elected for treatment with definitive chemoradiation and underwent CT and MRI simulation. Pretreatment dental evaluation was performed.

The patient completed successfully 7 weeks of concurrent radiation and cisplatin chemotherapy. The cumulative dose of radiation was 7,000 cGy to gross disease, 6,125 cGy to the uninvolved larynx,

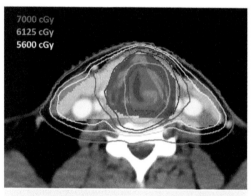

Fig. 11.1 Axial image from the radiation treatment plan showing isodose lines conforming to 7,000-, 6,125-, and 5,600-cGy target volumes.

and 5,600 cGy to bilateral cervical nodal levels II to IV (▶Fig. 11.1).

Simultaneous integrated boost technique was used with 35 daily fractions. Treatment was planned and delivered using image-guided volumetric modulated arc therapy (a type of intensity-modulated radiotherapy) with 6 MV photons and daily cone-beam CT guidance. The patient received all seven planned doses of weekly cisplatin at 40 mg/m^2 with routine IV hydration and antiemetics including ondansetron and dexamethasone. He developed grade 3 mucositis and grade 2 dysphagia, nausea, vomiting, and dysgeusia. These side effects led to inadequate oral intake with a weight loss of 24 pounds (12% body weight), so that a temporary nasogastric tube was placed. His pain was controlled with gabapentin, oxycodone, and a fentanyl patch. He also developed grade 3 dysphonia by the end of the treatment. The nasogastric tube was removed at 3 weeks posttreatment. He required frequent IV hydration and magnesium repletion for 6 weeks posttreatment.

Flexible laryngoscopy revealed that the patient had a complete clinical response to treatment (▶Fig. 11.2a, b).

The patient also successfully stopped smoking. At 3 months posttreatment, CT of the neck with IV contrast demonstrated decreased volume of the glottic mass and posttreatment changes (▶Fig. 11.3b). Subsequent PET/CT demonstrated non-FDG (fluorodeoxyglucose) avid posttreatment changes with only physiologic FDG uptake in the larynx (▶Fig. 11.3c).

At 12 months posttreatment, the patient had no evidence of disease and noted mild dysphagia, dysphonia, and lymphedema of the anterior neck. He was only partially compliant with SLP follow-up and swallowing exercises. He underwent physical therapy for the lymphedema with partial improvement.

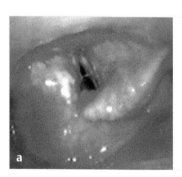
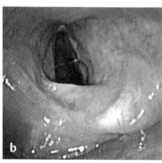

Fig. 11.2 Flexible laryngoscopy images of left glottic cancer before (a) and 12 months after (b) treatment with definitive concurrent chemoradiation.

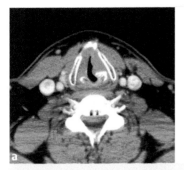 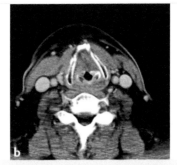 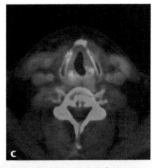

Fig. 11.3 Axial images from CT of the neck with contrast before **(a)** and 3 months after **(b)** treatment with definitive chemoradiation. The left glottic mass involved the paraglottic space. After treatment, the mass was reduced in volume with associated posttreatment edema. **(c)** PET after treatment showed only physiologic fluorodeoxyglucose uptake in the larynx.

11.2 Discussion

Accurate staging and functional assessment are critical in the evaluation of patients with glottic cancer. Treatment options typically include surgical or nonsurgical management for patients with stage T1 to T3 cancer, whereas total laryngectomy is strongly favored for patients with stage T4a cancer or severe baseline laryngeal dysfunction. For early glottic cancer (stage T1–T2 N0), patients may be treated with larynx-preserving or definitive radiotherapy with similar, excellent outcomes. TLM is often favored for unilateral stage T1aN0 cancer to preserve function of the vocal cord. Definitive radiotherapy is often favored for bilateral cancer (stage T1b) or cancer involving the supraglottis (stage T2). In this setting, radiotherapy is typically delivered using two opposed lateral beams to the larynx alone (not neck nodes) using a hypofractionated regimen of 6,300 to 6,525 cGy in 28 to 29 fractions.[2,3]

For intermediate-stage glottic cancers (T3 or N+), treatment options typically include definitive chemoradiotherapy, total laryngectomy, or in select cases partial laryngectomy.

Total laryngectomy remains the gold standard against which all organ preservation techniques are measured and, by removing the larynx and thus separating inspiration from swallowing, is associated with a lower incidence of late toxicity. In Surveillance, Epidemiology and End Results Program (SEER) Medicare data, surgery appears to be associated with improved survival, which may be a result of a lower odds of late pneumonia in surgical patients, which was associated with the greatest risk of death at

5 years.[4,5] However, total laryngectomy is disfiguring and results in a permanent tracheostoma, which has functional and psychological consequences.[6]

Surgical techniques that preserve the larynx (hemilaryngectomy, supraglottic laryngectomy, and supracricoid laryngectomy) preserve voice, avoid a tracheostoma, and offer the potential to avoid chemotherapy and to use radiation therapy (RT) in the adjuvant setting, with survival rates reported to be similar to that following total laryngectomy.[1] Larynx conservation surgery requires the patient to use compensatory strategies to protect the airway, and is associated with a high incidence of dysphagia and aspiration, but with careful patient selection a low incidence of morbidity and severe treatment-related complications, which is critical to a successful outcome.[7,8] Intelligible speech is preserved, but severe dysphonia results, which may impact patient-reported emotional, physical, and functional outcomes.[9] Compared to total laryngectomy, supracricoid laryngectomy is associated with an initial protracted period of swallowing difficulties and swallowing therapy, but speech intelligibility is rated as similar.[10] When medical and anatomic considerations are taken into account, less than one-third of patients are suitable candidates for larynx conservation surgery.[11]

Nonsurgical larynx preservation approaches for intermediate-stage cancer of the glottis include concurrent chemoradiation, neoadjuvant (induction) chemotherapy followed by radiation, and RT alone. Based on the results of a meta-analysis of chemotherapy added to standard local curative treatment in more than 17,000 patients with cancer of the head and neck[12] and prospective randomized controlled trials in larynx cancer,[13,14, 15]concurrent chemoradiation has been shown to offer a significant advantage over the approaches of induction or radiation alone for preserving the larynx and achieving locoregional control.

The Veterans Affairs (VA) Laryngeal Cancer Study, published in 1991, demonstrated equivalent survival for advanced cancer of the larynx treated with total laryngectomy or with induction chemotherapy followed by radiation, allowing for laryngectomy in nonresponders.[13] Salvage laryngectomy was ultimately performed for 56% of patients with T4 cancer, compared to 29% for T1 to T3 cancer, and was more frequently associated with glottic than supraglottic subsite, and with gross cartilage invasion than no cartilage invasion.[13] This higher local failure rate for T4 cancers led to the exclusion of high-volume T4 cancers (penetration through cartilage or into deep tongue musculature) from subsequent randomized trials and therefore combined chemoradiation larynx preservation approaches were limited to selected T4a cancers. By contrast, the data for intermediate-stage larynx cancer indicate equivalent survival outcomes with excellent locoregional control. Favorable results of chemoradiation were demonstrated in the Radiation Therapy Oncology Group (RTOG) Trial 91–11, which largely excluded T4 cancers and demonstrated improved locoregional control rates with concurrent chemoradiation therapy.[14] These data established larynx preservation with chemoradiation as a standard of care for intermediate-stage larynx cancers.

Concurrent cisplatin and radiation is endorsed in guidelines[16] as the recommended nonsurgical approach for larynx preservation based on high-level evidence and is the most commonly used approach in the United States. The RTOG 91–11 U.S. Intergroup trial of 547 patients directly compared the three approaches; concurrent cisplatin and RT, induction cisplatin/fluorouracil followed by RT, and RT alone in patients with locally advanced cancer of the glottis or supraglottis.[14,15] Most patients had stage III cancer, stage distribution was 79% T3, 50% N0, and 21% N1, and thus the results are applicable to this case of T3N0 cancer of the glottis. The long-term results of RTOG 91–11 showed that overall survival was similar with all three approaches but concurrent treatment was associated with a 54% relative risk reduction of laryngectomy compared with RT alone (hazard ratio [HR]: 0.46; 95% confidence interval [CI]: 0.30–0.71; $p < 0.001$) and a 42% risk reduction compared to induction

chemotherapy (HR: 0.58; 95% CI: 0.37–0.89; $p = 0.005$). Surprisingly, induction chemotherapy added to RT had no effect on laryngectomy rate compared to treatment with RT alone. The difference in local and locoregional control followed a similar pattern demonstrating clear superiority of concurrent chemoradiation. Less acute in-field toxicity is observed with the induction approach and with RT alone, and these treatment options may be preferred based on individual patient characteristics and the expertise of the treating team. The induction approach is preferred in some geographic regions outside of North America based on a series of induction trials conducted in Europe.[17,18,19] Treatment-related late toxicity is a concern with larynx preservation with surgery or with concurrent chemoradiation. The late-effects toxicity grading system (NCI/RTOG/UICC) may be inadequate to discriminate differences among treatment groups following radiotherapy or combined chemotherapy and radiotherapy. For example, there were no differences in the incidence of laryngopharyngeal/esophageal and soft-tissue late toxicity occurring between treatment groups in the RTOG 91–11 trial and no difference in speech and swallowing function assessments. However, the 10-year follow-up report of RTOG 91–11 found an increase in non-cancer-related deaths in patients treated with concurrent chemoradiation beyond 5 years.[15] This unexplained outcome could possibly be a consequence of unrecognized late toxicity. High crude rates of late laryngeal and pharyngeal dysfunction were reported in a combined analysis of multisite RTOG chemoradiation trials.[20] The data in all of these reports come from trials performed over two decades ago using two-dimensional RT. Whether the risk of late effects is the same today with the use of modern radiation techniques and aggressive supportive care including speech and swallowing therapy is not known. It is clear that patient selection is a key factor for achieving an optimal result of surgical or nonsurgical organ preservation.

Cisplatin is the radiosensitizer recommended for administration concurrent with RT. Carboplatin is recommended for patients with medical contraindications to cisplatin. There are insufficient data to support the use of any other radiosensitizer. Prospective clinical trials in cancer of the larynx have used once every 3 weeks. high-dose (100 mg/m²) cisplatin administered every three weeks once every three weeks during the course of RT. Alternative weekly dosing (40 mg/m²) has come into practice to reduce the risk of nephrotoxicity, ototoxicity, nausea/vomiting, and to insure adequate prehydration of patients treated in the outpatient setting. The weekly schedule has been studied in nasopharyngeal cancer and the two schedules appear to have equivalent efficacy. In the treatment of non-nasopharyngeal cancer, there is a clinical impression of equivalent efficacy of the two dosing schedules when a minimum total dose of 200 mg/m^2 is given. This has led to the frequent use of weekly cisplatin dosing in clinical practice. A recent meta-analysis of 52 studies (4,209 patients) of concurrent cisplatin and RT for definitive or adjuvant treatment of head and neck cancer revealed that there was no difference in overall survival or response rate among patients treated with weekly or high-dose cisplatin.[21] The weekly regimen in the definitive treatment setting was associated with higher treatment compliance and significantly less severe and life-threatening (grades 3 and 4) myelosuppression (leucopenia, neutropenia), nephrotoxicity, and nausea/vomiting. In the adjuvant setting, investigators at the Tata Memorial Hospital randomized 300 non-nasopharyngeal cancer patients to weekly (30 mg/m^2) cisplatin or every 3-week, high-dose (100 mg/m^2) cisplatin and RT.[22] There was a significant difference in the cumulative 2-year locoregional control rate, 58.5% versus 73% favoring 3-weekly cisplatin but no significant difference in median progression-free or overall survival outcomes. Toxicity was substantially higher with the high dose treatment. No other randomized non-nasopharyngeal cancer studies have been reported. Additional prospective studies addressing this question are unlikely given the resources that would be required to power a trial to show a small difference or noninferiority of the weekly low-dose schedule. Moreover, cisplatin efficacy is totally dose dependent, not schedule dependent. Thus, at present, a weekly dose of 40 mg/m^2 is viewed as a potentially safe and equally effective alternative to three-weekly high-dose treatment as was used in the case presented.

Baseline functional assessment is very important in the discussion of treatment options for patients with intermediate-stage glottic cancers, and multidisciplinary dialogue is critical. In the case presented here, the patient attended a multidisciplinary clinic including SLP, and he was found to have excellent baseline swallow function and moderate baseline dysphonia. Given these factors, as well as his young age, limited comorbidities, and availability of appropriate support and expertise, the multidisciplinary team anticipated a relatively high likelihood of successful larynx preservation. His occupational voice demand and personal preferences were also taken into account in his treatment decision.

Radiation techniques for treatment of intermediate- or advanced-stage glottic cancers are more complex than those for early-stage glottic cancers, requiring intensity-modulated radiotherapy with many beams or several continuous arc beams. The dose is typically approximately 70 Gy to gross disease, with lower doses to at-risk areas of the larynx, pharynx, and neck. Bilateral neck nodes should be included in the treatment volume, even for clinically node-negative patients. Conventional fractionation is preferred with approximately 2 Gy per fraction to limit the risk of late toxicities. Image guidance should be utilized when available. Whenever possible, the radiation plan should spare the parotid and submandibular glands, pharyngeal constrictors, and oral cavity.

11.3 Tips

- Patients with severe baseline dysphagia are at high risk after chemoradiation for long-term gastrostomy dependence and aspiration. It is important to emphasize these risks in the discussion of treatment options with these patients.
- Patient selection for surgery must take into account the extent of the cancer as well as the impact of aspiration and voice on function. Patients with poor pulmonary function and preoperative aspiration may be better served with total laryngectomy, which eliminates the risk of aspiration and permits safe swallowing, with voicing possible using tracheoesophageal puncture.
- Careful evaluation of preoperative imaging and staging laryngoscopy are critical before embarking on larynx-preservation surgery; subglottic and extralaryngeal extension are contraindications to supracricoid laryngectomy.
- Early and frequent involvement of SLP is important in baseline speech and swallow evaluation, counseling regarding exercises and compensatory strategies, and monitoring dysphagia during and after treatment.
- Patients with normal baseline swallowing function may not benefit from prophylactic gastrostomy, as maintaining oral intake during treatment is predictive for improved long-term swallow function. However, the need for enteral nutritional support must be monitored closely.

11.4 Traps

- Be careful in assessing vocal cord mobility and imaging involvement of the pre-epiglottic or paraglottic fat (stage T3 vs. T2). Given the significant differences in surgical and nonsurgical treatment recommendations for these stages, as well as the differences in radiotherapy techniques for T3 vs. T2 tumors, the distinction is critical. Similar caution is recommended in assessing subglottic extension, which is a contraindication to partial laryngectomy.
- Fiberoptic examination during radiotherapy is recommended to assess for edema, particularly if any new respiratory symptoms are reported. In the setting of acute edema, a methylprednisolone taper may help prevent the need for urgent tracheostomy.

References

[1] Laccourreye H, Laccourreye O, Weinstein G, Menard M, Brasnu D. Supracricoid laryngectomy with cricohyoidopexy: a partial laryngeal procedure for selected supraglottic and transglottic carcinomas. Laryngoscope. 1990; 100(7):735–741

[2] Yamazaki H, Nishiyama K, Tanaka E, Koizumi M, Chatani M. Radiotherapy for early glottic carcinoma (T1N0M0): results of prospective randomized study of radiation fraction size and overall treatment time. Int J Radiat Oncol Biol Phys. 2006; 64(1):77–82

[3] Marciscano AE, Charu V, Starmer HM, et al. Evaluating post-radiotherapy laryngeal function with laryngeal videostroboscopy in early stage glottic cancer. Front Oncol. 2017; 7:124

[4] Gourin CG, Dy SM, Herbert RJ, et al. Treatment, survival, and costs of laryngeal cancer care in the elderly. Laryngoscope. 2014; 124(8):1827–1835

[5] Gourin CG, Starmer HM, Herbert RJ, et al. Short- and long-term outcomes of laryngeal cancer care in the elderly. Laryngoscope. 2015; 125(4):924–933

[6] Lisan Q, George N, Hans S, Laccourreye O, Lemogne C. Post-surgical disfigurement influences disgust recognition: a case-control study. Psychosomatics. 2018; 59(2):177–185

[7] Benito J, Holsinger FC, Pérez-Martín A, Garcia D, Weinstein GS, Laccourreye O. Aspiration after supracricoid partial laryngectomy: incidence, risk factors, management, and outcomes. Head Neck. 2011; 33(5):679–685

[8] Lips M, Speyer R, Zumach A, Kross KW, Kremer B. Supracricoid laryngectomy and dysphagia: A systematic literature review. Laryngoscope. 2015; 125(9):2143–2156

[9] Zacharek MA, Pasha R, Meleca RJ, et al. Functional outcomes after supracricoid laryngectomy. Laryngoscope. 2001; 111(9):1558–1564

[10] Dworkin JP, Meleca RJ, Zacharek MA, et al. Voice and deglutition functions after the supracricoid and total laryngectomy procedures for advanced stage laryngeal carcinoma. Otolaryngol Head Neck Surg. 2003; 129(4):311–320

[11] Mendenhall WM, Parsons JT, Mancuso AA, Stringer SP, Cassisi NJ. Radiotherapy for squamous cell carcinoma of the supraglottic larynx: an alternative to surgery. Head Neck. 1996; 18(1):24–35

[12] Pignon JP, le Maître A, Maillard E, Bourhis J; MACH-NC Collaborative Group. Meta-analysis of chemotherapy in head and neck cancer (MACH-NC): an update on 93 randomised trials and 17,346 patients. Radiother Oncol. 2009; 92(1):4–14

[13] Wolf GT, Fisher SG, Hong WK, et al; Department of Veterans Affairs Laryngeal Cancer Study Group. Induction chemotherapy plus radiation compared with surgery plus radiation in patients with advanced laryngeal cancer. N Engl J Med. 1991; 324(24):1685–1690

[14] Forastiere AA, Goepfert H, Maor M, et al. Concurrent chemotherapy and radiotherapy for organ preservation in advanced laryngeal cancer. N Engl J Med. 2003; 349(22):2091–2098

[15] Forastiere AA, Zhang Q, Weber RS, et al. Long-term results of RTOG 91–11: a comparison of three nonsurgical treatment strategies to preserve the larynx in patients with locally advanced larynx cancer. J Clin Oncol. 2013; 31(7):845–852

[16] Forastiere AA, Ismaila N, Lewin JS, et al. Use of larynx-preservation strategies in the treatment of laryngeal cancer: American Society of Clinical Oncology Clinical Practice Guideline Update. J Clin Oncol. 2018; 36(11):1143–1169

[17] Lefebvre JL, Andry G, Chevalier D, et al; EORTC Head and Neck Cancer Group. Laryngeal preservation with induction chemotherapy for hypopharyngeal squamous cell carcinoma: 10-year results of EORTC trial 24891. Ann Oncol. 2012; 23(10):2708–2714

[18] Henriques De Figueiredo B, Fortpied C, Menis J, et al; EORTC Head and Neck Cancer and Radiation Oncology Cooperative Groups. Long-term update of the 24954 EORTC phase III trial on larynx preservation. Eur J Cancer. 2016; 65:109–112

[19] Janoray G, Pointreau Y, Garaud P, et al. Long-term results of a multicenter randomized phase III trial of induction chemotherapy with cisplatin, 5-fluorouracil, + docetaxel for larynx preservation. J Natl Cancer Inst. 2015; 108(4):djv368

[20] Machtay M, Moughan J, Trotti A, et al. Factors associated with severe late toxicity after concurrent chemoradiation for locally advanced head and neck cancer: an RTOG analysis. J Clin Oncol. 2008; 26(21):3582–3589

[21] Szturz P, Wouters K, Kiyota N, et al. Weekly low-dose versus three-weekly high-dose cisplatin for concurrent chemoradiation in locoregionally advanced non-nasopharyngeal head and neck cancer: a systemic review and meta-analysis of aggregate data. Oncologist. 2017; 22(9):1056–1066

[22] Noronha V, Joshi A, Patil VM, et al. Once-a-week versus once-every-3-weeks cisplatin chemoradiation for locally advanced head and neck cancer: a phase III randomized noninferiority trial. J Clin Oncol. 2018; 36(11):1064–1072

12 Locally Intermediate Glottic Cancer: Vertical Partial Laryngectomy

Rogério A. Dedivitis, Mario Augusto F. Castro

Abstract

Radiotherapy, laser endoscopic excision, and partial laryngectomy are the options in the treatment and of the moderate-stage cancer of the larynx. The decision must consider the patient's expectations. For the case described here, vertical technique (hemilaryngectomy) and the horizontal technique (horizontal supracricoid laryngectomy) may be recommended. The main advantage of the hemilaryngectomy is the maintenance of the hemilarynx structures not involved by the carcinoma. Probably the cases presenting microscopic infiltration of the thyroid cartilage for cancer would be eligible for transoral laser resection. Vertical laryngectomies are still a good option in cases where endoscopic surgery does not suffice or when it is not available, such as in some developing countries. The need for the reconstruction of the endolarynx by using flaps and grafts allows for a better glottic coaptation. The oncologic outcome is less favorable in cancer extending beyond the confines of the vocal folds, in which supracricoid laryngectomy can be performed.

Keywords: laryngectomy, laryngeal cancer, carcinoma, squamous cell, reconstructive techniques, voice

12.1 Case Report

A 76-year-old Caucasian male, retired stevedore, presented with a 4 month history of progressive dysphonia, followed by episodes of choking on liquids. He stated that he smoked one pack of cigarettes a day for 45 years as well as drinking alcohol socially. He also stated that he was hypertensive and was taking enalapril and atorvastatin for dyslipidemia.

At the time of the consultation, the patient was healthy and presented with hoarseness, with and little vocal range. No abnormalities were found on oroscopy and cervical palpation. A direct laryngoscopy revealed an ulcer-ated infiltrative lesion on the entire right vocal fold, which extended to the anterior commissure, with no involvement of the right vocal fold. The lesion did not extend

to the infraglottis, ventricle, or ipsilateral arytenoid (▶ Fig. 12.1) The mobility of the left vocal fold was reduced and Reinke's edema present.

For a better deeper evaluation of the extension of the lesion, an MRI scan was performed which demonstrated an infiltrative irregular lesion of the right vocal fold, with heterogeneous contrast enhancement, with partial invasion of the paraglottic space. The lesion infiltrated the anterior commissure, but the ipsilateral arytenoid was preserved. There were no signs of extension to the left vocal fold (▶ Fig. 12.2).

Microlaryngeal surgery for better staging and biopsy was carried out under general anaesthesia. The anatomopathological result showed a moderately differentiated squamous cell carcinoma.

The patient underwent a hemilaryngectomy, with the removal of the wedge of thyroid cartilage in en bloc resection of the cancer, respecting oncological margins in depth in the paraglottic space. Both arytenoids were preserved. Prior to the beginning of the hemilaryngectomy, a protective tracheostomy was performed, at the fifth tracheal ring out of the operative field. For the performance of the hemilaryngectomy, the skin was incised over the thyroid cartilage and the subplatysmal flap was raised. With the opening of the median raphe and exposure of the thyroid

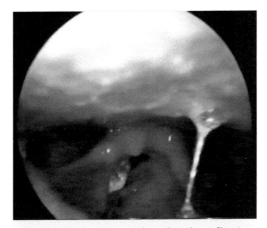

Fig. 12.1 The laryngoscopy showed an ulcer-infiltrative lesion involving the right vocal fold and anterior commissure.

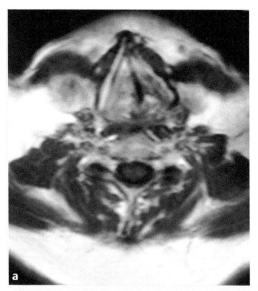
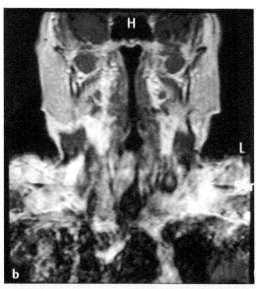

Fig. 12.2 (a,b) MRI scan, in transverse and coronal planes demonstrating a lesion of the left vocal fold and partial invasion of the paraglottic space.

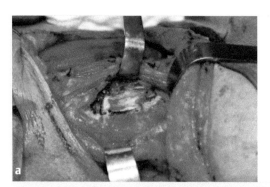
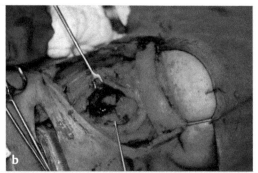

Fig. 12.3 Surgical field of the hemilaryngectomy. (a) Exposure of the thyroid cartilage, with the incision marking. (b) Thyroid cartilage separated laterally, allowing for the verification of the cancer on direct view.

cartilage, the fascia and the perichondrium were incised. Thyrotomy was performed vertically, at a distance of 4 mm from the midline contralateral to the cancer and at least 3 mm anterior to the posterior border of the ipsilateral thyroid cartilage. Entry into the larynx was performed by opening the cricothyroid membrane. The thyroid cartilage was retracted laterally and the oncological margins in the mucosa between 2 and 3 mm of the cancer were carefully delimited under direct view. The frozen section report confirmed that the margins were free. The internal perichondrium of the thyroid cartilage wing was removed together with the surgical specimen which included the epiglottic petiole was included in the specimen, since the anterior commissure was found to be invaded by the cancer. The mucosa of the pyriform sinus was mobilized medially to cover the exposed ipsilateral arytenoid (▶ Fig. 12.3).

After the cancer resection was completed, the left vocal fold was reconstructed with a bipedicled flap of the ipsilateral sternohyoid muscle (Bailey's flap), keeping the cranial and caudal pedicles. The flap was 1.5-cm thick and was kept in place by the pedicles, with no need for fixation. A fixation point of the contralateral vocal fold at the epiglottic petiole formed a neocommissure.

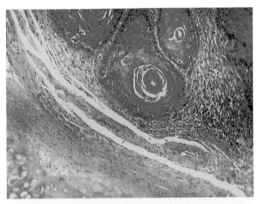

Fig. 12.4 Histopathological aspect, showing the tumor adjacent to cartilage. Cartilage in the inferior region and well-differentiated squamous cell carcinoma, with formation of keratin pearls, present in the upper field next to the perichondrium of the thyroid cartilage, however, with no invasion (high magnification [HE], ×10).

The histopathological report showed well-differentiated squamous cell carcinoma adjacent to the thyroid cartilage, but with no invasion (▶ Fig. 12.4).

The patient progressed satisfactorily and the tracheostomy was occluded on the second postoperative day; the cannula was removed 24 hours later, and the patient was discharged. The nasoenteral feeding tube was retained for a total of 5 days, after the reintroduction of purée on the third postoperative day. Patient's airway was adequate and the voice was rough.

12.2 Discussion

Radiotherapy, laser endoscopic excision, and vertical partial laryngectomies in selected cases have been successfully used in the treatment of the early-stage larynx carcinoma. In recent years, despite the new radiotherapy techniques and chemotherapy, surgery still presents the best oncological results.[1]

The decision between surgery or radiotherapy treatment in larynx cancer must consider the patient's clinical condition, their acceptance of the tracheostomy, even temporarily, expectations in terms of vocal results, as well as their own needs.

Regarding voice quality, when comparing parameters of acoustic analysis between laser endoscopic surgery and radiotherapy, these parameters revealed that there was no significant difference between patients treated with laser endoscopic surgery and those treated with radiotherapy.[3]

In 1956, Leroux-Robert described the partial frontolateral surgery technique. The opposite vocal fold had to be inserted ventrally. Normally, an anterior synechia occurs. Depending on the degree of damage to the anterior commissure, the frontolateral laryngectomy was simply anterior frontal or extended, more or less, to include the opposite hemilarynx.[4]

For the case described here, not only the vertical technique (hemilaryngectomy) but also the horizontal technique (supracricohyoidea laryngectomy) can be recommended. The main advantage of hemilaryngectomy is maintenance of the hemilarynx structures not involved by the cancer, leading to good results in decannulation, as well as in swallowing.

Microscopic infiltration of the thyroid cartilage was found in all 30 cases analyzed in a series.[5] In other study, four cases (8.3%) with microscopic infiltration of the thyroid cartilage were found.[6] A general prevalence of invasion of the thyroid cartilage of 8.5% was verified.[7] The rate of cartilaginous invasion was 3.7% of cases.[8] Another paper reported the rates of 5.4% in cases restricted to glottis and 32% in cases with supraglottic extension.[9]

Probably the cases presenting microscopic infiltration of the thyroid cartilage for cancer would be eligible for transoral laser microresection. In a series of 23 patients with T1 or T2 glottic cancer with involvement of the anterior commissure, none showed local recurrence after performing endoscopic microresection.[10] In 263 patients with T1/T2 glottic cancer undergoing laser microresection, the recurrence rate was 16% with involvement of the anterior commissure and 7% with uninvolved anterior commissure.[11]

Bilateral lesions and T2 lesions were more frequently associated with infiltration or tumor adjacency to cartilage in comparison with unilateral lesions.[6]

Despite not being widely used presently, vertical laryngectomy continues to be a good option in cases where endoscopic surgery does not suffice, with, in these cases, the maintenance of important structures being viable, in addition to the possibility of the reconstruction of the compromised vocal fold using several techniques.

Although Olsen and DeSanto stated in 1990 that larynx reconstruction of the after hemilaryngectomy is not necessary, the majority of authors emphasize it. The need for the reconstruction of the endolarynx by using flaps and grafts allows for a better glottic coaptation. There are several endolarynx reconstruction techniques, such as the use of the external perichondrium of the thyroid cartilage, cervical fascia, strap muscle, transposition of the tendon of the digastric muscle, thyroid cartilage, transposition of the epiglottic cartilage, and flap of the ventricular band.[12]

Bailey's publication in 1966 reports that during a partial laryngectomy with laryngoplasty, the author's first aim was complete removal of the cancer and the second was to maximize the preservation of breathing, phonation, and sphincter function of the larynx. The bipedicled sternohyoid muscle flap with perichondrium was used in an attempt to reline the larynx with adequate superficial tissue and a certain quantity of mass to provide support for the vocal and vestibular folds, with satisfactory preservation of the function of the larynx. The muscle filled the lack of tissue on one side of the larynx and provided support against which the opposite vocal fold could be adducted, permitting a better voice and more competent laryngeal sphincter; the muscular flap, in the interior of the larynx, tended to exert a lateral force, resisting an interior migration or collapsing in the thyroid cartilage blade. The muscle keeps some tonus or may suffer atrophy and fibrosis.[13]

Local recurrence following conservation laryngectomy for early glottis tumors was considered an important issue. A series of 416 patients with T1/T2N0Mo glottis carcinomas was evaluated. Among 42 patients who underwent the vertical partial approach, no local recurrence was observed when the cancer was confined to the middle third of the mobile vocal fold. On the other hand, local failure was verified in 8/111 (7.2%) patients with cancer confined to one mobile vocal fold. If some decreased mobility is related to a bulky cancer with deep invasion, the local recurrence rate is low, in comparison to true impaired vocal fold mobility, in which a more extensive thyroarytenoid muscle and paraglottic space invasion are found. The outcome is less favorable in cancers extending beyond the confines of the vocal folds.[14] In such cases, one surgical conservation option is the supracricoid laryngectomy with cricohyoidoepiglottopexy.[15] However, in our case, we considered that such approach would remove a large amount of tissue free of tumor in the contralateral side and this was the rationale for performing a vertical excision.

12.3 Tips

- The vertical partial laryngectomy is recommended for T2 cancer of the entire vocal fold, with or without extension to the anterior commissure, supra or infraglottis, paraglottic space, and the vocal process of the arytenoid.
- The infraglottic extension anteriorly of up to 10 mm and posteriorly of up to 5 mm also allows for the recommendation for hemilaryngectomy with partial resection of the cricoid cartilage.
- Always use some reconstruction technique for the vocal fold.
- Start the procedure with a protective tracheostomy.
- When closing the larynx, do not forget to fix the remaining vocal fold to the epiglottic petiole, forming a neocommissure.
- Inform the patient that every partial laryngectomy has the possibility to be extended to become total in the intraoperative stage.
- Discuss at length with the patient the expectations for vocal results, considering the other types of treatment, including radiotherapy.

12.4 Traps

- Be careful with the staging! A T1b cancer that infiltrates the thyroid cartilage becomes a T4a. Thus, it is important to perform a complementary image examination (CT or MRI).
- Inadequate exposure can compromise surgical success.
- The respiratory function is an essential factor in the hemilaryngectomy. Be cautious with elderly patients and those with obstructive chronic pulmonary diseases.
- Invasion of the pre-epiglottic space is a contraindication to hemilaryngectomy.
- The insertion of the nasoenteral tube should be performed before the laryngectomy in order to minimize the risk of fracturing the thyroid cartilage by excessive manipulation.

References

[1] Wigand ME, Steiner W, Stell PM. Functional partial laryngectomy conservation surgery for carcinoma. 1st ed. Erlangen, Germany: Springer-Verlag; 1984

[2] Biacabe B, Crevier-Buchman L, Hans S, Laccourreye O, Brasnu D. Vocal function after vertical partial laryngectomy with glottic reconstruction by false vocal fold flap: durational and frequency measures. Laryngoscope. 1999; 109(5):698–704

[3] Abdurehim Y, Hua Z, Yasin Y, Xukurhan A, Imam I, Yuqin F. Transoral laser surgery versus radiotherapy: systematic review and meta-analysis for treatment options of T1a glottic cancer. Head Neck. 2012; 34(1):23–33

[4] Leroux-Robert J. Indications for radical surgery, partial surgery, radiotherapy and combined surgery and radiotherapy

for cancer of the larynx and hypopharynx. Ann Otol Rhinol Laryngol. 1956; 65(1):137–153

[5] Rifai M, Khattab H. Anterior commissure carcinoma: I-histopathologic study. Am J Otolaryngol. 2000; 21(5):294–297

[6] Sava HW, Dedivitis RA, Gameiro GR, et al. Morphological evaluation of the thyroid cartilage invasion in early glottic tumor involving the anterior commissure. In press

[7] Hartl DM, Landry G, Hans S, et al. Thyroid cartilage invasion in early-stage squamous cell carcinoma involving the anterior commissure. Head Neck. 2012; 34(10):1476–1479

[8] Szyfter W, Leszczyńska M, Wierzbicka M, Kopeć T, Bartochowska A. Value of open horizontal glottectomy in the treatment for T1b glottic cancer with anterior commissure involvement. Head Neck. 2013; 35(12):1738–1744

[9] Ulusan M, Unsaler S, Basaran B, Yılmazbayhan D, Aslan I. The incidence of thyroid cartilage invasion through the anterior commissure in clinically early-staged laryngeal cancer. Eur Arch Otorhinolaryngol. 2016; 273(2):447–453

[10] Pearson BW, Salassa JR. Transoral laser microresection for cancer of the larynx involving the anterior commissure. Laryngoscope. 2003; 113(7):1104–1112

[11] Steiner W, Ambrosch P, Rödel RM, Kron M. Impact of anterior commissure involvement on local control of early glottic carcinoma treated by laser microresection. Laryngoscope. 2004; 114(8):1485–1491

[12] Olsen KD, DeSanto LW. Partial vertical laryngectomy: indications and surgical technique. Am J Otolaryngol. 1990; 11(3):153–160

[13] Bailey BJ. Partial laryngectomy and laryngoplasty: a technique and review. Trans Am Acad Ophthalmol Otolaryngol. 1966; 70(4):559–574

[14] Laccourreye O, Weinstein G, Brasnu D, Trotoux J, Laccourreye H. Vertical partial laryngectomy: a critical analysis of local recurrence. Ann Otol Rhinol Laryngol. 1991; 100(1):68–71

[15] Laccourreye H, Laccourreye O, Weinstein G, Menard M, Brasnu D. Supracricoid laryngectomy with cricohyoidoepiglottopexy: a partial laryngeal procedure for glottic carcinoma. Ann Otol Rhinol Laryngol. 1990; 99(6, pt 1):421–426

13 Locally Intermediate Glottic Cancer: Supracricoid Laryngectomy with CHEP

Antonio Augusto T. Bertelli, Antonio J. Gonçalves

Abstract

Locally intermediate glottic cancer may be treated by larynx preservation with chemoradiation or conservation laryngeal surgery. Supracricoid laryngectomy (SCL) is very useful for glottic and supraglottic tumors classified as T3 that do not extend to the subglottis and some selected T4a with limited extra laryngeal spread. At least one functional arytenoid must be preserved during this procedure. This technique allows voice rehabilitation and the removal of tracheostomy, bringing a better quality of life when compared to patients who have a total laryngectomy. It may be performed even in elderly patients provided that the patient has good pulmonary function and a multidisciplinary team are available for successful rehabilitation. SCL may be used as rescue surgery post radiotherapy in selected cases but with more frequent complications. When compared to chemoradiation, SCL has similar overall and disease-free survival rates, but with fewer patients requiring total laryngectomy due to recurrence or lack of rehabilitation.

Keywords: larynx cancer, partial laryngectomy, horizontal laryngectomy, conservation laryngeal surgery, larynx preservation

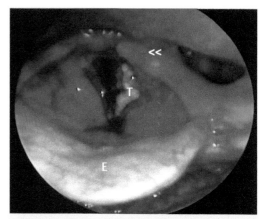

Fig. 13.1 Initial laryngoscopy which revealed a tumor (T) arising from the left vocal fold, extending to the left ventricle and vestibular fold, anterior commissure, and anterior third of the right vocal fold. The left arytenoid (<<) and left hemilarynx were fixed the epiglottis (E) is free of tumor.

13.1 Clinical Case

A 73-year-old Caucasian male, retired metallurgist presented to our clinic complaining of progressive hoarseness for 10 months. In the last month, he has noticed difficulty in breathing during physical efforts. He was a 25 pack-year cigarette smoker who had stopped smoking 30 years ago, a social alcohol drinker, and had no comorbidities except for a history of a partial gastrectomy 32 years ago for peptic ulcer. The Karnofsky's performance status was 70. Physical examination did not reveal any enlarged cervical lymph nodes. Laryngoscopy revealed an ulcerated lesion in the left vocal fold extending the anterior commissure to the anterior third of the right vocal fold, left ventricular fold, left ventricle, and with fixation of the ipsilateral arytenoid (▶ Fig. 13.1). Biopsies taken at the time of the endoscopy revealed an epidermoid carcinoma.

Computed tomography demonstrated left paraglottic space involvement but no extension to the subglottis (▶ Fig. 13.2). Initial staging was T3N0M0. A supracricoid laryngectomy (SCL) and cricohyoidoepiglottopexy (CHEP) with preservation of the right arytenoid and left a selective neck dissection (levels II–IV) were performed (▶ Fig. 13.3). The patient was discharged on postoperative day 5, without complications. The cancer was a grade 2 epidermoid carcinoma, measuring 2.5 × 2.0 × 1.5 cm, without vascular or neural invasion, with free margins, and without metastasis to the neck. Pathological staging was pT3pN0. No adjuvant therapy was advised. He did well with speech therapy, and has developed a well-tolerated hoarse voice, with no dysphagia. The tracheostomy tube was removed after 38 days and the feeding tube after 48 days. At 2 years after surgery, he is free of cancer (▶ Fig. 13.4) and fully rehabilitated.

13.2 Discussion

The supracricoid partial laryngectomy was described by Piquet et al in 1974, based on a technique developed by Majer and Rieder in 1959.[1]

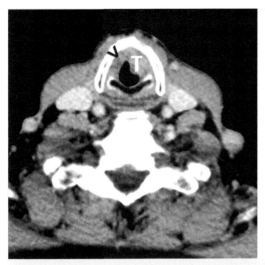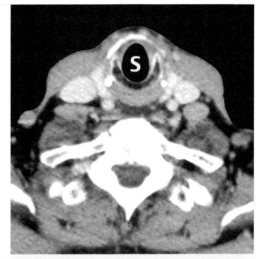

Fig. 13.2 Axial computed tomography with intravenous contrast showing (*left*) tumor (T) Evolving the left paraglottic space crossing the midline (>) and (*right*) no subglottis extension (S).

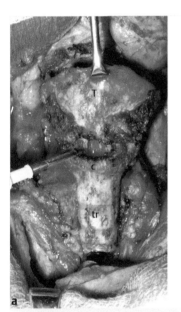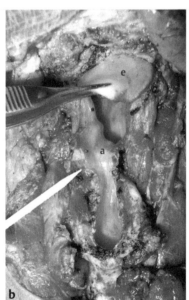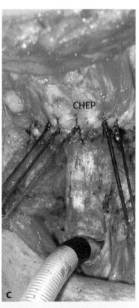

Fig. 13.3 Intraoperative photos of the supracricoid laryngectomy with cricohyoidoepiglottopexy. (a) Opening the cricothyroid membrane; cricoid (c), thyroid cartilage (T) and trachea (tr) below. (b) After resection, remaining right arytenoid (a), cricoid (c) and epiglottis (e). (c) Cricohyoidoepiglottopexy (CHEP).

Laccourreye et al in the 1990s promoted its use for the treatment of glottic cancer in Europe,[2] but the technique became popular in the Americas only in recent years.[1,3] Adaptations of this technique have been made for cancer of the supraglottis and hypopharynx.[4]

SCL consists of resection of the whole thyroid cartilage, starting from the cricoid to the base of the epiglottis, preserving one or two arytenoid cartilages, which have intact mobility and innervation, allowing for removal of the entire paraglottic spaces, and avoiding opening the larynx close to the cancer.[1] The epiglottis may be resected, if necessary. The remaining is reconstructed using the CHEP or cricohyoidopexy (CHP), e.g., fixation of the cricoid to the hyoid bone.[1,2,3] While preserving at

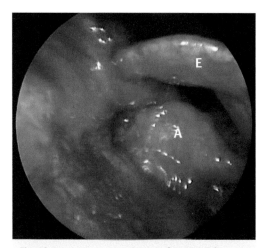

Fig. 13.4 Laryngoscopy at 2 years after SCL with cricohyoidoepiglottopexy for T3N0M0 glottic carcinoma demonstrating mobile arytenoid (A) and epiglottis (E).

least one functional arytenoid cartilage allows the rehabilitation of speech and deglutition, preserving the cricoid allows breathing, and the removal of the tracheostomy.[2]

Although SCL presents considerable advantages, when compared to total laryngectomy, the indications should be very must be very strict: the posterior commissure must be free of cancer and the subglottic extension should not reach the upper border of the cricoid cartilage. There should be very limited or no extralaryngeal spread,[5] at least one functional arytenoid cartilage must be preserved, and the patient's pulmonary function must be adequate. The patient's sychosocial condition, which is fundamental for a good rehabilitation must also be considered.[1]

SCL has been used for the treatment of glottic and supraglottic cancers, which do not invade the subglottis and preserve at least one mobile arytenoid.[1,2,3,4,5,6] Recently, this operation has been used, for post radiotherapy salvage of selected cases, obtaining promising oncologic and functional results,[7] with the advantages, compared to total laryngectomy, of maintaining the breathing function without tracheostomy and larynx phonation, resulting in a better quality of life.[4]

Alternatives to total laryngectomy have been sought for treatment of cancer of the larynx, without compromising oncological results.[6] SCL seems to be a good alternative, as long as its indications are seriously employed.[1]

Oncological local control is the main objective of larynx conservation surgeries,[5,6] since regional and distant metastatsis are rare unless there is local recurrence.[1] Rehabilitation of patients submitted to SCL poses another challenge. It is known that a better rehabilitation is related to the technique used. For instance, CHEP with preservation of both arytenoid cartilages results in an easier and faster rehabilitation while postoperative radiotherapy makes rehabilitation more difficult.[7,8,9] Women usually have a more difficult rehabilitation, possibly due to the smaller anteroposterior diameter of the larynx.[1] The average time for removal of the nasoenteral tube and tracheostomy, in the literature, takes place approximately 1 month postoperative.[1,2,3,4,5,6]

Although SCL was originally contraindicated in the elderly patient, recent studies suggest that open partial laryngectomies are safe even in very old patients, as demonstrated in this case, but with a higher risk of complications.[9]

Recently, a classification for open partial horizontal laryngectomies was proposed by the European Laryngological Society based on the inferior margin of resection.[8,10] Type I is the supraglottic laryngectomy, type II is the SCL, and type III is supratrachueal laryngectomy.

The rate of larynx preservation of SCL varies between 80 and 95%, as well as 5-year overall and disease free survival.[1,4,6] Considering patients submitted to total laryngectomy, and those submitted to larynx preservation with radiotherapy and chemotherapy for advanced cancers, local control and survival rates are very similar, but usually patients receiveing chemoradiation receive a total laryngectomy more because of recurrence or lack of adequate rehabilitation.[11]

13.3 Tips and Traps

- Conservation laryngeal surgery, such as SCL, has good functional and oncological outcomes, better than larynx preservation with chemoradiotherapy in some settings, especially outside clinical trials.
- more patients submitted to chemoradiotherapy for larynx preservation require a total laryngectomy for recurrences or failure of rehabilitation compared to those receiving conservation laryngeal surgery.
- SCL removes the entire thyroid cartilage with both paraglottic spaces and both vocal folds.

- Preservation of at least one functional laryngeal unit, one mobile arytenoid with its intact inervation, is fundamental for successful rehabilitation.
- Inferior and superior laryngeal nerves should be preserved to keep the arytenoid mobile and with its sensation.
- Cancer extending to the subglottis is the major contraindication for SCL; in such cases, supratracheal laryngectomy may be performed.
- Poor pulmonary function can lead to death if aspiration occurs after SCL.
- A multidisciplinary team is vital for successful rehabilitation.

References

[1] Gonçalves AJ, Bertelli AA, Malavasi TR, Kikuchi W, Rodrigues AN, Menezes MB. Results after supracricoid horizontal partial laryngectomy. Auris Nasus Larynx. 2010; 37(1):84–88

[2] Laccourreye O, Brasnu D, Périé S, Muscatello L, Ménard M, Weinstein G. Supracricoid partial laryngectomies in the elderly: mortality, complications, and functional outcome. Laryngoscope. 1998; 108(2):237–242

[3] Lima RA, Freitas EQ, Kligerman J, et al. Supracricoid laryngectomy with CHEP: functional results and outcome. Otolaryngol Head Neck Surg. 2001; 124(3):258–260

[4] Adamopoulos G, Yiotakis J, Stavroulaki P, Manolopoulos L. Modified supracricoid partial laryngectomy with cricohyoidopexy: series report and analysis of results. Otolaryngol Head Neck Surg. 2000; 123(3):288–293

[5] Succo G, Crosetti E, Bertolin A, et al. Benefits and drawbacks of open partial horizontal laryngectomies, part B: intermediate and selected advanced stage laryngeal carcinoma. Head Neck. 2016; 38(suppl 1):E649–E657

[6] Succo G, Crosetti E, Bertolin A, et al. Benefits and drawbacks of open partial horizontal laryngectomies, part A: early- to intermediate-stage glottic carcinoma. Head Neck. 2016; 38(suppl 1):E333–E340

[7] Makeieff M, Venegoni D, Mercante G, Crampette L, Guerrier B. Supracricoid partial laryngectomies after failure of radiation therapy. Laryngoscope. 2005; 115(2):353–357

[8] Succo G, Peretti G, Piazza C, et al. Open partial horizontal laryngectomies: a proposal for classification by the working committee on nomenclature of the European Laryngological Society. Eur Arch Otorhinolaryngol. 2014; 271(9):2489–2496

[9] Crosetti E, Caracciolo A, Molteni G, et al. Unravelling the risk factors that underlie laryngeal surgery in the elderly. Acta Otorhinolaryngol Ital. 2016; 36(3):185–193

[10] Rizzotto G, Crosetti E, Lucioni M, Succo G. Subtotal laryngectomy: outcomes of 469 patients and proposal of a comprehensive and simplified classification of surgical procedures. Eur Arch Otorhinolaryngol. 2012; 269(6):1635–1646

[11] Hartl DM, Ferlito A, Brasnu DF, et al. Evidence-based review of treatment options for patients with glottic cancer. Head Neck. 2011; 33(11):1638–1648

14 Transoral Robotic Surgery for Advanced Laryngeal Cancer

Young Min Park, Se-Heon Kim

Abstract

Transoral robotic surgery (TORS) of glottic cancer was performed for the first time in 2009, and its usefulness in patients with laryngeal cancer has been reported. TORS is similar to transoral laser microsurgery in that it proceeds through the oral cavity, but it allows more precise surgery because two robotic arms can move freely within a narrow space. Application of TORS in treatment of laryngeal carcinoma has mainly been performed for early laryngeal cancer, but treatment results have also recently been reported for advanced laryngeal cancer. Induction chemotherapy was performed in patients with locally advanced laryngeal cancer to reduce tumor volume, and residual tumor was removed by TORS with excellent outcomes. These new treatment modalities are aimed at improving quality of life after treatment by preserving organ function. Based on pathologic information obtained after surgery in our trial, 20% of patients survived NED (no evidence of disease) without further radiation therapy, and the remaining patients received adjusted radiation doses based on pathologic adverse features. In these patients, we expect that long-term complications may be reduced by radiotherapy.

Keywords: laryngeal cancer, induction chemotherapy, transoral robotic surgery

14.1 Introduction

In cases of locally advanced T3 and T4 laryngeal cancer, appropriate treatment methods are controversial because there is no reliable study comparing treatment outcomes of various treatment modalities.[1] T3 tumors have traditionally been treated with total laryngectomy as a single treatment modality, but partial laryngectomy is performed in some cases.[2] Radiation (RT) alone has a 50% lower local control rate than surgery in T3 disease.[3] Accordingly, concurrent chemoradiotherapy (CRT) is recommended for conservative laryngeal surgery or for bulky T3 tumors rather than RT alone. T4 tumors usually undergo total laryngectomy, followed by adjuvant RT or CRT, and definitive CRT may be performed for long-term preservation in limited cases. Although nonsurgical organ preservation trials can be performed for long-term preservation with T4 tumors, preserved organs may not remain functional after RT. If edema persists 6 months after radiation, remaining or recurrent disease should be suspected.[4]

The comparable oncologic outcome of transoral laser microsurgery has been reported only in cases of experienced operators with selective T3 and T4 tumors.[5] Park et al performed transoral robotic surgery (TORS) of glottic cancer for the first time in 2009 and reported its usefulness in patients with laryngeal cancer.[6] TORS is similar to transoral laser microsurgery in that it proceeds through the oral cavity, but it allows for precise surgery because two robotic arms can move freely within a narrow space. The use of TORS to treat laryngeal carcinoma has mainly been performed in early laryngeal cancer, but recently, treatment results have also been reported in advanced laryngeal cancer.[7] Induction chemotherapy was performed in patients with locally advanced laryngeal cancer to reduce tumor volume, and residual tumor was removed by TORS with excellent outcomes.[7] New treatment modalities are aimed at improving patient quality of life after treatment through preservation of organs and function.

14.2 Schematic Overview of Treatment Protocol (TORS Combined with Induction Chemotherapy)

Patients with locally advanced laryngeal cancer and resectable nodal disease were considered for the treatment protocol. Induction chemotherapy was performed for three cycles before surgery, and TORS was performed in patients with more than partial response. Mutilating surgery or definitive concurrent chemoradiation therapy (CCRTx) was performed in patients without response to induction chemotherapy. In patients who received

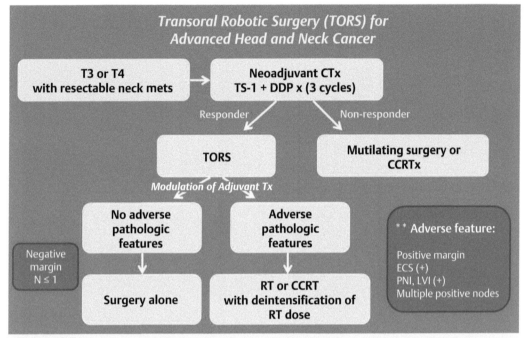

Fig. 14.1 Clinical trial design. Only patients with T3 and T4a lesions (resectable neck metastases) were included. All patients underwent three cycles of neoadjuvant chemotherapy (TS-1 and cisplatin). Chemotherapy response was evaluated after each cycle; responders completed the third cycle and then underwent transoral robotic surgery. Adjuvant therapy was scheduled based on pathological information. Mutilating surgery or concurrent chemoradiotherapy was scheduled for nonresponders.

TORS, use of additional adjuvant chemotherapy was determined based on the results of pathologic examination of specimens obtained after surgery. In the case of pathologic N ≤ 1 with negative margins, treatment consisted of only surgery (▶Fig. 14.1).

14.3 Selection of Patients for Treatment Protocol

Indications for this treatment protocol are as follows: (1) patients with T3 or T4 laryngeal cancer who were histologically diagnosed with squamous cell carcinoma; (2) patients who had not undergone previous surgery, chemotherapy, or radiotherapy; and (3) patients with Eastern Cooperative Oncology Group performance status below 2. The following patients were considered to have relative contraindications: (1) patients who could not undergo radical resection of the lesion with TORS, (2) patients with distant metastasis, (3) patients who were not expected to have good

follow-up compliance, and (4) patients with poor transoral exposure due to poor mouth opening.

14.4 Induction Chemotherapy Protocol

The chemotherapy regimen consisted of cisplatin (70 mg/m^2) by intravenous infusion on day 1 and TS-1 (combination of gimeracil 5.8 mg/m^2, oteracil 19.6 mg/m^2, and tegafur 20 mg/m^2) through oral route on days 1 through 14, which was repeated every 21 days. When myelosuppression appeared, chemotherapy was delayed for 1 week until leukocyte and platelet counts recovered. After two cycles of neoadjuvant chemotherapy, the response was evaluated by imaging studies and endoscopy based on Response Evaluation Criteria in Solid tumors. The largest tumor and neck mass diameter was measured to verify the response. TORS was performed on patients with more than partial response. Patients with less than partial response were considered for conventional surgery or definitive CCRTx (▶Fig. 14.1).

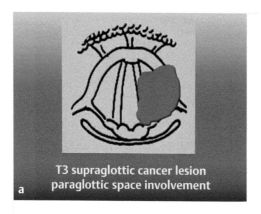

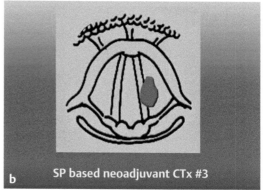

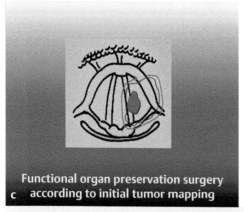

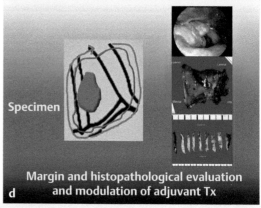

Fig. 14.2 Schematic view of neoadjuvant chemotherapy plus transoral robotic surgery in patients with T3 supraglottic cancer. **(a)** Tumor originated from right aryepiglottic fold with paraglottic space invasion. **(b)** After three cycles of neoadjuvant chemotherapy, tumor size decreased significantly. **(c)** Primary lesion was initially video recorded via rigid or flexible endoscopy. Resection margins (*blue line*) were mapped based on the pretreatment dimensions (*red line*) rather than on dimensions of reduced tumors after neoadjuvant chemotherapy. **(d)** Pathologic specimen was analyzed for margin status and other adverse pathologic features.

14.5 Operative Procedure

All patients underwent imaging studies, including CT, MRI, and PET, to assess the extent of disease. The extent of the primary lesion was recorded on video files captured via rigid or flexible endoscope. Based on the above data, the extent of resection was mapped based on the range of the pretreatment lesion rather than on reduced tumor volume after induction chemotherapy (▶ Fig. 14.2). Case 1 was a 54-year-old man with T3N0M0 aryepiglottic fold cancer. The tumor measured 1.7 cm by MRI, and right vocal cord palsy was detected on rigid endoscopy. After induction chemotherapy, the tumor shrunk and vocal cord mobility recovered. The residual tumor was removed through TORS.

On pathologic examination of the specimen, the surgical margin was negative and other adverse pathologic features were not observed. Therefore, the patient received surgery alone without radiotherapy, and there was no evidence of disease on the last visit (▶ Fig. 14.3).

14.6 Adjuvant Treatment

Adjuvant treatment (radiation therapy [RTx] or CCRTx) was performed for the following adverse pathologic features: positive margin, extracapsular nodal spread (ECS), perineural invasion (PNI), lymphovascular invasion (LVI), and multiple metastatic lymph nodes. Adjuvant treatment was started 4 to 6 weeks after surgery.

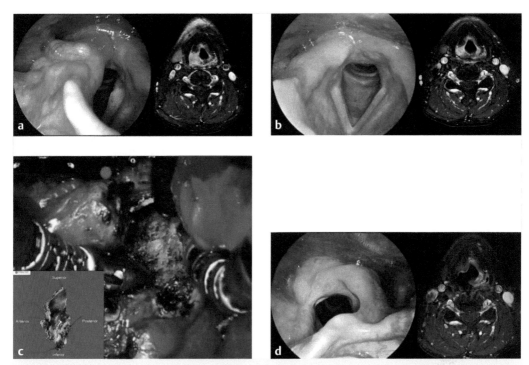

Fig. 14.3 Case 1 was a 54-year-old man with T3N0M0 aryepiglottic fold cancer. **(a)** The tumor measured 1.7 cm by MRI, and right vocal cord palsy was detected on rigid endoscopy. **(b)** After neoadjuvant chemotherapy, the tumor shrunk and vocal cord mobility was recovered. **(c)** Residual tumor was removed through transoral robotic surgery. On pathologic examination of the specimen, surgical margin was negative and other adverse pathologic features were not observed. **(d)** Therefore, the patient received surgery alone without radiotherapy and was alive with no evidence of disease.

Table 14.1 TNM classification of patients

T stage			N classification			Total
	0	1	2a	2b	2c	
3	5	3	0	3	4	15
4	0	0	0	0	0	0
Total	5	3	0	3	4	15

Note: Stage III: 53.5%; stage IV: 46.6%.

14.7 Treatment Outcomes

This clinical trial using induction chemotherapy and TORS included 15 patients with laryngeal cancer. The primary laryngeal cancer lesions were the true vocal cord in five patients, aryepiglottic fold in five patients, epiglottis in three patients, and false vocal cord in two patients. By TNM (*t*umor size, *n*ode involvement, and *m*etastasis status) stage, 15 patients (100%) had T3 tumors, 8 patients (53.5%) had stage III tumors, and 7 patients (46.6%) had stage IV tumors (▶Table 14.1). All patients were male, and the mean age was 67 years. The pathologic diagnosis of all patients was squamous cell carcinoma. Other patient information is summarized in ▶Table 14.2.

Here, we describe representative cases of patients who participated in this study. The first case was a 54-year-old male diagnosed with T3N0M0 aryepiglottic fold cancer. A 1.7-cm tumor originated from the right aortoesophageal fistula, and right vocal fold paralysis was observed. After induction chemotherapy, tumor size decreased and right vocal cord movement was restored. The residual cancer was removed through TORS. Pathologic examination of the surgical specimen confirmed negative margins, and other adverse pathologic features were not observed (▶ Fig. 14.2). ▶ Fig. 14.4 summarizes the entire treatment process of five patients with advanced laryngeal cancer. All of these patients showed partial response to induction chemotherapy. Upon pathologic examination of specimens after operation, three patients showed negative margins and node-free disease. These patients did not receive adjuvant therapy

after surgery, and there was no evidence of disease on the last visit. The two remaining patients showed positive margins and nodal metastasis on pathologic examination of surgical specimens. Therefore, they received adjuvant therapy.

After induction chemotherapy, 15 patients showed more than partial response. There were no cases of stable or progressive disease. All patients tolerated induction chemotherapy, and residual tumors were removed by TORS after induction chemotherapy. Lesions were removed through the oral cavity without additional external incisions. Eight patients (53%) had negative margins on postoperative pathologic examination, and the remaining seven patients (46%) had positive margins. All patients underwent secondary intention healing after TORS without additional reconstructive procedures. Fifteen patients underwent elective tracheotomy for postoperative airway, and 14 patients successfully underwent decannulation. The mean duration from tracheotomy to decannulation was 11.5 days. Patients tolerated oral ingestion 11.1 days postoperatively, on average. The functional outcome swallowing scale (FOSS) score described by Salassa was used to assess subjective swallowing function, and 86% of patients showed favorable results (13%).[8] Only two patients had feeding tube dependence at the last follow-up (▶ Table 14.3). During the perioperative period, one patient developed postoperative pneumonia that required medical treatment. There were no serious side effects

Table 14.2 Clinical information of all patients

Characteristics	No. of patients (%)
Sex	
Male	15 (100)
Female	0 (0)
Age, mean (range), y	67.2 (54–80)
Primary subsite	
True vocal cord	5 (33)
Aryepiglottic fold	5 (33)
Epiglottis	3 (20)
False vocal cord	2 (13)
Histopathology	
Squamous cell carcinoma	15 (100)

Sex/ Age	Primary	Initial Image	Induction CTx	Response	After ICTx	Operation	Pathology	F/U
M/65	AEF(L) (cT3N1M0)		회 (TS-1/Cisplatin)	Better than partial response		TORS. partial laryngectomy(L).LND(L)	Invasive SCCa 0.8*0.2cm ECS(−) / Margin: Free Node: Free	NED
M/67	AEF(R) (cT3N2M0)		3회 (TS-1/Cisplatin)	Better than partial response (80%)		TORS. SPL(R). LND(B)	SCCa, MD 1.1*0.6cm ECS(−) / Margin: Free Node: Free	NED
M/56	AEF(R) (cT3N0M0)		2회 (TS-1/Cisplatin)	Better than partial response		TORS. SPL(R). LND(R)	Invasive SCCa, 0.6*0.2cm ECS(−) / Margin: Free Node: Free	NED
M/80	AEF(R) (cT3N1M0)		5회 (TS-1/Cisplatin)	Better than partial response		TORS. SPL(R). mRND(R)	SCCa, MD 1.6*1.2cm ECS(−) / Margin: (+) Node: 1/65	NED
M/67	FVC(L) (cT3N0M0)		3회 (TS-1/Cisplatin)	Better than partial response		TORS. SPL(L). LND(L)	SCCa, MD 1.4*0.03cm ECS(−) / Margin: (+) Node: 1/30	NED

Fig. 14.4 Summary of treatment outcome for five other enrolled patients. After neoadjuvant chemotherapy, eight patients exhibited partial responses. All patients underwent transoral robotic surgery with simultaneous neck dissection to remove residual tumors that had shrunk after neoadjuvant chemotherapy. Three patients had negative surgical margins and three patients had positive surgical margins. Two patients exhibited adverse pathological features (multiple metastatic lymph nodes or extracapsular nodal spread). Adjuvant therapy was customized based on these pathological data. At last follow-up, all eight patients were alive with no evidence of disease.

related to surgery. Voice status was evaluated through acoustic waveform analysis. After transoral partial laryngectomy, jitter was significantly increased compared to other variables (▶Fig. 14.5).

The median follow-up period was 21.5 months (range: 4–91 months). At the time of final evaluation, the locoregional failure rate was 20% (3 of

Table 14.3 Functional outcomes

Measure	No. of patients (%)
Decannulation (d)	11.5
Return to oral diet (d)	11.1
FOSS score	
0–2 (favorable)	12 (80)
3–4 (unfavorable)	1 (6)
5 (tube dependence)	2 (13)

15 patients). One (2.9%) patient developed distant metastasis. Recurrent disease was treated with salvage surgery, RTx, chemotherapy, or combined modalities. The 5-year overall survival rate of patients with laryngeal cancer was 50.5%, while the 5-year disease-free survival rate was 53.7% (▶Fig. 14.6). Of all 15 patients, 12 had adverse features observed on pathologic specimens and were treated further (▶Table 14.4). Three patients did not undergo further adjuvant treatment after induction chemotherapy and TORS.

14.8 Consideration

The National Comprehensive Cancer Network guideline (2016) recommends RT or CCRTx ranging from 66 to 70 Gy in patients with laryngeal cancer and complete response or partial response after induction chemotherapy. Following this

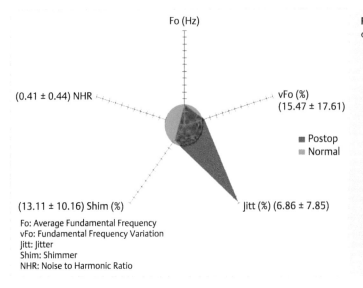

Fig. 14.5 Acoustic waveform analysis of patients.

Fo: Average Fundamental Frequency
vFo: Fundamental Frequency Variation
Jitt: Jitter
Shim: Shimmer
NHR: Noise to Harmonic Ratio

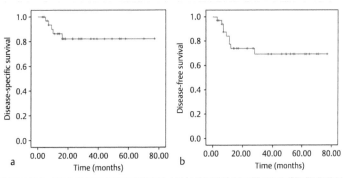

Fig. 14.6 Kaplan–Meier curves: disease-specific survival (a) and disease-free survival (b).

Table 14.4 Treatment outcomes

Measure	No. of patients (%)
Margin status	
Negative	8 (53)
Positive	7 (46)
Extracapsular nodal spread	
Yes	3 (20)
No	12 (80)
Lymphovascular invasion	
Yes	3 (20)
No	12 (80)
Perineural invasion	
Yes	3 (20)
No	12 (80)
Adjuvant therapy	
CCRTx	9 (60)
RTx	3 (20)
Surgery alone	3 (20)

Abbreviations: CCRTx, concurrent chemoradiation therapy; RTx, radiation therapy.

guideline can result in the following problems. First, tumor cell clones remaining after induction chemotherapy are more likely to show cross-resistance in RT, which reduces the efficiency of added RT.[9,10] According to previous reports, 28% of patients with complete response after induction chemotherapy had no tumor cells histologically, and the standard radiation dose of RT was unnecessary in these patients.[11] Because of these problems, the current guideline needs to be individualized to reflect patient characteristics. The total dose of RTx could be tailored based on pathologic specimen evaluation. In this study, we reduced the volume of locally advanced laryngeal cancer by induction chemotherapy and removed residual tumor through TORS minimally invasive surgery. By removing lesions through the mouth without additional external incisions, patients recovered rapidly after surgery and had preserved function of the larynx. Surgical removal of the remaining treatment-resistant tumor cell clones after induction chemotherapy can maximize the effect of added RT. Additional tailored treatment was possible based on pathologic information obtained after surgery, such as adjusting the RT dose. Based on pathologic information obtained after surgery, 20% of patients survived NED without further RTx, and the remaining patients had radiation doses adjusted based on adverse pathologic features. In these patients, we expect radiotherapy to reduce long-term complications.

References

[1] Licitra L, Bernier J, Grandi C, et al. Cancer of the larynx. Crit Rev Oncol Hematol. 2003; 47(1):65–80
[2] Kirchner JA, Som ML. Clinical significance of fixed vocal cord. Laryngoscope. 1971; 81(7):1029–1044
[3] Harwood AR, Bryce DP, Rider WD. Management of T3 glottic cancer. Arch Otolaryngol. 1980; 106(11):697–699
[4] Ward PH, Calcaterra TC, Kagan AR. The enigma of postradiation edema and recurrent or residual carcinoma of the larynx. Laryngoscope. 1975; 85(3):522–529
[5] Hinni ML, Salassa JR, Grant DG, et al. Transoral laser microsurgery for advanced laryngeal cancer. Arch Otolaryngol Head Neck Surg. 2007; 133(12):1198–1204
[6] Park YM, Lee WJ, Lee JG, et al. Transoral robotic surgery (TORS) in laryngeal and hypopharyngeal cancer. J Laparoendosc Adv Surg Tech A. 2009; 19(3):361–368
[7] Park YM, Keum KC, Kim HR, et al. A clinical trial of combination neoadjuvant chemotherapy and transoral robotic surgery in patients with T3 and T4 laryngo-hypopharyngeal cancer. Ann Surg Oncol. 2018; 25(4):864–871
[8] Salassa JR. A functional outcome swallowing scale for staging oropharyngeal dysphagia. Dig Dis. 1999; 17(4):230–234
[9] Park YM, Lee SY, Park SW, Kim SH. Role of cancer stem cell in radioresistant head and neck cancer. Auris Nasus Larynx. 2016; 43(5):556–561
[10] Shirai K, Saitoh JI, Musha A, et al. Clinical outcomes of definitive and postoperative radiotherapy for stage I-IVB hypopharyngeal cancer. Anticancer Res. 2016; 36(12):6571–6578
[11] Yang L, Chen WK, Guo ZM, et al. Long-term survival of induction chemotherapy plus surgery and postoperative radiotherapy in patients with stage IV hypopharyngeal cancer. Anticancer Drugs. 2010; 21(9):872–876

15 Locally Advanced Supraglottic Cancer: Larynx Preservation by Transoral Laser Microsurgery

Petra Ambrosch, Claudia Schmalz

Abstract

Transoral laser microsurgery (TLM) is now accepted in the treatment of early cancer of the supraglottis, as recent clinical practice guidelines confirm. However, there is ongoing debate as to whether TLM is appropriate for the management of locally advanced cancer of the supraglottis. We discuss diagnostic and management challenges in the clinical context of the case of a 78-year-old male patient with several comorbidities. The case presentation is followed by a review of the current literature. Our plan of management and the oncologic and functional outcomes following treatment are described.

Keywords: supraglottic cancer, transoral laser microsurgery, larynx preservation, oncologic outcomes, functional outcomes

15.1 Case Presentation

The following case presentation was approved by the ethics committee of the Medical Faculty of Kiel University (D 418/18) and consented by the patient. A 78-year-old retired male presented with a 3-month history of dysphagia and odynophagia with no associated dyspnea or stridor. He was a current smoker of 20 cigarettes per day for 50 years, and he had stopped drinking alcohol in the 1980s. His Eastern Cooperative Oncology Group performance status was 2, and he had several comorbidities. He suffered from chronic obstructive pulmonary disease (COPD), insulin-dependent type 2 diabetes mellitus, diabetic nephropathy with impaired renal function (glomerular filtration rate [GFR]: 60 mL/min), moderate sensorineural hearing loss, hypertension, coronary heart disease, and severe peripheral vascular disease resulting in an above-knee amputation 4 years ago. He was wheelchair dependent.

At flexible laryngoscopy, a tumor was detected involving the epiglottis, both ventricular folds, and the aryepiglottic fold on the left with extension to the mucosa above the arytenoid cartilage. Both vocal folds were mobile. (▶Fig. 15.1, ▶Fig. 15.2). Microlaryngoscopy revealed the tumor extension described earlier and with superficial involvement of the postcricoid mucosa with no extension beyond the midline. The ventricle of Morgagni was uninvolved on both sides. Panendoscopy excluded a second primary cancer in the head and neck sites, lung, and esophagus. There were no palpable cervical lymph nodes. Biopsy revealed moderately differentiated squamous cell carcinoma (SCC). Ultrasound-guided fine-needle aspiration cytology from enlarged lymph nodes in level IIa bilateral was positive for SCC. CT scan of the larynx demonstrated a supraglottic tumor with infiltration of the pre-epiglottic space, the ventricular folds, and the left aryepiglottic fold. There were no signs of tumor extension to the paraglottic space at the glottic level, no signs of cartilage infiltration, or infiltration of the base of the tongue. One enlarged lymph node in level IIa (left 12-mm diameter, right 10-mm diameter), with central necrosis suspicious for metastatic disease was diagnosed

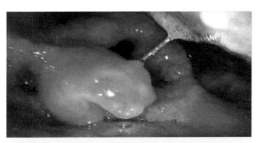

Fig. 15.1 Preoperative laryngoscopic view of the larynx. Supraglottic carcinoma involving epiglottis, left aryepiglottic fold, and both ventricular folds.

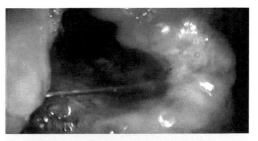

Fig. 15.2 Preoperative laryngoscopic view of the larynx. Higher magnification.

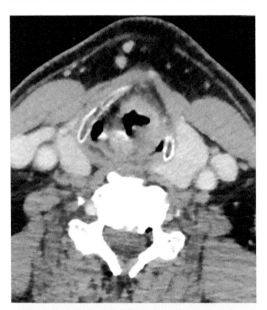

Fig. 15.3 Axial computed tomography scan of the larynx, showing infiltration of the pre-epiglottic space and left aryepiglottic fold.

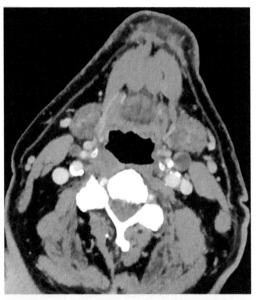

Fig. 15.4 Axial computed tomography scan of the neck, showing enlarged lymph nodes with central necrosis in level IIa bilaterally.

bilaterally (▸Fig. 15.3, ▸Fig. 15.4). CT scan of the lungs was unremarkable, as was the ultrasound examination of the abdominal organs.

The diagnosis was locally advanced SCC of the supraglottic larynx. The clinical stage according to the seventh edition of the Union for International Cancer Control (UICC) TNM (*tumor size, node involvement, and metastasis status*) classification system was cT3cN2cM0, UICC stage IVa.

15.2 Discussion

15.2.1 Treatment Options

Transoral laser microsurgery (TLM) is now accepted for the treatment of early cancer of the supraglottis, as a recent clinical practice guideline confirms[1] and there is consensus that a single-modality treatment should be performed. In patients with locally advanced cancer of the supraglottics, several treatment options are available. The surgical treatment options are total laryngectomy or supraglottic laryngectomy (SGL), either by open-neck or by a transoral approach with the CO_2 laser (TLM), for the treatment of the primary cancer. With limited metastases to the neck, the surgical treatment of the regional lymphatics consists in bilateral selective neck dissection of levels II to IV (SND II–IV).[2]

Depending on the histopathologic findings regarding resection margins and the status of the neck nodes, adjuvant radiotherapy or chemoradiotherapy of the primary site and both sides of the neck might be indicated. The nonsurgical treatment options are radiotherapy alone, induction chemotherapy followed by radiotherapy, and concurrent chemoradiotherapy. Well-recognized issues to be considered when selecting a particular treatment option are accurate staging of the disease, the general health of the patient, and prospects for a good functional outcome.

The Surgical Options

Success of a surgical approach to larynx preservation depends on complete resection of the cancer (R0 resection), experience of the surgeon, and appropriate patient selection. The key issue to address when considering surgical options is the anatomic extent of the cancer. Standard SGL includes the resection of the epiglottis together with the pre-epiglottic fat and both ventricular folds. The vocal folds and both arytenoid cartilages are preserved. The resection can be extended to the aryepiglottic fold (medial wall of the piriform sinus), one arytenoid cartilage, one vocal fold, and/or the postcricoid area. The resection can be done either open through the neck or by the TLM approach. In open resections, the supraglottic portion of the thyroid cartilage is removed but in endoscopic resections it is usually preserved. Contraindications for open-neck and endoscopic SGL in T3 supraglottic cancer are bilateral vocal cord fixation, bilateral paraglottic space invasion, and/or invasion of the inner cortex of the thyroid cartilage at the glottic level.

In case the cancer is amenable to SGL, it must be determined whether a potential candidate is likely to compensate for the functional impairments caused by the operation. Because smoking and alcohol abuse are the major risk factors for supraglottic cancer, many patients also suffer from other tobacco-associated diseases, such as COPD. Age older than 70 years and severe comorbid diseases may exclude patients with a cancer otherwise amenable to partial resection from the operation. All authors who have reported on TLM of supraglottic cancers agree that swallowing rehabilitation proceeds more quickly and has better outcomes than open-neck SGL.[3,4] The rate of secondary total laryngectomy for persistent aspiration after open-neck SGL is in the range of 3.5–12.5%.[3] Due to considerable surgery-associated morbidity and postoperative functional impairment, open-neck SGL often does not qualify as a treatment option, particularly in elderly patients with preexisting poor pulmonary function. However, from clinical experience and reports in the literature, it is known that with TLM the indication for surgery can be extended to that patient group. After TLM, 95% of these patients are reported to have adequate swallowing function without the need for a gastrostomy tube.[5,6,7,8,9] The reason for this observation is that the endoscopic approach is less invasive, tracheostomy is usually not necessary and TLM does not interfere with the elevation of the larynx and the mobility of the base of tongue during swallowing. Preservation of complete glottic closure is helpful and the sensory innervation might be better by preservation of the internal branches of the superior laryngeal nerves.

There is evidence from single center cohort studies that the oncologic outcomes following TLM are comparable to open-neck SGL and to total laryngectomy. Steiner's group retrospectively reviewed 104 patients with pT3 cancers of the supraglottis. The 5-year overall, recurrence-free, and disease-specific survival rates were 67, 68, and 84%, respectively, thus comparable to open-neck SGL. The 5-year local control rate was 77.3% and the larynx preservation rate was 92% (97 of 104 patients).[6] Grant et al[10] reported on a series of 38 patients with supraglottic carcinoma (T1/T2 22 patients, T3/T4 16 patients). The 2-year local control rate was 97%. Ambrosch et al[5] treated 50 patients with pT3 supraglottic carcinomas (40 stage III, 10 stage IV) with TLM. The 5-year larynx preservation rate was 96%. The 5-year recurrence-free survival rate was 71%. All patients were on an unrestricted oral diet after removal of the feeding tube. Special swallowing training was not required. Peretti et al[7] reported on a series of 56 patients treated with TLM, among them 20 patients with pT3 supraglottic lesions. In 21 of 22 patients larynx preservation was achieved, the 5-year disease-free survival rate was 76.3%. Vilaseca et al[8] treated 96 patients with T3 cancer of the supraglottis. The 5-year local control rate, overall, and disease-specific survival rates were 69.8, 45.8, and 61.8%, respectively. Vilaseca et al[9] in a follow-up publication, published the up-to-now largest series including 128 patients with pT3 and 25 patients with pT4a cancer of the supraglottis treated with TLM. The 5-year laryngectomy-free survival with preserved function was 74.5%, and the 5-year overall and disease-specific survival rates were 55.6 and 47%, respectively. Recently, Ambrosch et al[11] reported a 5-year larynx preservation rate of 89% for pT3 and a 5-year disease-free survival rate of 64% for stage III and IVa supraglottic carcinomas treated with TLM.

TLM is associated with lower morbidity than open surgery and the functional results with respect to swallowing function and voice are optimal, when TLM is used as single modality. The need for postoperative adjuvant radiotherapy or chemoradiotherapy increases morbidity. Adjuvant radiotherapy is not indicated for patients with complete removal of the primary cancer and histopathologically cancer-free cervical lymph nodes. Adjuvant (chemo)radiotherapy is indicated for patients in whom microscopic residual cancer is assumed to be present at the primary site (R1 resection), in patients with more than one lymph node positive for cancer and in patients with lymph node metastases having extracapsular spread.[12,13] Whether postoperative radiotherapy after open-neck SGL and TLM has an adverse effect on laryngeal function is controversial. We did not see that patients receiving postoperative radiotherapy with maximum doses of 60 Gy to the larynx were more likely to need lifelong gastrostomy tube feeding or were more likely to develop airway obstruction due to persisting laryngeal edema.

The Nonsurgical Options

The radiation therapy oncology group (RTOG) 91–11 trial compared induction chemotherapy with radiotherapy in responders with concurrent chemoradiotherapy with high-dose cisplatin and with conventionally fractionated radiotherapy alone.[14] That landmark study demonstrated improved locoregional control and preservation of the larynx in the concurrent chemoradiotherapy arm. Today in many cancer centers, concurrent chemoradiotherapy has become the standard nonsurgical treatment for larynx preservation, despite its toxicity. Even though more than 80% of the patients in the RTOG 91–11 trial had a Karnofsky index greater than 90, only 70% of patients were able to complete the entire concurrent chemoradiotherapy protocol due to toxicity. Eighty-two percent of patients suffered from grade 3 and 4 toxicity and 5% died due to therapy-related complications. In summary, therapy-related mortality is significantly higher when organ-preservation protocols are used than after primary surgical treatment. Long-term results of the RTOG 91–11 trial were published in 2013.[15] It was remarkable that in the concurrent chemoradiotherapy arm late deaths unrelated to larynx cancer occurred. The cause of death in these patients is not known but it was speculated that some might be due to late toxicity such as swallowing dysfunction and (silent) aspiration.[15]

A significant number of patients with cancer of the larynx, have comorbidities that preclude the use of high-dose cisplatin. The criteria for clinical trials regularly exclude these patients to avoid interacting effects and very little is known about nonsurgical larynx preservation strategies in these patients.

15.2.2 Suggested Approach to Treatment

In our patient with locally advanced cancer of the supraglottis, the initial consideration was whether he was suitable for surgical or nonsurgical larynx preservation or whether total laryngectomy should be recommended. The anatomic extent and endoscopic accessibility of the tumor allowed TLM-extended SGL. The metastases to the neck nodes were found to be resectable. His age, general condition, and comorbidities, however, limited the acceptability of a treatment protocol with high-dose chemotherapy as well as

organ-preserving surgery, making total laryngectomy a reasonable recommendation. However, the patient declined total laryngectomy. Therefore, a combined approach consisting of TLM, bilateral SND, and—depending on histopathological findings—adjuvant radiotherapy or chemoradiotherapy remain as treatment options. The decision of our multidisciplinary tumor (MDT) board to recommend TLM/SND and postoperative radiotherapy rather than concurrent chemoradiotherapy was based on the comorbidities making the patient most probably unable to receive high-dose cisplatin and to tolerate full-course radiotherapy with 70 Gy. The patient himself opted for surgery and postoperative radiotherapy. He was very motivated and confident in his ability to succeed with swallowing rehabilitation.

15.2.3 Treatment and Posttreatment Course

The patient received TLM-extended SGL and bilateral SND II to IV. The operation was performed using the technique previously described.[16] The resection included the epiglottis and pre-epiglottic fat, both ventricular folds, left aryepiglottic fold, mucosa of the postcricoid area, as well as the mucosa covering the left arytenoid cartilage. The resection is not classifiable according to the European Laryngological Society (ELS) classification system for supraglottic resections.[16] The postoperative course was uneventful. The patient received a nasogastric feeding tube and had planned extubation the day after surgery. Tracheostomy was not necessary.

The histopathologic examination of the resected specimens from the larynx showed an SCC with infiltration of the pre-epiglottic fat, both ventricular folds, the mucosa covering the arytenoid, and the postcricoid region. The maximum depth of invasion with 6 mm was found in the petiole area of the epiglottis. Multiple biopsies from the laryngeal remnant were free of cancer that R0 resection was assumed. The neck dissection specimens from the left side showed 3 positive out of 31 examined nodes, one with extra capsular spread (ECS), and from the right side 2 positive out of 24 examined nodes. The postoperative TNM stage was pT3pN2c(5/55, ENS+)M0G2L0V0Pn0pR0, UICC stage IVa.

Adjuvant treatment was recommended by the MDT board due to the finding of multiple lymph node metastases in the neck, one with ECS. In cases with pN2 disease and metastases with ECS, most authors agree that adjuvant radiotherapy is necessary for adequate regional control.[2,18] It is not as clear which patient groups would benefit from chemoradiotherapy after surgery. The very similarly designed European Organisation for Research and Treatment of Cancer (EORTC)[11] and RTOG trials,[13] both published in 2004, supported the concept that postoperative radiotherapy and concurrent cisplatin for high-risk resected head and neck cancer improves locoregional control and disease-free survival compared with postoperative radiotherapy alone. The long-term results of the RTOG 9501 trial, however, show no statistically significant difference for locoregional control and disease-free survival.[19] The subgroup analysis demonstrated that patients with metastases with ECS and/or positive resection margins seemed to benefit from concurrent chemoradiotherapy. This was the rationale for our MDT board to recommend adjuvant chemoradiotherapy.

Our patient received adjuvant concurrent chemotherapy with intensity-modulated radiotherapy (60 Gy in 30 fractions over 6 weeks) and cisplatin (133 mg/m², which is 66% of 200 mg/m²)

to reduce the radiation dose to the uninvolved constrictor muscles and the parotid glands (▶ Fig. 15.5). During treatment, he required temporary percutaneous endoscopic gastrostomy feeding for nutritional support. He was referred to our speech and swallowing rehabilitation program, and the tube was removed 6 weeks after treatment.

However, 60 months after completion of treatment at the age of 83 years, he was diagnosed with a second primary. CT-guided fine-needle aspiration cytology revealed SCC. PET-CT scan revealed a segment 3 tumor in the lung with one positive node at the lung hilum. There were no suspicious findings in larynx, pharynx, or the neck.

Surveillance up to 64 months after completion of treatment shows that the patient remained disease free (▶ Fig. 15.6, ▶ Fig. 15.7). His swallowing is almost normal and his diet is normal. He does not have a tracheostomy and his voice is normal (recording of posttherapeutic voice can be found on the DVD). There are no late toxicities. He reports a very good health-related quality of life. Using the EORTC QoL HN43 Module,[20] we were able to gain information about several aspects of his actual quality of life, at that point time. He does not have any impairment

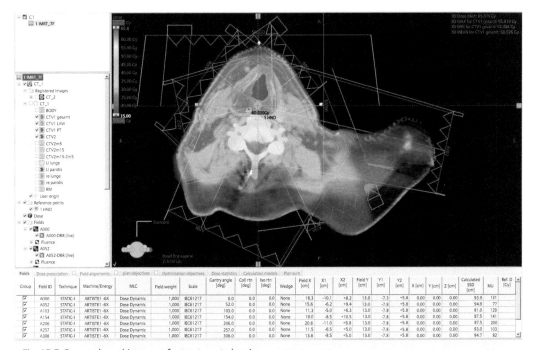

Fig. 15.5 Dose-volume histogram for treatment planning.

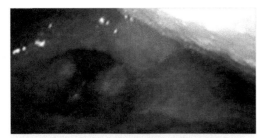

Fig. 15.6 Larynx in respiration, 64 months following transoral laser microsurgery, bilateral selective neck dissection, and adjuvant radiochemotherapy.

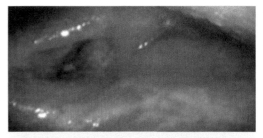

Fig. 15.7 Larynx in phonation, 64 months following transoral laser microsurgery, bilateral selective neck dissection, and adjuvant radiochemotherapy.

in his body image or his social contacts. He does not have any skin or shoulder problems, no problems with special senses, and no weight loss. He does not suffer anxiety even having gone through several treatments. There are minor impairments ("not a lot") regarding dry mouth.

15.3 Conclusion

The treatment of elderly patients and patients with comorbidities with locally advanced supraglottic cancer is challenging. Patients need not to be excluded from larynx preservation if TLM and adjuvant radiotherapy is performed. Careful pretreatment evaluation and treatment in a multidisciplinary expert team is mandatory for success.

15.4 Tips

- Cutting through the cancer is essential. The surgeon follows and removes the cancer, individually adapted to cancer spread.
- Tracheostomy should be avoided whenever possible. It immobilizes the larynx and delays swallowing rehabilitation.
- Cancer of the upraglottis involving the petiole might have infiltrated the pre-epiglottic space. Microscopic invasion is possible, even in the absence of radiologic evidence. The pre-epiglottic fat should always be resected completely. This does not negatively influence long-term functional outcomes.
- Given the significant toxicities, adjuvant chemoradiotherapy should only be considered for high-risk patients with microscopically positive margins and/or lymph node metastases with extracapsular spread.

15.5 Traps

- Accurate staging of the disease is the prerequisite for treatment success.
- Inadequate endoscopic exposure is the main limitation for TLM.
- Contraindications for TLM in T3 cancer of the supraglottis are bilateral vocal cord fixation, bilateral paraglottic space invasion, and/or invasion of the inner cortex of the thyroid cartilage at the glottic level.

References

[1] Forastiere A, Ismaila N, Lewin JS, et al. Use of larynx-preservation strategies in the treatment of laryngeal cancer: American Society of Clinical Oncology clinical practice guideline update. J Clin Oncol. 2017; 36(11):1143–1169

[2] Ambrosch P, Kron M, Pradier O, Steiner W. Efficacy of selective neck dissection: a review of 503 cases of elective and therapeutic treatment of the neck in squamous cell carcinoma of the upper aerodigestive tract. Otolaryngol Head Neck Surg. 2001a; 124(2):180–187

[3] Ambrosch P, Fazel A. Functional organ preservation in laryngeal and hypopharyngeal cancer. GMS Curr Top Otorhinolaryngol Head Neck Surg. 2011; 10:Doc02

[4] Peretti G, Piazza C, Cattaneo A, De Benedetto L, Martin E, Nicolai P. Comparison of functional outcomes after endoscopic versus open-neck supraglottic laryngectomies. Ann Otol Rhinol Laryngol. 2006; 115(11):827–832

[5] Ambrosch P, Rödel R, Kron M, Steiner W. Die transorale Lasermikrochirurgie des Larynxkarzinoms. Eine retrospektive Analyse von 657 Patientenverläufen. Onkologe. 2001b; 7:505–512

[6] Canis M, Ihler F, Martin A, Wolff HA, Matthias C, Steiner W. Results of 226 patients with T3 laryngeal carcinoma after treatment with transoral laser microsurgery. Head Neck. 2014; 36(5):652–659

[7] Peretti G, Piazza C, Penco S, et al. Transoral laser microsurgery as primary treatment for selected T3 glottic and supraglottic cancers. Head Neck. 2016; 38(7):1107–1112

[8] Vilaseca I, Bernal-Sprekelsen M, Luis Blanch J. Transoral laser microsurgery for T3 laryngeal tumors: prognostic factors. Head Neck. 2010; 32(7):929–938

[9] Vilaseca I, Blanch JL, Berenguer J, et al. Transoral laser microsurgery for locally advanced (T3–T4a) supraglottic squamous cell carcinoma: sixteen years of experience. Head Neck. 2016; 38(7):1050–1057

[10] Grant DG, Salassa JR, Hinni ML, Pearson BW, Hayden RE, Perry WC. Transoral laser microsurgery for carcinoma of the supraglottic larynx. Otolaryngol Head Neck Surg. 2007; 136(6):900–906

[11] Ambrosch P, Gonzalez-Donate M, Fazel A, Schmalz C, Hedderich J. Transoral laser microsurgery for supraglottic cancer. Front Oncol. 2018; 8:158–167

[12] Bernier J, Domenge C, Ozsahin M, et al; European Organization for Research and Treatment of Cancer Trial 22931. Postoperative irradiation with or without concomitant chemotherapy for locally advanced head and neck cancer. N Engl J Med. 2004; 350(19):1945–1952

[13] Cooper JS, Pajak TF, Forastiere AA, et al; Radiation Therapy Oncology Group 9501/Intergroup. Postoperative concurrent radiotherapy and chemotherapy for high-risk squamous-cell carcinoma of the head and neck. N Engl J Med. 2004; 350(19):1937–1944

[14] Forastiere AA, Goepfert H, Maor M, et al. Concurrent chemotherapy and radiotherapy for organ preservation in advanced laryngeal cancer. N Engl J Med. 2003; 349(22):2091–2098

[15] Forastiere AA, Zhang Q, Weber RS, et al. Long-term results of RTOG 91–11: a comparison of three nonsurgical treatment strategies to preserve the larynx in patients with locally advanced larynx cancer. J Clin Oncol. 2013; 31(7):845–852

[16] Steiner W, Ambrosch P. Endoscopic Laser Surgery of the Upper Aerodigestive Tract. Stuttgart: Thieme; 2000

[17] Remacle M, Hantzakos A, Eckel H, et al. Endoscopic supraglottic laryngectomy: a proposal for a classification by the working committee on nomenclature, European Laryngological Society. Eur Arch Otorhinolaryngol. 2009; 266(7):993–998

[18] Strojan P, Ferlito A, Langendijk JA, Silver CE. Indications for radiotherapy after neck dissection. Head Neck. 2012; 34(1):113–119

[19] Cooper JS, Zhang Q, Pajak TF, et al. Long-term follow-up of the RTOG 9501/intergroup phase III trial: postoperative concurrent radiation therapy and chemotherapy in high-risk squamous cell carcinoma of the head and neck. Int J Radiat Oncol Biol Phys. 2012; 84(5):1198–1205

[20] Singer S, Araújo C, Arraras JI, et al; EORTC Quality of life and the EORTC Head and Neck Cancer Groups. Measuring quality of life in patients with head and neck cancer: update of the EORTC QLQ-H&N Module, phase III. Head Neck. 2015; 37(9):1358–1367

16 Locally Intermediate Supraglottic Cancer: Radiotherapy

Giuseppe Sanguineti, Alessia Farneti, Laura Marucci

Abstract

The present case of T3N0 cancer of the supraglottic larynx highlights some of the issues related to nonsurgical organ-preservation strategies. In particular, we discuss the importance of pretreatment functional evaluation, proper patient staging and, the role of chemotherapy in addition to radiotherapy and its timing, as well as some of the planning/ technical issues of radiotherapy. Unfortunately, the majority of clinical data on organ preservation with nonsurgical approaches have been obtained in patients who were candidates for total laryngectomy and without a formal evaluation of pretreatment laryngeal function, limiting their applicability to current practice. Highly destructive/extensive/ circumferential cancers, even if still staged as T3, may not be good candidates for laryngeal preservation and patients should be specifically counseled. Regarding the role of chemotherapy, its addition to radiotherapy has been shown to provide improved organ preservation rates over radiotherapy alone, though the timing of the chemotherapy remains controversial. For a T3N0 cancer of the supraglottis, radiotherapy should deliver a definitive dose to the larynx and cover electively the neck at levels II to IV bilaterally. Intensity-modulated radiotherapy allows the dose of radiation to organs outside the target to be minimized and the one on structures that are (even only partially) "embedded" within the target (and its expansion at planning), such as the constrictor muscles and the thyroid gland, to be "controlled."

Keywords: radiotherapy, chemotherapy, organ preservation, IMRT

16.1 Case Report

A 71-year-old cigarette smoker without significant comorbidities and with a 6-month history of progressive dysphonia was referred to our clinic. He denied dysphagia, pain, and weight loss. He recently consulted an Otolaryngologist who found an ulcerative lesion in the right supraglottic larynx. Physical examination revealed an approximately 2-cm ulcerative lesion involving the entire right false cord associated with edema and reduced mobility of the right hemilarynx was noted. The glottis and the right piriform sinus was unremarkable. (▶Fig. 16.1).

A biopsy was taken, which revealed nonkeratinizing squamous cell carcinoma. He completed the locoregional staging with an MRI, which demonstrated a 3-cm lesion centered in the right false vocal cord, involving the paraglottic space without erasion of the thyroid cartilage erosion. There were no signs of contralateral spread or involvement of either the pre-epiglottic space (PES) or the arytenoid (▶Fig. 16.2).

The neck was negative on both palpation and imaging. The lesion was staged as cT3N0M0 (CT chest). The patient discontinued smoking shortly after the diagnosis was made. Before deciding treatment options, the patient underwent a speech pathologist examination (FEES) that revealed no signs of penetration/aspiration. Moreover, the patient was cleared for both a conservation surgical approach (pulmonary function tests) and chemotherapy. Therefore, after multidisciplinary discussion, the patient was offered two options: supracricoid laryngectomy + bilateral elective neck dissections or definitive chemoradiotherapy. The patient opted for the latter.

A CT scan with the head hyperextended was obtained at simulation. The patient was instructed

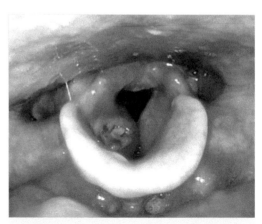

Fig. 16.1 The laryngoscopy showed an ulcerative-infiltrative lesion centered in the right false vocal cord.

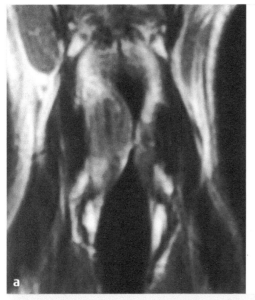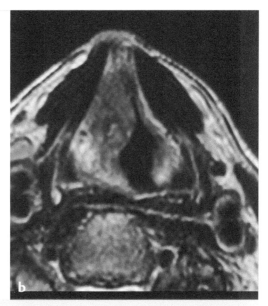

Fig. 16.2 Coronal and axial MRI scan (fast spin echo [FTE] T2) showing a lesion of the right false vocal cord invading the left paraglottic space. The thyroid cartilage is unremarkable.

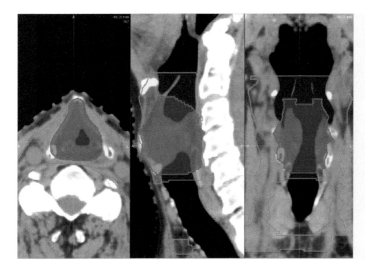

Fig. 16.3 Planning CT showing the two clinical target volumes, CTV58.1 (*blue*) and CTV70 (*red*).

to breathe quietly and to avoid swallowing. The entire larynx and levels II to IV on both sides were contoured. The prescription doses were 70 and 58.1 Gy for the volume containing macroscopic and microscopic disease, respectively, in 35 fractions (▶ Fig. 16.3).

Seven-field intensity-modulated radiotherapy (IMRT) with 6-MV photons were used to deliver at least 95% of the prescription dose to at least 95% of the target volumes expanded isotropically by 5 mm to planning target volumes (PTVs).

The resulting dose distribution is reported in ▶ Fig. 16.4.

The dose to the following organs was constrained (goal): parotids (V30 < 50%); spinal cord + 2 mm (Dmax 0.1 mL: 44 Gy), brain (Dmax 1 mL: 60 Gy), brainstem (Dmax 0.1 mL: 54 Gy), brachial plexuses (Dmax 0.1 mL: 60 Gy), upper gastrointestinal (GI) mucosa (out-Dmax 1 mL: 30 Gy; in-V66.5 < 64 mL). The right upper panel of ▶ Fig. 16.4 illustrates the achieved dove volume histograms for selected organs at risk.

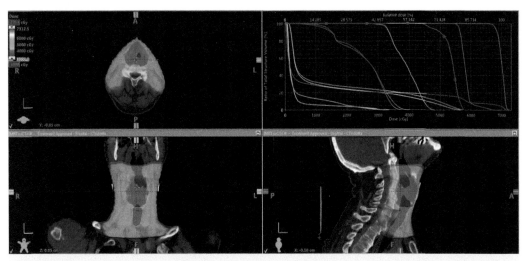

Fig. 16.4 Dose distribution on the three planes showing the higher dose to the larynx while electively treating both necks-levels II to IV. In the right upper quadrant, the dose volume histogram is reported: PTV70 (*red*), PTV58.1 (*light blue*), left brachial plexus (*pink*), right brachial plexus (*green*), cord and cord + 2 mm (*deep blue*), right parotid gland (*turquoise*), left parotid gland (*light green*), upper GI mucosa (*violet*), brain (*green*), and brainstem (*yellow*).

The treatment was delivered with daily image guidance throughout cone-beam CTs. Concomitant chemotherapy consisted of cisplatin, 100 mg/m² on days 1, 21, and 42.

The patient completed treatment as planned despite grade 3 (confluent) mucositis and grade 2 skin toxicity. The patient kept eating by mouth and parenteral/enteral feeding was not needed despite an about 8% weight loss from baseline.

A reevaluation physical examination is awaited 6 weeks after treatment end as well as a repeated MRI shortly there after.

16.2 Discussion

Patients with a functional larynx with a T3 cancer of the supraglottis (false cord and paraglottic space) are potentially eligible for organ preservation. This can be achieved by both surgical and nonsurgical treatment approaches without jeopardizing overall survival[1]; in this specific case, after being cleared for both, the patient opted for a nonsurgical approach.

Due to the lack of randomized studies, it is unclear whether partial (conservation) surgery would yield better outcomes compared to over nonsurgical alternatives. Since most of the data obtained by radiotherapy (RT) ± chemotherapy have involved patients eligible for total laryngectomy (TL), but

not partial surgery, in 2009 the Larynx Preservation Consensus Panel recommended selecting only patients eligible for TL for clinical trials of laryngeal preservation.[2] Nevertheless, we currently offer both options to properly selected patients.

Once a nonsurgical approach is selected, the next issues are whether chemotherapy should be part of the treatment strategy and which would be the best timing. There is level I evidence supporting the use of chemotherapy in addition to RT over conventionally fractionated (CF) RT alone, with cisplatin as the drug of choice in this setting.[2] However, in a subset analysis of the meta-analysis of chemotherapy for head and neck cancer, patients older than 70 years of age did not benefit from the addition of chemotherapy to RT.[3] However, since this is hypothesis generating rather than conclusive evidence, we still offer chemotherapy to patients older than 70 years if their general health allows. Alternatively, hyperfractionated (HF) RT, which is also supported by level I evidence over CF-RT in locally advanced head and neck cancer,[4] represents a reasonable choice for patients who want to maximize the chance of organ preservation and who are not candidates for chemotherapy.

Regarding timing of chemotherapy, based on the long-term results of the Radiation Therapy Oncology Group (RTOG)/NRG study 91–11, the latest American Society of Clinical Oncology (ASCO) guidelines still favor concomitant chemoradiotherapy over induction chemotherapy followed by RT based on a presumed higher chance of larynx preservation[1] though this is controversial.[5]

Regarding the RT technique, for a T3N0 supraglottic carcinoma, RT typically targets the site of the primary cancer to full dose and covers electively the neck, levels II to IV. In this setting, the inclusion of level IIB is somewhat controversial,[6] and it was incompletely treated in the era of 3D conformal RT.[7] The use of IMRT is justified by a better control of the dose outside of the target region, namely the parotid glands and the mucosa, and a more comprehensive coverage of the selected neck levels. In our definition of the upper GI mucosa,[8] which includes/overlaps with the middle/inferior constrictor muscles besides the whole oral cavity and oropharynx, the dose to the portions overlapping with the PTV is controlled as a secondary objective (after target coverage), while the dose outside the PTV is tentatively limited to 30 Gy, thereby reducing the risk of severe acute toxicity (mucositis and dysphagia).[9,10]

16.3 Tips

- Proper local imaging[11] is mandatory and highly destructive/extensive/circumferential lesions, even if still staged as T3 and not associated with a "dysfunctional" larynx,[2] may not be good candidates for laryngeal preservation[1]; once treated with nonsurgical organ preservation, these lesions are more likely to result in worse functional outcomes due to scarring/edema after treatment: give patient realistic and "adjusted" functional expectations.
- Most of the data from the early trials on organ preservation did not include a functional evaluation of the larynx at baseline that nowadays is mandatory: preserve only the function larynx.
- Adequate patient hydration (1.5–2 L of liquids per day) during chemoradiotherapy is essential.
- To minimize the risk of long-term swallowing problems, patients are usually advised to keep the swallowing muscles "alive" by eating by mouth or by prophylactic swallowing exercises.
- Avoid breaks/gaps during the course of treatment.
- Suspicious cervical lymph nodes[12] may be prescribed a dose level between 50 and 70 Gy, typically 63 Gy in 35 fractions.

16.4 Traps

- Beware of the long-term extramortality of concomitant chemoradiotherapy[13] and the need for long-term evaluation of laryngeal function to rule out (chronic) aspiration.
- Persistent mild/severe laryngeal edema after treatment completion is a diagnostic challenge and may mask tumor persistence/recurrence; imaging such as MR or PET-CT may help in this setting[14]; moreover, even if a timely diagnosis of persistent/recurrent disease is essential, repeated biopsies should be used cautiously due to the risk of necrosis of the larynx.[15]
- In thin patients, check the dose in the anterior part of the larynx (anterior commissure, PES) and use bolus accordingly to avoid underdosing.
- Check thyroid function baseline every 6 months and give replacement therapy as necessary.

References

[1] Forastiere AA, et al. Use of Larynx-Preservation Strategies in the Treatment of Laryngeal Cancer: American Society of Clinical Oncology Clinical Practice Guideline Update. J Clin Oncol. 2017:JCO2017757385

[2] Lefebvre JL, Ang KK; Larynx Preservation Consensus Panel. Larynx preservation clinical trial design: key issues and recommendations-a consensus panel summary. Int J Radiat Oncol Biol Phys. 2009; 73(5):1293–1303

[3] Pignon JP, Bourhis J, Domenge C, Designé L. Chemotherapy added to locoregional treatment for head and neck squamous-cell carcinoma: three meta-analyses of updated individual data. MACH-NC Collaborative Group. Meta-Analysis of chemotherapy on head and neck cancer. Lancet. 2000; 355(9208):949–955

[4] Lacas B, Bourhis J, Overgaard J, et al; MARCH Collaborative Group. Role of radiotherapy fractionation in head and neck cancers (MARCH): an updated meta-analysis. Lancet Oncol. 2017; 18(9):1221–1237

[5] Licitra L, Bonomo P, Sanguineti G, et al. Different view on larynx preservation evidence-based treatment recommendations. J Clin Oncol. 2018; 36(13):1376–1377

[6] Sezen OS, Kubilay U, Haytoglu S, Unver S. Frequency of metastases at the area of the supraretrospinal (level IIB) lymph node in laryngeal cancer. Head Neck. 2007; 29(12):1111–1114

[7] Sanguineti G, Culp LR, Endres EJ, Bayouth JE. Are neck nodal volumes drawn on CT slices covered by standard three-field technique? Int J Radiat Oncol Biol Phys. 2004; 59(3):725–742

[8] Becker M, Burkhardt K, Dulguerov P, Allal A. Imaging of the larynx and hypopharynx. Eur J Radiol. 2008; 66(3):460–479

[9] Sanguineti G, Endres EJ, Gunn BG, Parker B. Is there a "mucosa-sparing" benefit of IMRT for head-and-neck cancer? Int J Radiat Oncol Biol Phys. 2006; 66(3):931–938

[10] Sanguineti G, Sormani MP, Marur S, et al. Effect of radiotherapy and chemotherapy on the risk of mucositis during

intensity-modulated radiation therapy for oropharyngeal cancer. Int J Radiat Oncol Biol Phys. 2012; 83(1):235–242

[11] Sanguineti G, Gunn GB, Parker BC, Endres EJ, Zeng J, Fiorino C. Weekly dose-volume parameters of mucosa and constrictor muscles predict the use of percutaneous endoscopic gastrostomy during exclusive intensity-modulated radiotherapy for oropharyngeal cancer. Int J Radiat Oncol Biol Phys. 2011; 79(1):52–59

[12] Rao NG, Sanguineti G, Chaljub G, Newlands SD, Qiu S. Do neck levels negative on initial CT need to be dissected after definitive radiation therapy with or without chemotherapy? Head Neck. 2008; 30(8):1090–1098

[13] Forastiere AA, Zhang Q, Weber RS, et al. Long-term results of RTOG 91–11: a comparison of three nonsurgical treatment strategies to preserve the larynx in patients with locally advanced larynx cancer. J Clin Oncol. 2013; 31(7):845–852

[14] Bae JS, Roh JL, Lee SW, et al. Laryngeal edema after radiotherapy in patients with squamous cell carcinomas of the larynx and hypopharynx. Oral Oncol. 2012; 48(9):853–858

[15] Fu KK, Woodhouse RJ, Quivey JM, Phillips TL, Dedo HH. The significance of laryngeal edema following radiotherapy of carcinoma of the vocal cord. Cancer. 1982; 49(4):655–658

17 Locally Intermediate Supraglottic Cancer: Supracricoid Laryngectomy with Cricohyoidopexy

Carlos N. Lehn, Fernando Walder

Abstract

The case of a 56-year-old patient with glottic and supraglottic carcinoma is presented as an example of supracricoid laryngectomy with cricohyoidopexy. The surgical technique is outlined, comprising the main steps to execute the procedure correctly. Important a natomical landmarks are presented and correlated with the steps of the technique. The goals of larynx preservation surgery are discussed after a brief introduction remembering the overindication of chemoradiation during the 1980s and 1990s. Indications and contraindications for the procedure are discussed and a series of tips are given, including the indications, limits for this surgery concerning the amount of subglottic extension, the importance in preserving both arytenoid cartilages whenever possible, reconstruction using sutures folding the hypopharyngeal mucosa, and the importance of frozen section intraoperative examination. Possible traps included the indication in patients with chronic obstructive pulmonary disease (COPD), previously irradiated patients, the insertion of the feeding tube before the closure of the pharynx, and the position of the skin incision for the tracheostomy.

Keywords: supracricoid laryngectomy, cricohyoidopexy, cancer, larynx

17.1 Case Report

A 56-year-old Caucasian male painter, presented with a history of dysphonia for 6 months, followed by cough and odynophagia. He smoked, two packs of cigarettes per day for the last 20 years, and was a moderate alcohol drinker. He had no comorbidities.

During the consultation the patient appeared to be healthy and had an obvious hoarse voice. No lesions were found in the nasal and oral cavities. Laryngoscopy revealed an ulcerated and infiltrative lesion involving the anterior commissure and the anterior half of both true vocal folds (▶Fig. 17.1). Superiorly, the lesion infiltrated the false vocal cords and the epiglottic petiole. Both vocal cords were mobile and the subglottis were not easily visible. There were no palpable lymph nodes and the laryngeal crepitation was present bilaterally.

Due to the difficulty in evaluating the subglottis, the patient underwent direct rigid laryngoscopy under general anesthesia for better evaluation of the lesion. This procedure revealed an extension of the tumor with a vegetative characteristic toward the subglottis on the right side (▶Fig. 17.2). Biopsies were taken and the histopathological examination showed a moderately differentiated squamous cell carcinoma.

The therapeutic proposal was a supracricoid laryngectomy (SCL) with cricohyoidopexy (CHP). A large horizontal cervical incision was performed with subplatysmal flaps to provide an operative field with good visualization of the structures.

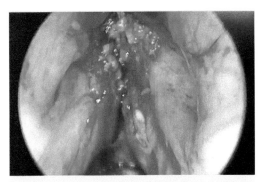

Fig. 17.1 Laryngoscopy demonstrating an ulcerated and infiltrative lesion involving the anterior commissure and two-thirds of both true and false vocal folds with extension to the petiole of the epiglottis.

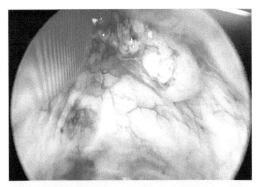

Fig. 17.2 Laryngoscopy demonstrating subglottic extension of the tumor of the right vocal fold.

The sternohyoid and omohyoid muscles were transected bilaterally at the superior border of the thyroid cartilage. The sternothyroid muscles were transected at the inferior border of the thyroid cartilage. A bilateral Tapia maneuver was then performed bilaterally by transecting the constrictors of the pharynx which released the pyriform sinuses.

The cricothyroid joint was then disarticulated in a subperichondrial plane being careful to preserve the recurrent laryngeal nerves. The isthmus of the thyroid gland was transected.

The periosteum of the hyoid bone was incised along its inferior aspect bilaterally allowing the release of the thyrohyoid membrane, hyoepiglottic membrane, and the pre-epiglottic space that will be removed with the specimen. The suprahyoid muscles were not transected. Using blunt dissection, the trachea was released along its anterior wall inferiorly to allow its upward motion at the time of the closure.

An entry to the larynx was made on the left side of the cricothyroid membrane (because there was evidence of subglottic extension on the right side). At this time, the orotracheal ventilation tube was removed and another one was inserted in the cricothyrotomy. A transvallecular horizontal approach was performed and the epiglottis was retracted anteriorly. Sections were carefully made along the pharyngoepiglottic and aryepiglottic folds for visualization of the tumor and clear margins.

From the superior aspect of the cricoid cartilage, incisions using scissors were made toward the arytenoid cartilages that were preserved by the vocal processes. The entire paraglottic space was then removed with the thyroid cartilage after using scissors were made connecting with the cricothyrotomy previously made and the specimen was removed (▶ Fig. 17.3).

Three sutures of 1 Vicryl were applied between the overlying retrocricoid mucosa to elevate the cricoid cartilage and made a pexy with the hyoid bone (▶ Fig. 17.4). The tracheostomy was placed at the level of the skin incision while the assistant tightened the central suture without tying it (▶ Fig. 17.5). No sutures were needed to close the pharynx.

The pathology report revealed a moderate differentiated squamous cell carcinoma with clear margins. The patient's postoperative course was satisfactory and the tracheostomy was plugged on the 20th postoperative day and removed on

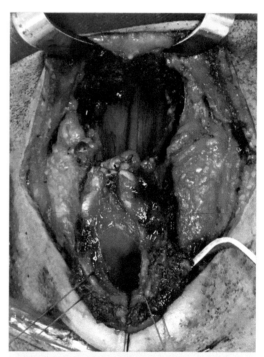

Fig. 17.4 The surgical field after removing the specimen. Three suspension sutures are placed through the cricoid cartilage and absorbable suture between the mucosa overlying the arytenoid cartilages and mucosa of the hypopharynx.

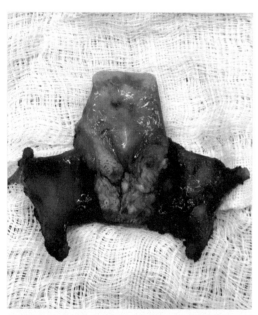

Fig. 17.3 Surgical specimen with the entire thyroid cartilage and epiglottis.

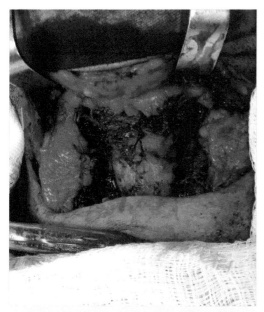

Fig. 17.5 Final aspect after the larynx suspension and closure.

the 25th day. The nasoenteral feeding tube was removed on the 31st day.

17.2 Discussion

Treatment of intermediate supraglottic or transglottic laryngeal squamous cell carcinoma can include many techniques with different therapeutic outcomes. Along with cancer control, quality of life is one of the main goals and, since it is a subjective aspect, the method of treatment should be chosen by the patient. Conservation surgery of the larynx was stimulated by Ogura et al[1] in the 1980s and their reports of partial and subtotal laryngectomies with similar results when compared to more radical approaches and with preservation of function.

During the period from mid-1980s to mid-1990s, chemoradiation therapy became almost the pattern for treatment of cancer of the larynx in intermediate stages. The search for organ preservation during this period was biased by some grade of overindication resulting in decreasing survival rates in that period according to database reviews.[2,3]

Among the therapeutic options, an alternative surgical technique that preserves the function and provides adequate oncologic control for T2 and T3 and even some T4 larynx cancer cases was

popularized by Laccourreye in France and Weinstein in the United States.[4,5] The SCL with CHP can be used even in cases with invasion of the pre-epiglottic space when partial horizontal supraglottic laryngectomy is not indicated and can replace total laryngectomy (in selected cases) with similar cure rates. One important point is that the presence of invasion of the pre-epiglottic space can be related to lymph node metastases, and in these cases neck dissection should be considered.[6]

The anterior commissure is always a concern when partial laryngectomies are considered as a therapeutic option. When this anatomic subsite is involved by the cancer, SCL allows histopathologic analysis of the entire region including the thyroid cartilage since microscopic invasion is difficult to be evaluated by mucosal extension and may be present in 20% of T2 cases.[7]

When compared in terms of oncologic results with total laryngectomy for N1 patients, the SCL has similar overall and disease-specific survival rates and is still safe for intermediate stage cancers.[8] Among the two techniques of reconstruction, CHP and cricohyoidoepiglottopexy (CHEP), each one with its specific indications, patients who underwent CHEP had better recovery due to the preservation of a larger amount of soft tissue, but both procedures are well tolerated and have good local control and disease-specific survival.[9] The mean decannulation and nasoenteral feeding tube removal time is significantly longer in CHP cases when compared to CHEP.[10]

Another issue is the extent of disease but when comparing the results of SCL with CHP for T2 and T3 cases, there are no significant differences for overall and disease-specific survival in 3 and 5 years, according to Topaloğlu et al.[11]

About the preservation of one or both arytenoid cartilages, some authors described higher bolus retention and aspiration in cases with arytenoid resection,[12] while more recent studies did not encounter functional differences.[13]

17.3 Tips

- Supracricoid laryngectomy with CHP is recommended treatment of T2 and T3 cancers even with invasion of the pre-epiglottic space.
- Subglottic extension up to 10 mm anteriorly and up to 5 mm posteriorly man need partial cricoid cartilage resection in some cases.
- Preserving both arytenoid cartilages, if possible, results in better swallowing outcomes.

- Sutures applied between the postcricoid hypopharyngeal mucosa and the arytenoids improve the functional results.
- Always use frozen section examination to assure clear margins.

17.4 Traps

- Avoid to suggest this procedure for elderly patients and those with chronic obstructive pulmonary disease.
- Functional results are poorer in patients who have been previously irradiated.
- Always insert the nasoenteral feeding tube before the surgery to avoid extension of the neck after the closure.
- The site of the skin incision for the tracheostomy must be higher to avoid tension after the closure.

References

[1] Ogura JH, Marks JE, Freeman RB. Results of conservation surgery for cancers of the supraglottis and pyriform sinus. Laryngoscope. 1980; 90(4):591–600

[2] Hoffman HT, Porter K, Karnell LH, et al. Laryngeal cancer in the United States: changes in demographics, patterns of care, and survival. Laryngoscope. 2006; 116(9, pt 2, suppl 111):1–13

[3] Nakayama M, Laccourreye O, Holsinger FC, Okamoto M, Hayakawa K. Functional organ preservation for laryngeal cancer: past, present and future. Jpn J Clin Oncol. 2012; 42(3):155–160

[4] Laccourreye H, Laccourreye O, Weinstein G, Menard M, Brasnu D. Supracricoid laryngectomy with cricohyoidopexy: a partial laryngeal procedure for selected supraglottic and transglottic carcinomas. Laryngoscope. 1990; 100(7):735–741

[5] Laccourreye O, Brasnu D, Merite-Drancy A, et al. Cricohyoidopexy in selected infrahyoid epiglottic carcinomas presenting with pathological preepiglottic space invasion. Arch Otolaryngol Head Neck Surg. 1993; 119(8):881–886

[6] Joo YH, Park JO, Cho KJ, Kim MS. Relationship between preepiglottic space invasion and lymphatic metastasis in supracricoid partial laryngectomy with cricohyoidopexy. Clin Exp Otorhinolaryngol. 2014; 7(3):205–209

[7] Prades JM, Gavid M, Dumollard JM, Timoshenko AT, Karkas A, Peoc'h M. Anterior laryngeal commissure: histopathologic data from supracricoid partial laryngectomy. Eur Ann Otorhinolaryngol Head Neck Dis. 2016; 133(1):27–30

[8] De Virgilio A, Fusconi M, Gallo A, et al. The oncologic radicality of supracricoid partial laryngectomy with cricohyoidopexy in the treatment of advanced N0-N1 laryngeal squamous cell carcinoma. Laryngoscope. 2012; 122(4):826–833

[9] Wang Y, Li X, Pan Z. Analyses of functional and oncologic outcomes following supracricoid partial laryngectomy. Eur Arch Otorhinolaryngol. 2015; 272(11):3463–3468

[10] Pinar E, Imre A, Calli C, Oncel S, Katilmis H. Supracricoid partial laryngectomy: analyses of oncologic and functional outcomes. Otolaryngol Head Neck Surg. 2012; 147(6):1093–1098

[11] Topaloğlu I, Bal M, Salturk Z. Supracricoid laryngectomy with cricohyoidopexy: oncological results. Eur Arch Otorhinolaryngol. 2012; 269(8):1959–1965

[12] Topaloglu I, Köprücü G, Bal M. Analysis of swallowing function after supracricoid laryngectomy with cricohyoidopexy. Otolaryngol Head Neck Surg. 2012; 146(3):412–418

[13] Kılıç C, Tunçel Ü, Kaya M, Cömert E, Özlügedik S. Swallowing and aspiration: how much is affected by the number of arytenoid cartilages remaining after supracricoid partial laryngectomy? Clin Exp Otorhinolaryngol. 2017; 10(4):344–348

18 Locally Advanced Glottic Cancer: Supracricoid Laryngectomy

Roberto A. Lima, Fernando L. Dias, Emilson Q. Freitas

Abstract

There are many treatment options for advanced or moderately advanced laryngeal squamous cell carcinoma (SCC). After the 1990s, chemoradiation has become the first choice of treatment for these cancers. However, other treatment options have evolved, mainly in Europe and Brazil. One good option for moderately advanced cancer of the larynx is supracricoid laryngectomy with cricohyoidoepiglottopexy (CHEP) or cricohyoidopexy (CHP). Organ preservation and local control with surgery are comparable to that of chemoradiation, although the voice is not functional in some cases. In this chapter, we discuss a patient with cT2N0M0 cancer of the glottis who has upgraded to T4N0M0 after reviewing the imaging studies. We discuss the surgical and nonsurgical treatment options. Trying to explain the advantages of this technique in treating advanced and moderately advanced laryngeal cancer, we present a comparison of vertical partial laryngectomy and supracricoid laryngectomy for patients with T2 glottic cancer, including local control and complications. We also discuss nonsurgical treatment options and other surgical options such as endoscopic laser resection. We suggest that supracricoid laryngectomy is a good treatment option in selected cases and also discuss the contraindications of the procedure.

Keywords: supracricoid, laryngectomy, partial, larynx, cancer

18.1 Case Report

A 59-year-old male, trader, presented to our hospital with a history of progressive hoarseness for 4 months. He smoked one pack of cigarettes per day for 25 years. He had no comorbidities and was able to climb six flights of stairs to his apartment every day.

At first medical consultation, he was in a good performance status presenting with hoarseness as the main symptom. During the routine oroscopy, no lesion was identified, and the examination of the neck did not reveal any enlarged lymph nodes neck. Videolaryngoscopy, with a 70-degree optic, revealed an infiltrative white lesion of the right vocal fold reaching the anterior commissure; with reduction of the mobility of the right vocal fold, the left vocal fold was normal (▶ Fig. 18.1). The disease was classified at this moment as cT2N0M0.

A CT scan was performed to evaluate the endolaryngeal extension A review of the scan disclosed a tumor invasion through the anterior commissure reaching to and destroying the thyroid cartilage (▶ Fig. 18.2); no neck metastasis was detected. The patient was reclassified as T4aN0M0. A squamous cell carcinoma was the histopathologic diagnosis obtained following a direct laryngoscopy and biopsy.

During our service tumor board, the patient was discussed and it was suggested that the patient be treated with supracricoid laryngectomy with cricohyoidoepiglottopexy (CHEP).

The patient underwent a bilateral lateral neck dissections, levels II to IV, and supracricoid laryngectomy with CHEP reconstruction. The entire thyroid cartilage was removed along with the paraglottic space and the vocal folds bilaterally sparing the arytenoid cartilage were (▶ Fig. 18.3).

The pathology from the surgical specimen (▶ Fig. 18.4) revealed squamous cell carcinoma with free margins, and focal destruction of the thyroid cartilage.

The reconstruction was with CHEP (▶ Fig. 18.5).

The patient had a good outcome without fistulas or infection. He was successfully decannulated after 15 days and began oral feeding at 21 days, with successful voice recovery at 16 days. The local control was successful during 60 months.

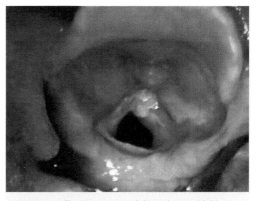

Fig. 18.1 Infiltrative cancer of the right vocal fold reaching the anterior commissure.

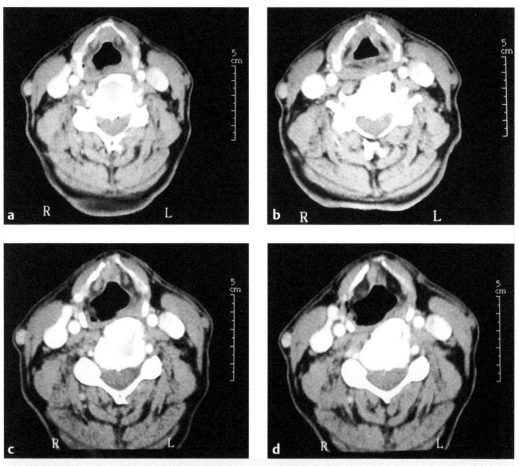

Fig. 18.2 (a–d) CT scan demonstrating invasion of the thyroid cartilage at the anterior commissure.

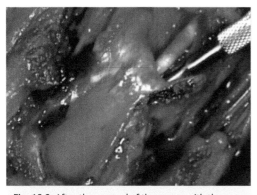

Fig. 18.3 After the removal of the cancer with the vocal folds and thyroid cartilage. Note the placement of the nasoenteral tube, and the two arytenoids.

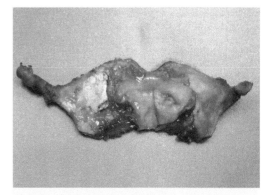

Fig. 18.4 Surgical specimen.

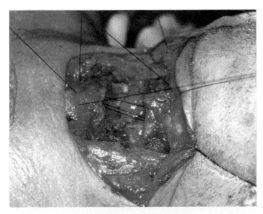

Fig. 18.5 Preparing the cricohyoidoepiglottopexy.

18.2 Discussion

The conventional surgical treatment for advanced squamous cell carcinoma of the laryngeal consists of total laryngectomy or total laryngectomy and postoperative radiotherapy.[1,2,3] Since a laryngectomy results in substantial loss of function and a high degree of morbidity, organ-preservation protocols with chemoradiation have been proposed to maintain the larynx function.[4,5]

Other surgical treatment options are near-total laryngectomy and supracricoid laryngectomy, which have been offered for patients with limited T3/T4 laryngeal cancer.[6,7,8,9]

Supracricoid laryngectomy with CHEP has been employed to treat glottic cancer with impaired vocal cords (T2) and selected cases of fixed vocal cords (T3/T4).[9,10,11]

According to Laccourreye et al[12] (▶Table 18.1), the local control and survival are better with supracricoid laryngectomy for T2 lesions.

The objective of preservation surgery for advanced cancer of the glottis is to achieve better local control while preserving the voice. A supracricoid laryngectomy with CHEP for the treatment of cancer of the glottis had its first reference in the English literature in 1990; 36 cases of CHEP were reported, mainly for T1 and T2 although cancers of the glottis; with a fixed vocal cord were excluded from this study.[13]

Jean-Jacques Piquet[14] in 1991, published a study of 104 patients with cancer of the glottis treated with CHEP, 77 patients with T2 cancer and 15 patients with T3 cancer. After these two publications, this technique gained international acceptance.

Most patients come to our Department for the first time with advanced cancer of the larynx. This has influenced our team to extend the CHEP indications for selected cases of T3/T4 cancer of the glottis. The 5-year survival for all stages reported in the literature is 75 to 95%.[10,13,14]

Lefèbvre and Chevalier[10] reported local recurrences in 4.8% and a 5-year overall survival of 76.8%; the most common cause of death was metachronous cancer. Chevalier et al[15] reported a 5-year actuarial local control and 5-year cause-specific survival rates for patients with a fixed vocal cord of 95.4 and 94.1%, respectively. Dufour et al[9] reported a 5-year actuarial local control of 91.4% for patients with endolaryngeal glottic and supraglottic T3 cancer. Eighty-one patients underwent CHEP and 37 patients cricohyoidopexy (CHP). In this publication, 100 patients had preoperative induction chemotherapy with cisplatin and fluorouracil.

Anatomopathological studies[16,17] indicated that the fixation of the vocal fold in cancer of the glottis resulted from invasion of the paraglottic space with extensive invasion of the thyroarytenoid muscle. Hirano et al[18] reported that the fixation of the vocal fold resulted from an extensive invasion of the thyroarytenoid muscle.

The survival rates reported in a series of T3 cancers treated by surgery ranges from 54 to 80%.[19,20]

The larynx-preservation protocols successfully preserve the larynx in 50 to 66%, regarding the extent and site of the disease.

Table 18.1 Comparison of vertical partial laryngectomy to supracricoid partial laryngectomy according to Laccourreye et al[12]

Glottic T2N0	Vertical partial laryngectomy (%)	Supracricoid laryngectomy (%)	p
10-y survival	46.2	66.4	0.019
10-y local control	69.3	94.6	0.001
Permanent tracheostomy	1.2	2.4	–
Completion laryngectomy	1.2	0.8	–

The Veterans Affairs Laryngeal Cancer Study Group[4] preserved the larynx in 101 of 166 patients (66%); 64% retained a functioning larynx. Another study carried out by Shirinian[5] reported 44% successful larynx preservation in 25 patients with cancer of the larynxstages III and IV. Lefèbvre and Chevalier[10] in a study with 207 patients who underwent CHEP preserved the larynx in 200. Ten (4.8%) presented local recurrences; 3 were salvaged with a completion laryngectomy and 7 were not salvaged. In the same study, 17 patients had stenosis and 7 required a permanent tracheostomy. Although only 16 patients were T3 cancer of the glottis, the overall larynx preservation rates were 96.6%, with 91.8% full-functioning larynx.

Endoscopic laser resection for T3 laryngeal cancer has been reported in the international literature as a laryngeal preservation option. Motta et al[21] in a study of 516 patients with cancer of the glottis treated by endoscopic laser resection reported only 7.1% with T3 carcinoma. Other published series[22,23] with more than 100 patients did not include T3 cancer of the glottis in the group of glottic cancers treated by endoscopic laser resection. Thirty-eight patients in our series[24] retained their larynx over a 5-year survival period. Our successful overall laryngeal preservation rate was 83.7%.

The differences in survival of patients with invasion of the laryngeal cartilage and exolaryngeal extension have been reported.[25] The occurrence of thyroid cartilage erosion or invasion by the cancer without reaching the exolaryngeal tissues have not been correlated with the prognosis.

A previous study at our institution demonstrated the importance of careful evaluation by imaging in the correct staging of cancer of the glottis.[26]

A previous study conducted in our Department revealed pathological cartilage invasion in a surgical specimen of 11 patients; this finding did not influence the survival rates.[24]

One controversy regarding the treatment of cancer of the glottis is the elective neck dissection associated with CHEP, because of the low rate of neck metastasis in this group of patients (9%).[15]

Previous publications[27] revealed a 10% incidence of occult neck metastasis in cancer of the glottis. In these publications, the overall rate of metastasis for cancer of the glottis was 22.2%, with extra capsular spread in 12 (37.5%) patients. Another option, instead of elective neck dissection associated with

CHEP for T3 tumors, is the watchful-waiting attitude; nevertheless, the rates of salvage neck dissection are as low as 11 to 56%.[28,29]

Successful decannulation with CHEP ranges from 93 to 98%.[30,31]

Naudo et al[32] reported a 9-day mean time to decannulation and found a relation between increased time with tracheostomy and advanced age and postoperative edema of the arytenoid. Bron et al[33] reported a 27-day mean time to decannulation; 62 patients with one arytenoid cartilage resected presented a mean time with tracheostomy of 29 days. Nine patients had no arytenoid resected, with a mean time to decannulation of 36 days.

18.3 Tips

- Supracricoid laryngectomy is a good surgical option to treat moderately advanced cancer of the glottic. Extension of the cancer to the arytenoids or subglottis is a contraindication, is extralaryngeal massive cancer.
- If there is a subglottic extension of less than 0.5 cm anteriorly, it is possible to so a supracricoid laryngectomy.
- Posterior subglottic extension is a contraindication to this procedure.
- In patients with T3/T4 cancer, lateral neck dissection should be considered.
- Good pulmonary function is very important for successful postoperative results.
- Advise the patient that the voice quality after the surgery will be weak and to swallow carefully.
- Instead of routine gastrostomy, patients can be fed after the surgery with nasoenteral tube.

18.4 Traps

- Never forget to incise the isthmus of the thyroid along with a pretracheal dissection to release the remaining larynx.
- Never forget to introduce the nasoenteral tube before CHP.
- Do a pexy carefully; remember, any rotation of the cricoid during the pexy can cause stenosis of the neoglottis.
- Do not initiate oral feeding before the patient is decannulated. Decannulation releases the neolarynx facilitating swallowing function.

References

[1] Mendenhall WM, Parsons JT, Stringer SP, Cassisi NJ, Million RR. Stage T3 squamous cell carcinoma of the glottic larynx: a comparison of laryngectomy and irradiation. Int J Radiat Oncol Biol Phys. 1992; 23(4):725–732

[2] DeSanto LW, Olsen KD, Perry WC, Rohe DE, Keith RL. Quality of life after surgical treatment of cancer of the larynx. Ann Otol Rhinol Laryngol. 1995; 104(10, pt 1):763–769

[3] Lassaletta L, García-Pallarés M, Morera E, Bernáldez R, Gavilan J. T3 glottic cancer: oncologic results and prognostic factors. Otolaryngol Head Neck Surg. 2001; 124(5):556–560

[4] Wolf GT, Fisher SG, Hong WK, et al; Department of Veterans Affairs Laryngeal Cancer Study Group. Induction chemotherapy plus radiation compared with surgery plus radiation in patients with advanced laryngeal cancer. N Engl J Med. 1991; 324(24):1685–1690

[5] Shirinian MH, Weber RS, Lippman SM, et al. Laryngeal preservation by induction chemotherapy plus radiotherapy in locally advanced head and neck cancer: the M. D. Anderson Cancer Center experience. Head Neck. 1994; 16(1):39–44

[6] Pearson BW, DeSanto LW, Olsen KD, Salassa JR. Results of near-total laryngectomy. Ann Otol Rhinol Laryngol. 1998; 107(10, pt 1):820–825

[7] Andrade RP, Kowalski LP, Vieira LJ, Santos CR. Survival and functional results of Pearson's near-total laryngectomy for larynx and pyriform sinus carcinoma. Head Neck. 2000; 22(1):12–16

[8] Laccourreye O, Salzer SJ, Brasnu D, Shen W, Laccourreye H, Weinstein GS. Glottic carcinoma with a fixed true vocal cord: outcomes after neoadjuvant chemotherapy and supracricoid partial laryngectomy with cricohyoidoepiglottopexy. Otolaryngol Head Neck Surg. 1996; 114(3):400–406

[9] Dufour X, Hans S, De Mones E, Brasnu D, Ménard M, Laccourreye O. Local control after supracricoid partial laryngectomy for "advanced" endolaryngeal squamous cell carcinoma classified as T3. Arch Otolaryngol Head Neck Surg. 2004; 130(9):1092–1099

[10] Lefèbvre J, Chevalier D. Supracricoid partial laryngectomy. Adv Otolaryngol Head Neck Surg. 1998; 12:1–15

[11] de Vincentiis M, Minni A, Gallo A, Di Nardo A. Supracricoid partial laryngectomies: oncologic and functional results. Head Neck. 1998; 20(6):504–509

[12] Laccourreye O, Laccourreye L, Garcia D, Gutierrez-Fonseca R, Brasnu D, Weinstein G. Vertical partial laryngectomy versus supracricoid partial laryngectomy for selected carcinomas of the true vocal cord classified as T2N0. Ann Otol Rhinol Laryngol. 2000; 109(10, pt 1):965–971

[13] Laccourreye H, Laccourreye O, Weinstein G, Menard M, Brasnu D. Supracricoid laryngectomy with cricohyoidoepiglottopexy: a partial laryngeal procedure for glottic carcinoma. Ann Otol Rhinol Laryngol. 1990; 99(6, pt 1):421–426

[14] Piquet JJ, Chevalier D. Subtotal laryngectomy with crico-hyoido-epiglotto-pexy for the treatment of extended glottic carcinomas. Am J Surg. 1991; 162(4):357–361

[15] Chevalier D, Laccourreye O, Brasnu D, Laccourreye H, Piquet JJ. Cricohyoidoepiglottopexy for glottic carcinoma with fixation or impaired motion of the true vocal cord: 5-year oncologic results with 112 patients. Ann Otol Rhinol Laryngol. 1997; 106(5):364–369

[16] Kirchner JA, Som ML. Clinical significance of fixed vocal cord. Laryngoscope. 1971; 81(7):1029–1044

[17] Olofsson J, Lord IJ, van Nostrand AW. Vocal cord fixation in laryngeal carcinoma. Acta Otolaryngol. 1973; 75(6):496–510

[18] Hirano M, Kurita S, Matsuoka H, Tateishi M. Vocal fold fixation in laryngeal carcinomas. Acta Otolaryngol. 1991; 111(2):449–454

[19] Foote RL, Olsen KD, Buskirk SJ, Stanley RJ, Suman VJ. Laryngectomy alone for T3 glottic cancer. Head Neck. 1994; 16(5):406–412

[20] Johnson JT, Myers EN, Hao SP, Wagner RL. Outcome of open surgical therapy for glottic carcinoma. Ann Otol Rhinol Laryngol. 1993; 102(10):752–755

[21] Motta G, Esposito E, Cassiano B, Motta S. T1–T2–T3 glottic tumors: fifteen years experience with CO_2 laser. Acta Otolaryngol Suppl. 1997; 527:155–159

[22] Rudert H, Werner JA. [Partial endoscopic resection with the CO_2 laser in laryngeal carcinomas. II. Results] Laryngorhinootologie. 1995; 74(5):294–299

[23] Steiner W. Results of curative laser microsurgery of laryngeal carcinomas. Am J Otolaryngol. 1993; 14(2):116–121

[24] Lima RA, Freitas EQ, Dias FL, et al. Supracricoid laryngectomy with cricohyoidoepiglottopexy for advanced glottic cancer. Head Neck. 2006; 28(6):481–486

[25] Fagan JJ, D'Amico F, Wagner RL, Johnson JT. Implications of cartilage invasion in surgically treated laryngeal carcinoma. Head Neck. 1998; 20(3):189–192

[26] Barbosa MM, Araújo VJ, Jr, Boasquevisque E, et al. Anterior vocal commissure invasion in laryngeal carcinoma diagnosis. Laryngoscope. 2005; 115(4):724–730

[27] Myers EN, Fagan JF. Management of the neck in cancer of the larynx. Ann Otol Rhinol Laryngol. 1999; 108(9):828–832

[28] Schramm VL, Jr, Myers EN, Sigler BA. Surgical management of early epidermoid carcinoma of the anterior floor of the mouth. Laryngoscope. 1980; 90(2):207–215

[29] Yuen APW, Ho CM, Wei WI, Lam LK. Analysis of recurrence after surgical treatment of advanced laryngeal carcinoma. J Laryngol Otol. 1995; 109(11):1063–1067

[30] Bussi M, Riontino E, Cardarelli L, Luce FL, Juliani E, Staffieri A. Cricohyoidoepiglottopexy: deglutition in 44 cases Acta Otorhinolaryngol Ital. 2000; 20(6):442–447

[31] Marioni G, Marchese-Ragona R, Ottaviano G, Staffieri A. Supracricoid laryngectomy: is it time to define guidelines to evaluate functional results? A review. Am J Otolaryngol. 2004; 25(2):98–104

[32] Naudo P, Laccourreye O, Weinstein G, Jouffre V, Laccourreye H, Brasnu D. Complications and functional outcome after supracricoid partial laryngectomy with cricohyoidoepiglottopexy. Otolaryngol Head Neck Surg. 1998; 118(1):124–129

[33] Bron L, Brossard E, Monnier P, Pasche P. Supracricoid partial laryngectomy with cricohyoidoepiglottopexy and cricohyoidopexy for glottic and supraglottic carcinomas. Laryngoscope. 2000; 110(4):627–634

19 Hemicricolaryngectomy with Tracheal Autotransplantation

Pierre R. Delaere, Vincent Vander Poorten

Abstract

Tracheal autotransplantation is a reconstructive technique that allows for organ-sparing treatment of selected patients with advanced cricoid cartilage chondrosarcoma and T2 or T3 laryngeal squamous cell carcinoma (SCC; unilateral T2 with impaired vocal fold mobility; T3 with subglottic extension and/or arytenoid cartilage fixation). For this particular group of patients, our tracheal autotransplantation technique provides excellent functional results for respiration, speech, and swallowing without compromising the oncologic outcome. This is particularly true for patients younger than 65 years and for those with cricoid chondrosarcoma.

Keywords: tracheal, autotransplantation, chondrosarcoma, squamous cell carcinoma

19.1 Case Report

A 54-year-old male patient presented with a T3N0 unilateral glottic squamous cell carcinoma (SCC) with involvement of the arytenoid and with infraglottic tumor extension. The lesion did not extend to the ventricle. Two years earlier, he received radiation therapy for a T1N0 glottic SCC. His pulmonary function test was within the normal range. The patient had no other comorbidities.

An extended hemicricolaryngectomy with tracheal autotransplantation was performed in this patient. An overview of the tumor extent and the amount of resection is depicted in ▶ Fig. 19.1.

19.1.1 First Operation

The operation began with a lateral selective neck dissection (levels II–IV)[1] with inclusion of one an ipsilateral thyroidectomy. A hemilaryngectomy with inclusion of half of the cricoid cartilage was performed (▶ Fig. 19.2).

After tumor resecting the cancer, the cervical trachea was wrapped with the radial forearm subcutaneous tissue and fascia with the aim of

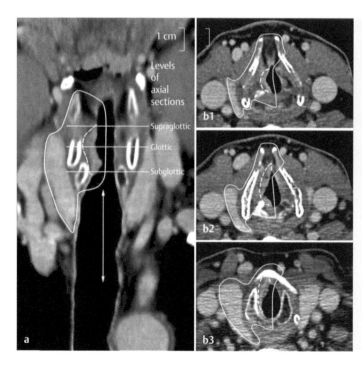

Fig. 19.1 Preoperative CT scan. Overview on CT scan of laryngeal tumor (*dotted line*) and the planned resection (*white contour lines*). (a) Coronal reformatted CT scan. The extended hemilaryngectomy defect involving up to one half of the cricoid cartilage will be reconstructed with the top 4 cm of the cervical trachea (*double arrow*). (b) Axial sections. b1, supraglottic level; b2, glottic level; b3, subglottic level.

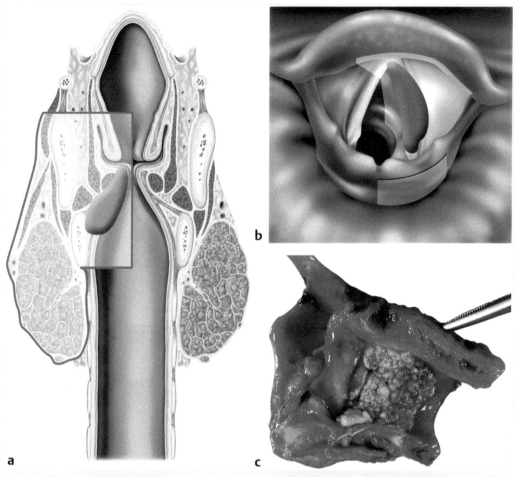

Fig. 19.2 Tumor resection for a right glottis squamous cell carcinoma with subglottic extension. **(a)** Artist's representation of resection on a coronal sectional view. **(b)** Endoscopic view. The anterior commissure was included in the resection because the squamous cell carcinoma reached the anterior commissure. The aryepiglottic fold remains preserved. **(c)** Resection specimen. Lateralized cancer with subglottic extension.

fabricating a transplantable tracheal patch, axially vascularized by the radial forearm flap (RFF) pedicle. The hemilaryngeal defect was repaired temporarily with the radial forearm skin paddle. A tracheostomy was necessary for respiration (▶Fig. 19.3).

The sphincteric function after resection was restored by closing the gap between preserved aryepiglottic fold and epiglottis at the side of resection and by using the skin paddle of the RFF as a buttress for apposition (▶Fig. 19.3a). The aryepiglottic fold allowed for a posterior midline reconstruction at the glottic and supraglottic level. After this intervention, the patient could close the

glottic chink during speech and swallowing. A CT scan after 2 weeks illustrates the first step in the reconstruction process (▶Fig. 19.4).

At this point, the tracheostomy remains necessary for respiration. In the immediate postoperative period, first the nurses and after a few days the patient aspirated his own secretions using the bedside hospital suction system. Frequent suctioning through the tracheostomy tube was indicated to evacuate pulmonary secretions. Oral alimentation was begun after 1 week.

The histopathological report confirmed a T3N0 SCC. Resection margins were tumor free.

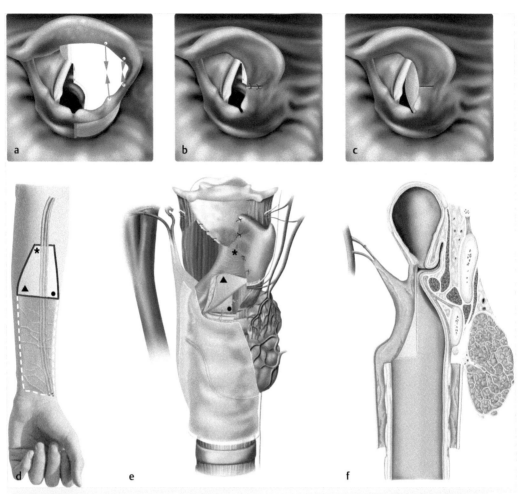

Fig. 19.3 Tracheal revascularization and temporary reconstruction. **(a–c)** Endoscopic representation after tumor resection and after closure (*arrows*; **a,b**) of the lateral gap between aryepiglottic fold and epiglottis. **(c)** Endoscopic representation after temporary reconstruction with forearm skin. **(d–f)** The radial forearm flap is designed with a paddle consisting of fascia and a paddle consisting of skin. The fascial paddle will serve for revascularization of the cervical trachea and the skin paddle will serve as temporary closure for the hemilaryngectomy defect. The forearm fascia **(d)** is wrapped around the 4-cm segment of cervical trachea **(e,f)**. The superior surface of the forearm fascia lies against the tracheal wall. The hemilaryngectomy defect is covered as a temporary measure until step 2 of the procedure using the cutaneous part of the revascularized free flap from the forearm. The first lateral site of the skin flap is sutured to the posterior laryngeal section margin of the cricoid cartilage from inferior (*black dot*) to superior. The second lateral side of the skin paddle is sutured to the anterior laryngeal section line from superior (*asterisk*) to the inferior (*triangle*) aspect. The lower edge (*triangle*) is not sutured into the laryngeal defect. An opening is left that served as a tracheostomy. The radial blood vessels are sutured to the neck vessels. The superior thyroid artery (end to end) and the internal jugular vein (end to side) are mostly used. A Gore-Tex membrane (*asterisk*; Preclude Pericardial Membrane, 0.1 mm, W.L. Gore and Associates, Inc. Flagstaff, AZ) is applied over the fascial-enwrapped trachea.

19.1.2 Second Operation

During the second-stage operation, 2 months after the first, the skin paddle was removed from the laryngeal defect and de-epithelialized. The cervical trachea was autotransplanted with an intact blood supply (i.e., the vascular pedicle of the RFF) to the hemilaryngeal defect. After tracheal autotransplantation, the continuity between the lower cervical trachea and the reconstructed larynx was still preserved. A small rim of membranous trachea was removed

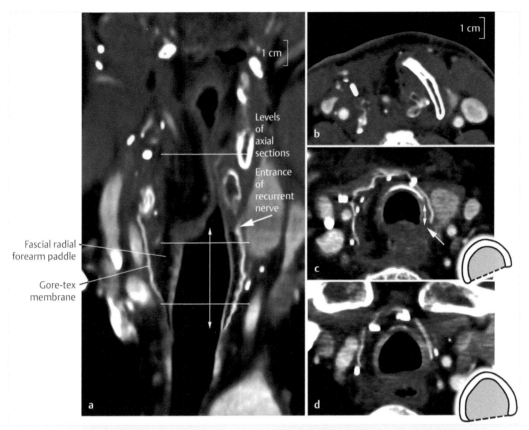

Fig. 19.4 CT scan after first operation. Overview on CT scan of tracheal revascularization and temporary larynx reconstruction. **(a)** Coronal reformatted CT scan. Levels of axial sections. *Arrow* indicates entrance of recurrent nerve. Double arrow indicates amount of cervical trachea to be used for larynx reconstruction. **(b)** Glottic level. A complete obliteration of the laryngeal lumen is visible at the glottic level. **(c)** Upper tracheal level. The double arrow shows a 1-cm segment of cervical trachea near the recurrent nerve (*position indicated with arrow*) that is not included in the autotransplant. Inset shows the amount of cartilaginous trachea that will be included in the autotransplant. **(d)** Lower tracheal level. Inset: At the lower tracheal level, the full amount of cartilaginous trachea will be included in the autotransplant.

to allow for easy end-to-end anastomosis. The stump of the lower cervical trachea was anastomosed posteriorly and laterally toward the cricoid cartilage and to the hemilaryngeal patch. The end-to-end anastomosis was performed without tension (▶ Fig. 19.5).

A CT scan after 2 weeks illustrates the situation following the second step of the reconstruction (▶ Fig. 19.6).

A tracheostomy was maintained between the reconstructed larynx and the mediastinal trachea. The patient was able to swallow puréed and semisolid food after 1 week. The patient swallowed most types of food by the end of the second week following surgery. The tracheostomy was closed under local anesthesia 4 weeks after the second intervention.

At the last follow-up visit 3 years after the intervention, the patient remained tumor free and he displayed a functional voice (voice with sufficient quality for a normal life and performance of all normal daily activities).

19.2 Discussion

Tracheal autotransplantation has been developed as a technique to reconstruct a functional larynx in patients undergoing extended hemilaryngectomy for selected laryngeal or cricoid tumors. Suitable tumors are the glottis SCC stage T2N0 to

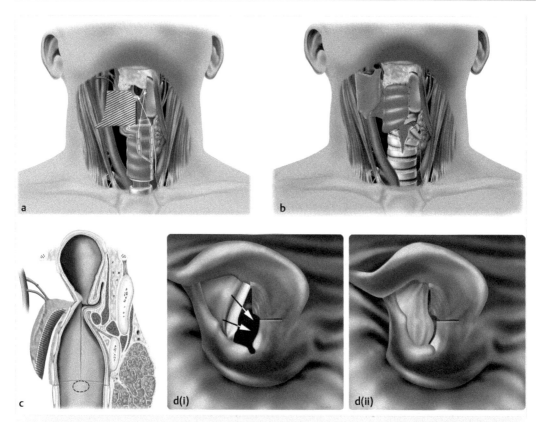

Fig. 19.5 Tracheal autotransplantation: steps during second operation. **(a)** The anterior, superior, and posterior suture lines between radial forearm flap and laryngeal remnant are opened and the skin paddle is completely separated from the laryngeal remnant. The revascularized trachea is isolated. The radial forearm skin flap is de-epithelialized (*shaded area*). The isolated tracheal patch is ready for transfer to the laryngeal defect (*arrows*). **(b)** The revascularized trachea is isolated and transplanted to the laryngeal defect. The skin paddle is removed from the defect and de-epithelialized. A tracheostomy remains between reconstructed larynx and mediastinal trachea. **(c)** Coronal sectional view after tracheal autotransplantation. Dotted line indicates the site of the tracheostomy. **(d)** Artist's representation of the endoscopic laryngeal view during inspiration and phonation (*arrows*) after hemilaryngectomy with tracheal autotransplantation.

T3N0 and lateralized cricoid chondrosarcomas, which cannot be treated through an endoscopic approach. Specifically, in patients with advanced unilateral chondrosarcomas of the cricoid and in those with unilateral glottic SCC T2 classified with impaired vocal fold mobility (former T2b) or T3 with subglottic extension (▶Fig. 19.1), and/or involvement of the cricoid, a more aggressive surgical resection than can be achieved by classical partial laryngectomy procedures is necessary. Whereas previously such patients had no other choice than to undergo a total laryngectomy, in the new approach, hemilaryngectomy secures complete tumor resection while the autotransplant aims to preserve laryngeal speech,

prevent a permanent tracheostomy, and maintain swallowing function.

Over the last decades, considerable interest has risen in the use of larynx preservation strategies for the treatment of laryngeal SCC. In addition to chemotherapy, radiotherapy, and chemoradiotherapy, transoral laser microsurgery (TLM) is increasingly being used.[2] However, these organ-sparing strategies have significant limitations. TLM is primarily indicated for the treatment of early-stage carcinoma of the glottis (without compromised vocal fold mobility and without subglottic extension). For resection of more advanced-stage glottis SCC and certainly for salvage resection of extended radiorecurrent glottic SCC, TLM is known to yield

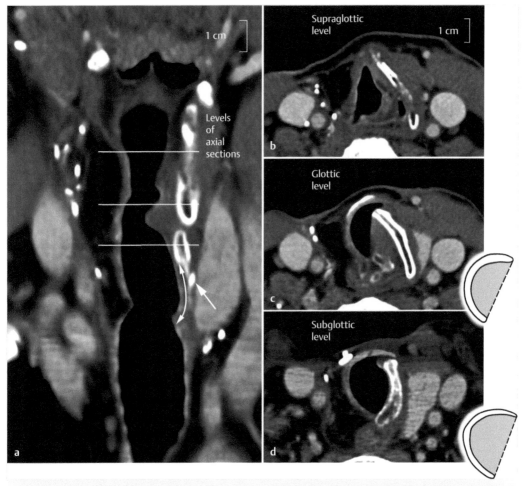

Fig. 19.6 CT scan after second operation. **(a)** Coronal reformatted CT scan. Levels of axial sections. Arrow indicates entrance of recurrent nerve into larynx. Curved double arrow indicates 1.5-cm segment of cervical trachea near the recurrent nerve. Straight double arrow indicates length of tracheal autotransplant. **(b)** Supraglottic level. **(c)** Glottic level. Inset shows the amount of cartilaginous trachea (full amount) minus 1-cm segment, which remains attached close to the entrance of the recurrent nerve (▶ Fig. 19.4c) included at the glottic level. **(d)** Subglottic level. Inset shows the amount of cartilaginous trachea (full amount) included at the subglottic level.

inferior local control rates.[3] In the treatment of cricoid chondrosarcomas, the use of radiotherapy and chemotherapy has proven not to be successful for advanced-stage tumors that involve 50% or more of the cricoid cartilage.[4] For such patients, the tracheal autotransplantation approach offers a valuable alternative to total laryngectomy.

The first human tracheal autotransplantation was performed in 1996 following extensive preclinical testing. Using this promising early work as a basis, we designed an optimized reconstructive autotransplant approach, involving a two-step procedure in which a segment of the cervical trachea is orthotopically provided with an independent vascular supply and subsequently used as an autograft to reconstruct the surgical hemilaryngectomy defect.[5,6,7,8] Having implemented this technique in our center in 2003, we have now treated a series of 30 patients with advanced cricoid cartilage chondrosarcoma or glottis SCC.[7] Tracheal autotransplantation proves to be a functional alternative for a total laryngectomy in selected cases of unilateral T2 (with impaired vocal fold mobility) or T3 glottic SCC and advanced chondrosarcoma of the cricoid cartilage. The technique provides excellent functional results regarding respiration, voice, and swallowing, without compromising the oncologic outcome, especially in patients ≤ 65 years old and patients with chondrosarcoma.[9]

19.3 Tips

- Tracheal autotransplantation allows for conservation laryngectomy for unilateral glottic cancer with vocal fold fixation and infraglottic extension reaching the superior aspect of the cricoid cartilage, two major contraindications for all "classic" conservation procedures.
- An extended hemilaryngectomy may be used for unilateral T2 to T3 glottic cancer with posterior subglottic extension greater than 5 mm but without extension into the ventricle.
- The resection can be extended toward the anterior third of the contralateral vocal fold for tumors reaching the anterior commissure.
- The maximal amount of removable tumor is shown in ▶ Fig. 19.2. The aryepiglottic fold, which can safely be preserved, will play a very important role in the restoration of the posterior larynx. It will allow for a posterior midline reconstruction at the glottic and supraglottic level.
- The sphincteric function after resection is restored by closing the gap between aryepiglottic fold and epiglottis at the side of resection (▶ Fig. 19.3).

19.4 Traps

- In order to achieve optimal oncological and functional outcomes, careful patient selection is of utmost importance. As the tracheal autotransplantation technique requires preservation of one cricoarytenoid unit, T2 or T3 laryngeal SCCs are considered possible candidates, provided that the tumor does not extend over the anterior commissure, which makes resection with safe margins while preserving a sufficient portion of the contralateral vocal fold impossible. This is a fundamental requirement for both primary and salvage cases.
- For advanced chondrosarcomas, limited extension over the anterior commissure is no contraindication for the autotransplant technique because no wide resection margins are aimed at.
- Apart from tumor location and extension, functional status and age are important factors that are taken into account when considering tracheal autotransplantation. Ideally, good candidates for this technique have a high or medium

performance status (WHO performance status classification categories 0, 1, or 2), have no restrictive or obstructive lung disease (except if due to the laryngeal tumor), and have stopped smoking prior to surgery.
- We found worse functional results in patients older than 65 years.
- A drawback of the tracheal autotransplantation technique is its complexity and the need for a two-stage approach. However, this two-stage approach provides additional safety, because it allows for reevaluation of the section margins before the definitive reconstruction, possibly helping with the oncological outcome. Notwithstanding its complexity, it is important to understand that this technique offers a functional alternative to a total laryngectomy for patients with advanced cricoid chondrosarcoma and for selected patients with extended glottic SCC, both in the primary and salvage settings.

References

[1] Ferlito A, Robbins KT, Shah JP, et al. Proposal for a rational classification of neck dissections. Head Neck. 2011; 33(3):445–450

[2] Lagha A, Chraiet N, Labidi S, et al. Larynx preservation: what is the best non-surgical strategy? Crit Rev Oncol Hematol. 2013; 88(2):447–458

[3] Ramakrishnan Y, Drinnan M, Kwong FNK, et al. Oncologic outcomes of transoral laser microsurgery for radiorecurrent laryngeal carcinoma: a systematic review and meta-analysis of English-language literature. Head Neck. 2014; 36(2):280–285

[4] Sauter A, Bersch C, Lambert KL, Hörmann K, Naim R. Chondrosarcoma of the larynx and review of the literature. Anticancer Res. 2007; 27(4C):2925–2929

[5] Delaere PR. Tracheal autotransplantation as a new and reliable technique for the functional treatment of advanced laryngeal cancer. Laryngoscope. 2003; 113(7):1244–1251

[6] Delaere P, Vander Poorten V, Vranckx J, Hierner R. Laryngeal repair after resection of advanced cancer: an optimal reconstructive protocol. Eur Arch Otorhinolaryngol. 2005; 262(11):910–916

[7] Delaere P, Goeleven A, Poorten VV, Hermans R, Hierner R, Vranckx J. Organ preservation surgery for advanced unilateral glottic and subglottic cancer. Laryngoscope. 2007; 117(10):1764–1769

[8] Delaere PR, Vranckx JJ, Dooms C, Meulemans J, Hermans R. Tracheal autotransplantation: guidelines for optimal functional outcome. Laryngoscope. 2011; 121(8):1708–1714

[9] Loos E, Meulemans J, Vranckx J, Poorten VV, Delaere P. Tracheal autotransplantation for functional reconstruction of extended hemilaryngectomy defects: a single-center experience in 30 patients. Ann Surg Oncol. 2016; 23(5):1674–1683

20 Locally Advanced Glottic Cancer: Supratracheal Laryngectomy

Giovanni Succo, Erika Crosetti

Abstract

Following the current European Laryngological Society (ELS) classification, supratracheal laryngectomy (STPL) or type III open partial horizontal laryngectomy (OPHL) is an OPHL aimed at resecting some intermediate to advanced glottic cancers with subglottic extension. Furthermore, type III OPHL represents the most extensive function sparing surgical option currently available in the surgical armamentarium. In selected patients, STPLs show promising long-term oncologic and functional outcomes, similar to those of supracricoid partial laryngectomy. The core indication for STPL is glottic/transglottic cT3 cancer with subglottic extension ≥10 mm from the free edge of the true vocal cord, calculated at its midline. Other local indications are cancer of the glottis (T2) tumors with anterior subglottic extension reaching the cricoid ring and some selected cT4a with limited anterior or lateral extralaryngeal extension. The application of STPL in the context of a modular surgical approach to the larynx affected by intermediate/advanced cancer can be considered a valid and effective therapeutic choice, not only in terms of oncologic results but also with regard to functional outcome. The main criticisms of STPL are poor voice quality outcomes, slight dysphagia with aspiration pneumonia, and soft-tissue laryngeal stenosis occurring in about 20% of cases.

Keywords: supratracheal laryngectomy, laryngeal cancer, glottic–subglottic cancer, partial laryngectomy, larynx, fixed arytenoid, cT3 glottic cancer, cT4a glottic cancer

20.1 Clinical Case 1

This patient was a 63-year-old male, in good general condition, with a Karnofsky index of 90, and who was a drinker and a cigarette smoker. Because of persistent dysphonia, he underwent laryngoscopic examination during which a suspected glottic neoplasm with subglottic extension was identified, with vegetating aspects, involving the right hemilarynx, with fixation of the true vocal cord (TVC) and arytenoid. No palpable lymph nodes were present. During the evaluation of the patient, neck MRI with surface coils (▶ Fig. 20.1) and CT scans were performed disclosing a glottic tumor with subglottic extension of about 10 to 12 mm from the free edge of the TVC measured at its midline, involvement of the superior and inferior paraglottic space, no involvement of the thyroid cartilage wing or the cricoid plate, apparent involvement of the anterior commissure, involvement of the cricoarytenoid joint, and absence of cervical and/or level VI pathologic lymph nodes. In the course of direct microlaryngoscopy, subglottic extension of about 12 mm was noted; posteriorly, the margin between the lesion and the posterior commissure was 3 mm. The pathological report on the biopsy sample revealed a squamous cell G2 carcinoma staged as glottic cT3N0. During the tumor board meeting, an open partial horizontal laryngectomy (OPHL) type III was proposed as the first therapeutic option or, as an alternative, concurrent chemoradiotherapy. The patient chose the partial laryngectomy option. A CO_2 fiber laser OPHL type IIIa + right cricoarytenoid unit (CAU) + selective neck dissection (SND; levels II–IV) + right tracheoesophageal groove dissection was carried out; all margins were free of cancer (>2 mm). During the resection, a supracricoid access was made demonstrating the insufficiency of safe margins with this approach (▶ Fig. 20.2); this is a clear example of the usefulness of OPHL type III in the modular surgical approach strategy using OPHLs.

Final staging based on biopsy specimen was glottic pT3N0 and there was no indication for adjuvant radiotherapy. The postoperative course was uncomplicated, swallowing recovery was conducted without cannula, and the patient was discharged 18 days after the operation, with the tracheostoma still open but occluded with a gauze dressing, which the patient removed during the night. The tracheostoma underwent a spontaneous closure within 30 days after the operation. Two years after surgery, the patient is free, manages to lead a normal life without tracheostomy, and his weight is stable. During this period, no episodes of aspiration pneumonia have been reported.

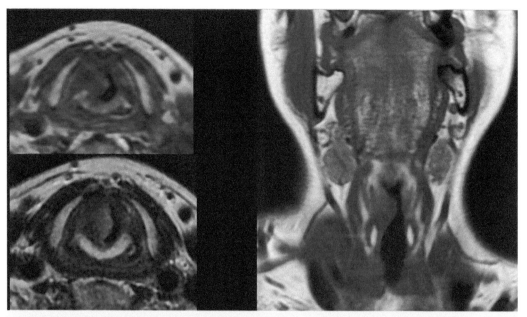

Fig. 20.1 MRI of the neck (axial + coronal view) demonstrates a T3 glottic cancer with subglottic extension, involvement of the superior and inferior space, no involvement of the thyroid cartilage wing or the cricoid plate, apparent involvement of the anterior commissure, and involvement of the right cricoarytenoid joint.

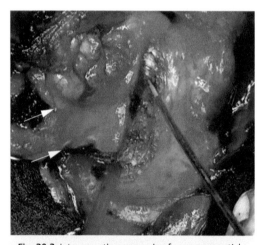

Fig. 20.2 Intraoperative conversion from open partial horizontal laryngectomy (OPHL) type IIa + arytenoid (ARY) to OPHL type IIIa + cricoarytenoid unit (CAU) performed by CO_2 fiber laser. (*White arrow* indicates the attempt to perform an OPHL type IIa → insufficient margins. *Yellow arrow* indicates the immediate conversion to OPHL type IIIa + CAU gaining a 1-cm margin).

20.2 Clinical Case 2

This was a 57-year-old male, in perfect general health, a current cigarette smoker, with a Karnofsky index of 100, and without any comorbidities. Because of persistent dysphonia, he underwent phoniatric examination during which an ulcerated glottic neoplasm with subglottic extension was discovered, involving the right hemilarynx, apparently extending from the anterior to the posterior commissure, and showing fixation of the TVC and arytenoid. No palpable lymph nodes were present. During the evaluation, MRI of the neck with surface coils (▶Fig. 20.3) was performed, demonstrating a glottic cancer with subglottic extension of about 15 mm from the free edge of the TVC at its midline, involvement of the superior and inferior paraglottic space, full-thickness involvement of the inferior aspect of the thyroid cartilage wing and possible involvement of the cricoid plate, apparent involvement of the anterior and posterior commissure, involvement of the cricoarytenoid joint, and absence of cervical and/or level VI pathologic lymph nodes. In the course of direct microlaryngoscopy, a subglottic extension of about 14 mm was noted; posteriorly, the margin between the lesion and the posterior commissure was approximately 3 mm. The pathological report on the biopsy sample revealed a squamous cell G2 carcinoma staged as glottic cT4aN0. During the tumor board meeting, a total laryngectomy + SND (levels II–IV + VI) + primary tracheoesophageal puncture (TEP) was proposed as the first

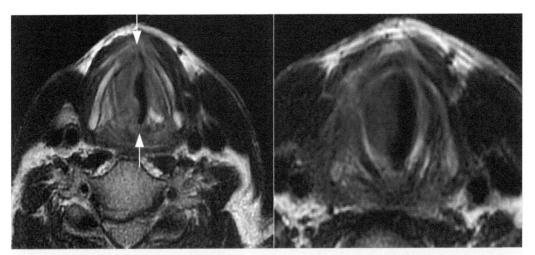

Fig. 20.3 Neck MRI (axial view) shows the glottic tumor with subglottic extension, involvement of the superior and inferior paraglottic space, full-thickness involvement of the inferior aspect of the thyroid cartilage wing and possible involvement of the cricoid plate, apparent involvement of the anterior and posterior commissure (*white arrows*), and involvement of the right cricoarytenoid joint.

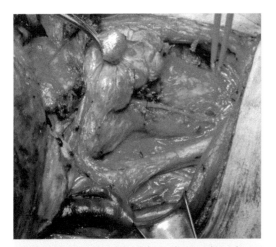

Fig. 20.4 Dissection of the right tracheoesophageal groove before performing open partial horizontal laryngectomy type IIIa + right cricoarytenoid unit.

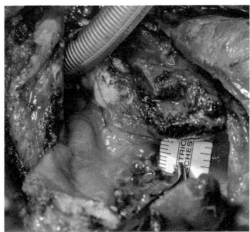

Fig. 20.5 Open partial horizontal laryngectomy type IIIa + right cricoarytenoid unit: the posterior margin of resection was close but free from cancer (2 mm).

therapeutic option, which the patient absolutely refused, expressly asking to be submitted to the therapeutic option allowing him the greatest guarantee of preservation of the larynx. Faced with the two options represented by concurrent chemoradiotherapy and OPHL type III, the patient chose the latter, considering also the potential better degree of freedom from total laryngectomy. After signing an informed consent that also included the option of an intraoperative conversion from partial to total laryngectomy based on the real

extent of the tumor, an OPHL type IIIa + right CAU + SND (levels II–IV) + right tracheoesophageal groove dissection (▶ Fig. 20.4) was carried out. The posterior margin of resection was close (▶ Fig. 20.5) but free from tumor (2 mm). Final staging of the specimen was pT4aN0 due to minimal thyroid cartilage and cricoid arch and plate involvement, there was no indication for adjuvant radiotherapy.

The postoperative course was uncomplicated, swallowing recovery was conducted without cannula, and the patient was discharged 14 days after the operation, with the tracheostoma still open but occluded with a gauze, which the patient removed during the night. The patient complained about the persistence of obstructive sleep apnea syndrome when he tried to keep the tracheostomy occluded during the night. This was studied by sleep endoscopy during which a double obstruction of the neoglottis was observed caused by a preexisting hypertrophy of the base of the tongue together with a mucosal flap of the hypopharyngeal mucosa on the side of the resected CAU. On two occasions, the patient was subjected to refinement of the base of the tongue and neoglottis by CO_2 laser and was definitively decannulated within 3 months postoperatively. Three years after surgery, the patient is cancer free, leads normal life without a tracheostomy, practices sports, his weight is stable, and he occasionally makes use of C-pap ventilation during the night. During this period, no episodes of aspiration pneumonia were reported.

20.3 Discussion

The main purpose of OPHL is the achievement of locoregional control of the cancer by means of a single therapy while sparing laryngeal functions and the maintenance of phonation, respiration, and swallowing by natural pathways, avoiding the need for tracheostomy, gastrostomy, or voice prosthesis. A model for a rational classification of OPHLs was proposed in 2014 by the European Laryngological Society (ELS) based on the craniocaudal extent of laryngeal resection. It defined three types: supraglottic laryngectomy (SGL; type I), supracricoid laryngectomy (SCL; type II), and supratracheal laryngectomy (STL; type III).[1]

Type II OPHLs are the most established solution for the treatment of intermediate- to advanced-stage laryngeal tumors affecting the glottis[2,3,4] however, a significant number of glottic/transglottic cancer are not in any way amenable to be safely treated by supracricoid laryngectomy (e.g., those with subglottic extension and cricoid involvement, or those classified as cT4a because of extralaryngeal extension through the thyroid cartilage and/or the cricothyroid membrane). For some of these intermediate to advanced laryngeal cancers with subglottic extension, STL (type III OPHL) is the most extensive function sparing surgical option. OPHL type III includes four procedures: STL with tracheohyoidoepiglottopexy ± extending to one CAU and STL with tracheohyoidopexy ± extending to one CAU. The CAU is represented by half of the

posterior cricoid plate with the corresponding arytenoid, and the intact ipsilateral inferior laryngeal nerve.

In 1972, Italo Serafini first described the procedure for a supratracheal partial laryngectomy (STPL).[5] Although the oncological results were interesting, allowing a good surgical radicality, the resulting functional outcomes were poor and the technique was soon abandoned. In 1996, Laccourreye et al[6] described a technical modification to the conventional supracricoid partial laryngectomy in order to remove the cricoid ring in the case of glottic tumors with anterior subglottic extension, and in 2005, Sparano et al[7] examined the preoperative clinical characteristics useful to predict safe inferior margins of glottic squamous cell carcinoma extending toward the cricoid cartilage when performing organ/function preservation surgery of the larynx. These studies opened the door for the development of the "functional" STL, which, as it currently stands, was described by Rizzotto et al in 2006.[8]

Type III OPHL represents a "functional" modification of Serafini's original technique: the procedure entails the resection of the entire glottic and subglottic sites, as well as the thyroid cartilage. Inferiorly, the limit of resection encompasses the cricoid ring and possibly a hemicricoid plate, reaching the first tracheal ring. The various type III OPHLs, as well as the type II OPHLs, differ from each other in the amount of resected supraglottis and in the posterolateral extension to possibly include one CAU. Laryngeal reconstruction is accomplished by either tracheohyoidoepiglottopexy (type IIIa OPHL)[9] or tracheohyoidopexy (type IIIb OPHL). For the type IIIa + CAU, the remaining portion of the epiglottis and the hyoid bone are both fixed to the trachea. For the type IIIb + CAU, the base of the tongue and the hyoid bone are fixed to the trachea.

For both type IIIa and IIIb OPHLs without CAU resection, the difference in reconstruction lies in the fact that the maneuvers for pyriform sinus remodeling are not necessary because the pyriform sinus mucosa is still adherent to the remnant half of the cricoid plate and the arytenoid.

The suspected presence of clinically positive cervical lymph nodes greater than cN1 is not considered to be an absolute contraindication. However, it should not represent, in general, a good indication for OPHL due to the probable need for postoperative RT or CRT. The tracheostomy will be included in the central portion of the incision later in the procedure. Since the procedure is indicated for locally advanced cancer and is used to achieve the maximum radicality possible, removal of all strap muscles is preferable in order to eliminate any microscopic disease. We have found that sacrificing these structures does not adversely affect functional recovery in terms of swallowing.

In addition to neck dissection, central compartment lymphatics from the hyoid bone to the thyroid isthmus, including the Delphian lymph nodes, are removed and sent for immediate histologic assessment using frozen sections. Positivity due to the presence of metastases to the Delphian lymph node, obviously in the absence of invasion of the laryngeal tracheal axis due to extra capsular extension, is a further indication for the use of type III OPHL allowing a block resection of the cricothyroid membrane, of the cricoid ring, and of the isthmus of the thyroid. For patients with inferior paraglottic space invasion with subglottic extension and arytenoid fixation, an ipsilateral tracheoesophageal groove dissection should be performed, given the high rate of occult metastasis in level VI. Eventual damage to the recurrent nerve on the same side does not present any further negative effects to laryngeal function because the corresponding functional unit, represented by the CAU, will then be completely removed.

20.4 Tips

The absence of major comorbidities and the ability to undergo a rigorous postoperative rehabilitation are general prerequisites for all partial laryngectomies.

The Karnofsky performance status index should be at least 80 (i.e., the patient is able to carry out normal activities, even though with difficulty). In addition to a Karnofsky index less than 80, exclusion criteria are severe diabetes mellitus, severe chronic obstructive pulmonary disease, or severe cardiac disease. Advanced age, even though historically, an age of 70 years has been an important cutoff for relative surgical indication of some partial laryngectomies, in our experience, it is no longer, in itself, an exclusion criterion.[10] After accurate selection of patients on the basis of the absence of important comorbidities and with a strong desire of the patient to avoid permanent tracheostomy, age is also considered along with the patient's general condition. Of course, the ideal candidates are younger patients with a good pulmonary function.

Some spreading patterns of laryngeal cancer cannot be safely managed by type II OPHLs, but can be treated successfully with a type III OPHL, whose current T-related indications have recently been reported.[11] The absolute contraindications for OPHL type III are (1) lesions extending to the base of the tongue or pyriform sinus; (2) lesions with major invasion of the pre-epiglottic space involving the hyoid bone, lesions involving the interarytenoid space, the posterior commissure, and both arytenoid cartilages; (3) extensive extralaryngeal spread of cancer involving the thyroid gland, strap muscles, cervical skin, internal jugular vein, or common carotid artery; (4) lesions reaching the first tracheal ring; and (5) N3 lymph node metastases.

An aid to the correct selection of patients eligible for this type of surgery is given by the anterior and posterior compartmentalization of the larynx, considering the transgression, or not, of an ideal "magic plane" passing before the vocal process of the arytenoid and perpendicular to the thyroid cartilage, together with subglottic extension of the cancer less than or greater than 10 mm at the free edge of the TVC measured at its midline and the presence/absence of functional data represented by arytenoid mobility.[12]

In summary, it can be stated that (1) every type of cancer that does not transgress the "magic plane" and without impairment of mobility of the arytenoid, even though it has subglottic extension toward or reaches the cricoid ring or has limited anterior extralaryngeal extension (anterior cT2 → early cT4a), can be successfully treated by OPHL type III as demonstrated by Laccourreye et al by applying the so-called cricotracheohyoidoepiglottopexy[6]; (2) in the case of a glottic tumor that transgresses the "magic plane", even with transglottic evolution and a fixed arytenoid (cT3) but with subglottic extension ≤10 mm at the free edge of the TVC measured at its midline, the risk of involvement of one or more anatomic elements of the CAU is low and, at most, focal in comparison to the cancer itself. The type II OPHL + ARY often achieves the goal of radical resection, but type III + CAU, with the resection extending downward for more than 1 cm, allows the surgeon to modulate the resection on the basis of the real extent of the cancer with safer margins; (3) in the subcategory of cancer with subglottic extension greater than 10 mm at the free edge of the TVC measured at its midline showing transgression of the "magic plane," even with transglottic evolution and fixed arytenoid (cT3), this latter aspect is linked not only to neoplastic evolution toward the thyroarytenoid and cricoarytenoid spaces (with the tendency for invasion of the cricoarytenoid joint [CAJ] and the lateral cricoarytenoid muscle) but also to evident subglottic evolution, with the possibility that the tumor involves the CAJ and the cricoid medially to laterally, puncturing the conus elasticus. In this pattern (posterior cT3 → early cT4a), the potential for extralaryngeal spread, laterally through the cricothyroid space and posteriorly through the cricoid, tends to be significant. As demonstrated by Brasnu et al,[13] involvement of one or more anatomic elements of the CAU is very high, equating this pattern to a T4a. In this case, the unique "rational" treatment is represented by total laryngectomy, which produces a complete and "en bloc" removal of all laryngeal musculature, intrinsic and extrinsic. In the case of categorical refusal of total laryngectomy by a patient, a conservative treatment through CRT or partial laryngectomy can be offered. The only proposable partial laryngectomy is an OPHL type IIIa + CAU, whose inferoposterior resection limits are the first tracheal ring and the retrocricoid mucosa. In this case also, the possibility of using a very precise cutting tool, such as a CO_2 fiber laser, used free hand in open surgery, allows all of the anatomic structures comprising the CAU to be understood. In particular, it allows great precision in the dissection and separation of very narrow anatomic layers, to check intraoperatively the eventual extralaryngeal extension and to determine whether a partial procedure needs to be converted into a total laryngectomy.

In conclusion, STL can be considered a valid surgical option among the function sparing therapeutic approaches to cancer of the larynx. The choice of a type III OPHL approach can be considered viable in comparison to chemoradiation protocols for some selected glottic and/or transglottic tumors with subglottic extension. Advantages can be obtained in terms of prognosis (better identification of upstaging and reduction in recurrence rate) and reduction in the rate of total laryngectomy, even at the expense of voice quality and the occurrence of sequelae, such as soft-tissue stenosis and chronic aspiration phenomena.[14]

The introduction of type III OPHL has opened new perspectives in the function sparing surgical approach to laryngeal cancer. Since extension of the resection both superior and inferior are possible in trying to spare laryngeal function, OPHL can be conducted following the principles of a modular surgical approach.

20.5 Traps

- Persistent slight dysphagia and aspiration pneumonia are still major complications in patients undergoing STPLs, while voice is significantly deteriorated, and generally quite hoarse and breathy.[15]
- In elderly patients (older than 70 years), CAU resection can have a clear negative impact, with poor recovery of swallowing.[16]
- Avoid using this procedure as a salvage surgery after failure of previous radiochemotherapy, due to the pattern of recurrence that is difficult to assess.
- After performing this type of surgery, be prepared to manage poor anatomical and/or functional results by corrective phonosurgery (laser and/or injective laryngoplasty).[17,18]
- If a more "extreme" type III OPHL is required upfront, ethical considerations must be taken into account. These cases are considered amenable to total laryngectomy and are therefore recommended for a nonsurgical organ sparing protocol. Hence, the patient must be clearly informed that the surgery will be converted to a total laryngectomy if resection margins from frozen sections are positive, thus excluding the concomitant chemoradiotherapy option (recommendation IIA in the current guidelines).
- Extreme caution must be taken when considering the OPHL option if the cancer clearly extends beyond the limits of the larynx, due to both the severity of the intervention and the necessity for adjuvant radiotherapy.

References

[1] Succo G, Peretti G, Piazza C, et al. Open partial horizontal laryngectomies: a proposal for classification by the working committee on nomenclature of the European Laryngological Society. Eur Arch Otorhinolaryngol. 2014; 271(9):2489–2496

[2] de Vincentiis M, Minni A, Gallo A, Di Nardo A. Supracricoid partial laryngectomies: oncologic and functional results. Head Neck. 1998; 20(6):504–509

[3] Mercante G, Grammatica A, Battaglia P, Cristalli G, Pellini R, Spriano G. Supracricoid partial laryngectomy in the management of T3 laryngeal cancer. Otolaryngol Head Neck Surg. 2013; 149(5):714–720

[4] Crosetti E, Garofalo P, Bosio C, et al. How the operated larynx ages. Acta Otorhinolaryngol Ital. 2014; 34(1):19–28

[5] Serafini I. Reconstructive laryngectomy Rev Laryngol Otol Rhinol (Bord). 1972; 93(1):23–38

[6] Laccourreye O, Brasnu D, Jouffre V, Couloigner V, Naudo P, Laccourreye H. Supra-cricoid partial laryngectomy

extended to the anterior arch of the cricoid with tracheo-crico-hyoido-epiglottopexy. Oncologic and functional results Ann Otolaryngol Chir Cervicofac. 1996; 113(1):15–19

[7] Sparano A, Chernock R, Feldman M, Laccourreye O, Brasnu D, Weinstein G. Extending the inferior limits of supracricoid partial laryngectomy: a clinicopathological correlation. Laryngoscope. 2005; 115(2):297–300

[8] Rizzotto G, Succo G, Lucioni M, Pazzaia T. Subtotal laryngectomy with tracheohyoidopexy: a possible alternative to total laryngectomy. Laryngoscope. 2006; 116(10):1907–1917

[9] Succo G, Crosetti E, Bertolin A, et al. Supratracheal partial laryngectomy with tracheohyoidoepiglottopexy (open partial horizontal laryngectomy type IIIa + cricoarytenoid unit): surgical technique illustrated in the anatomy laboratory. Head Neck. 2017; 39(2):392–398

[10] Rizzotto G, Crosetti E, Lucioni M, et al. Oncologic outcomes of supratracheal laryngectomy: critical analysis. Head Neck. 2015; 37(10):1417–1424

[11] Succo G, Bussi M, Presutti L, et al. Supratracheal laryngectomy: current indications and contraindications. Acta Otorhinolaryngol Ital. 2015; 35(3):146–156

[12] Succo G, Crosetti E, Bertolin A, et al. Treatment of T3–T4a laryngeal cancer by open partial horizontal laryngectomies: prognostic impact of different pT

subcategories. Head Neck. 2018:(e-pub ahead of print). 10.1002/hed.25176

[13] Brasnu D, Laccourreye H, Dulmet E, Jaubert F. Mobility of the vocal cord and arytenoid in squamous cell carcinoma of the larynx and hypopharynx: an anatomical and clinical comparative study. Ear Nose Throat J. 1990; 69(5):324–330

[14] Schindler A, Fantini M, Pizzorni N, et al. Swallowing, voice, and quality of life after supratracheal laryngectomy: preliminary long-term results. Head Neck. 2015; 37(4):557–566

[15] Schindler A, Pizzorni N, Fantini M, et al. Long-term functional results after open partial horizontal laryngectomy type IIa and type IIIa: a comparison study. Head Neck. 2016; 38(suppl 1):E1427–E1435

[16] Benito J, Holsinger FC, Pérez-Martín A, Garcia D, Weinstein GS, Laccourreye O. Aspiration after supracricoid partial laryngectomy: incidence, risk factors, management, and outcomes. Head Neck. 2011; 33(5):679–685

[17] Lucioni M, Bertolin A, Lionello M, et al. Transoral laser microsurgery for managing laryngeal stenosis after reconstructive partial laryngectomies. Laryngoscope. 2017; 127(2):359–365

[18] Bergamini G, Alicandri-Ciufelli M, Molteni G, et al. Rehabilitation of swallowing with polydimethylsiloxane injections in patients who underwent partial laryngectomy. Head Neck. 2009; 31(8):1022–1030

21 Locally Advanced Glottic Cancer: Total Laryngectomy and Voice Prostheses

Michiel W.M. van den Brekel, Marije J.F. Petersen

Abstract

Patients with advanced cancer of the larynx should be adequately counseled about the different treatment options (radiotherapy, chemoradiotherapy, or a total laryngectomy), in terms of both overall survival and expected quality of life. Patients with a T4 cancer have higher overall survival rates after a primary total laryngectomy, although an increasing number of patients are treated with organ-preservation protocols. Rehabilitation is crucial in obtaining a good voice and quality of life.

Keywords: advanced cancer of the larynx, total laryngectomy, voice prosthesis, pharyngocutaneous fistula

21.1 Case Report

A 66-year-old male patient was referred to our outpatient clinic at the Netherlands Cancer Institute in Amsterdam with progressive dysphonia during the previous 3 months. The referring Otolaryngologist identified a lesion suspicious for squamous cell carcinoma, which was proved by biopsy. In the Netherlands, head and neck oncology care is centered in dedicated head and neck centers, so the patient was referred to us. The patient had a history of smoking cigarettes but had stopped 10 years ago. He used alcohol moderately. Besides taking oral medication for his diabetes, he was otherwise healthy and had no prior surgery. Adult Comorbidity Evaluation 27 (ACE-27) comorbidity score was 1.

Videolaryngoscopy with stroboscopy revealed a red, irregular right true vocal cord, with no mucosal wave pattern but only slightly diminished mobility (▶ Fig. 21.1). The tumor seemed limited to the true vocal cord and was clinically staged as T2N0.

Though clinically thought to be a relatively small cancer, CT scan demonstrated a bulky tumor of the right vocal cord, crossing the anterior commissure to the left vocal cord (▶ Fig. 21.2). The tumor expanded outside the thyroid cartilage on both sides and there was obliteration of adipose tissue between the thyroid cartilage and strap muscles.

There was no subglottic extension and no suspicious lymph nodes were seen. The maximal diameter was 4.3 cm.

Direct laryngoscopy under anesthesia showed a nonulcerative tumor extending from the anterior commissure toward the anterior two-thirds of the right true vocal cord and anterior first one-third part of the left vocal cord. On the right surface, the cancer grew into the sinus of Morgagni and toward the false vocal cord. Via the anterior commissure, there was extension toward the laryngeal side of the epiglottis. No subglottic extension was noted. The cancer was staged as T4aN0 transglottic.

After discussing the results in our multidisciplinary Tumor Board meeting, the results were shared with the patient. The three options of total laryngectomy (TL) plus adjuvant radiotherapy (RT), concomitant chemoradiotherapy (CRT), and primary RT were discussed, where he was informed that TL + RT was associated with the highest overall survival. Based on the expected higher overall survival after TL, he opted for the surgery.

Two weeks later, he underwent a TL with selective neck dissection of levels II to IV bilateral, sparing the sternocleidomastoid muscle, internal jugular vein, and the spinal accessory nerve. After general anesthesia and perioperative administration of cefazolin and metronidazole, a modified

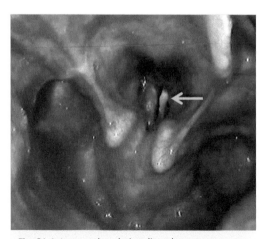

Fig. 21.1 Image taken during direct laryngoscopy showing the cancer on the right vocal cord (*arrow*).

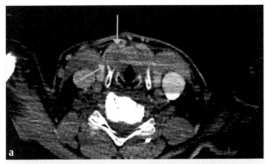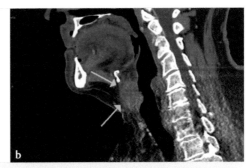

Fig. 21.2 (a) CT scan preoperatively demonstrating the bulging of the thyroid on the right side (*arrow*). There is obliteration of the fat plane between thyroid and strap muscles and invasion/displacement of the paraglottic fat. **(b)** Coronal plane showing subglottic extension until 15 mm below the true vocal cords and the infiltration caudally of the pre-epiglottic fat (*arrow*).

Gluck–Sorenson incision was made and a separate incision for the stoma was created 2 cm beneath the incision line. The dissection was carried deep from the platysma muscle creating cranial and caudal myocutaneous flaps. The right neck dissection was carried out first. The anterior border of the sternocleidomastoid muscle was used as a reference point and the great auricular nerve was found and spared. The sternocleidomastoid muscle was skeletonized and the omohyoid muscle was identified. Dissection proceeded to the posterior edge of the sternocleidomastoid muscle where the deep cervical muscles and the cervical plexus were identified. the deep cervical muscles and the cervical plexus. Carefully dissecting all fatty tissue over the plexus and muscle and over the internal Jugular vein, Carotid artery and Vagal nerve we proceeded in dissecting the specimen towards to the larynx. The internal Jugular vein, the Accessory nerve and Hypoglossal nerve were spared. A similar procedure was performed on the left side. There was some chyle leakage caudally, which stopped after clipping the thoracic duct. The strap muscles were subsequently dissected. The superior thyroid arteries on both sides were dissected and the thyroid gland isthmus was left on the specimen, but both lateral lobes were separated from the larynx and preserved.

The hyoid bone was then skeletonized at the cranial side and the pharyngeal constrictor muscles were seperated from the posterior edge of the thyroid. The trachea was divided in a horizontal plane below the second tracheal ring. The tracheal tube was removed and a new ventilation tube was placed in the trachea. The larynx was then opened in the vallecula and the larynx was removed preserving as much of the mucosa as oncologically safe. The wound was irrigated with distilled water and the patient was re-draped.

The trachea, with an intact third tracheal cartilage ring, was meticulously sutured into the skin, making sure the cartilage was covered with skin. Using the Vega puncture set, a Provox Vega 22.5-Fr-width, 8-mm-long voice prosthesis (VP) was placed. A pharynx protector, puncture needle, and guidewire allowed for an easy placement of the VP. To prevent spasm, a myotomy of the upper esophageal constrictor muscle was performed, as well as a myotomy of the sternal head of the sternocleidomastoid to create a flat stoma in the neck. A nasogastric feeding tube was inserted. The pharynx was closed with absorbable Vicryl 3–0 sutures in two layers in a T-shape. The mucosa was sutured with inversion of the mucosa (Connell type) and subsequently a hemiclosure of the crico- and thyropharyngeal muscles from one side over the suture line was performed, after which fibrin glue was placed on the suture line. The lobes of the thyroid gland were sutured on the neopharynx to model a flat stoma. Two drains were placed through separate incisions, making sure the drains were not lying over the pharyngeal closure. The skin was then closed in two layers. An adhesive with heat and moister exchanger (HME) was placed and no cannula was used postoperatively. The patient was monitored for one night in the intensive care unit.

Initially, the patient experienced an uncomplicated recovery; only minor shrinkage of the stoma occurred for which he received a LaryTube silicon cannula. After 24 hours, the patient started drinking water and after 48 hours a liquid diet was started. However, a barium swallow examination

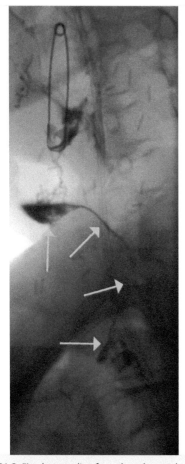

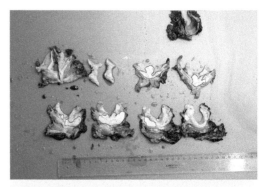

Fig. 21.4 Slices of the larynx clearly showing how the bulk of the tumor is situated in the cartilage and not in the submucosa.

Fig. 21.3 Fistula extending from the submental pocket toward the voice prosthesis (*arrow*).

on postoperative day 7, revealed extraluminal contrast fluid at the superior suture line. Oral intake was then stopped and antibiotics treatment started. A second barium-swallowing examination on day 14 showed a fistula tract to the stoma (▶ Fig. 21.3). The patient was treated conservatively with nothing per mouth and a cuffed cannula. Six days later, the barium swallow examination was repeated that showed only a small sinus tract. After another 6 days, the barium swallow examination showed complete recovery and the patient was able to resume oral intake and start voicing. A few days later, he was able to consume a full diet and produce intelligible sound with his VP and was discharged from the hospital.

The histopathological report revealed a moderately differentiated squamous cell carcinoma invading the cartilage and extending extralaryngeal but without perineural or vascular invasion growth. Resection margins were free from cancer and no cervical lymph node metastases were found. Staging was pT4N0 according to the TNM-7. ▶ Fig. 21.4 illustrates how only a small portion of the cancer was growing in the laryngeal lumen and the bulk of the cancer is situated in the cartilage and beyond. This explains why the patient had only minor complaints and clinically the cancer was staged as a T2 glottis cancer of the larynx. The patient received adjuvant RT on the larynx using intensity-modulated radiotherapy (IMRT) in 33 fractions of 2 Gy to the laryngeal area and 46 Gy electively to the neck.

21.1.1 Quality of Life

The patient tolerated the RT very well without any toxicities. He maintained oral intake and an adequate voice. Since his surgery, he had five VP replacement for transprosthetic leakage and his median device lifetime was 46 days. Because of this limited lifetime, he was offered an Acti-Valve light, which is still in situ now counting 261 days. He uses Provox ExtraBase FlexiDerm adhesives that generally stay on for 1 day with an HME (▶ Fig. 21.5). He cannot use an automatic speaking valve because the adhesive does not tolerate the pressure.

As part of our standard care, several quality-of-life questionnaires such as the European Quality of Life-5 Dimensions 5 level questionnaire (EQ-5D-5L),[1] the Voice Handicap Index-10 (VHI-10),[2] and the swallowing screening tool (EAT-10)[3] were given to the patient before treatment and 3 months, 6, months, and 1 year after treatment. On the EQ-5D, a standardized

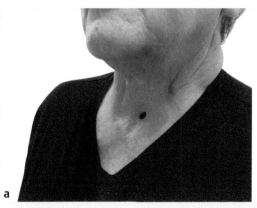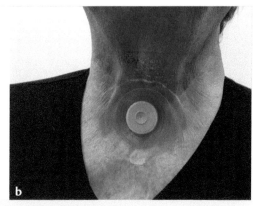

Fig. 21.5 Stoma of the patient without **(a)** and with adhesive and heat and moisture exchanger **(b)**.

measure of health status, he scored a self-rated health status of 80/100 preoperatively, which increased to 100/100 3 months postoperatively. Six months after treatment, he is very independent, still walking on average 2 hours per day. He does have some trouble being fast and witty in big groups but still is satisfied with his voice, physical functioning, and social functioning. His voice was evaluated using the VHI-10, an instrument to quantify patients' perception on their voice handicap. The scores ranges from 0 (no problems at all) to 40 (having trouble on all aspects all the time). Preoperatively he scored 22/40, which decreased to 3/40, 3 months postoperatively. One year after treatment, his health status scored 100/100 and his VHI-10 decreased to 2/40, only scoring that because sometimes people ask him what is wrong with his voice. The patient did not report any swallowing problems on the EAT-10 questionnaire before treatment nor 1 year after treatment.

21.2 Discussion

In this case report, we discussed a 66-year-old patient with a glottic T4N0M0 carcinoma who underwent a primary TL and adjuvant RT. Although we see a declining use of primary surgery for advanced larynx cancer since the introduction of CRT in the 1990s,[4,5] it is still a valid treatment strategy for advanced cancer. In fact, the proclaimed equal survival results, as published by the veterans affairs (VA) trial, were later reconsidered and showed that in fact T4 cancers achieved higher overall survival when treated with primary TL.[6] This finding has been confirmed by two national studies' evaluation trends in treatment and overall survival in larynx and hypopharynx cancer;

for both groups, T4 tumors reached highest overall survival figures following TL when compared to organ-preservation strategies.[7,8]

The treatment choice between TL and organ preservation is, however, a difficult task for both patient and physician and does not depend only on the highest expected overall survival. Expected functional outcome and patient preferences play an important role as well. One of the first studies on this difficult trade-off question was published in 1981 by McNeil et al, who investigated the attitude toward quantity and quality of life following a TL or primary RT among 37 healthy volunteers. In this study, despite considerably higher overall survival after TL (60 vs. 30–40%), 20% of the volunteers still opted for RT when theoretically confronted with this dilemma.[9] More recently, Hamilton et al performed a similar study and concluded that in fact *larynx preservation* may not be the only consideration, though in current practice, a TL seems to be reserved only for salvage reasons.[10] In a subsequent study, they compared the attitude of patients with cancer of the head and neck to that of the head and neck multidisciplinary team. While both groups preferred CRT with optimal outcome, staff members rated the functional outcomes following CRT or TL different than patients, underlining the importance of the involvement of the patient in clinical decision-making.[11] To conclude, values of patients and physicians might differ, and assumptions regarding treatment preference should be made only after adequate counseling. The use of specific patient decision aids, developed to give easy, accessible, and trusted patient information regarding the different treatment options, could play a role in future shared decision-making.[12]

21.2.1 Postoperative Care

Postoperatively this patient showed a fistula on a barium swallow radiograph. It was not a typical pharyngocutaneous fistula (PCF) as it tracked from a submental pocket ventrally along the pharynx toward the stoma. The incidence of PCFs lies between 3 and 66% and is the most common complication observed after TL.[13] Predictive factors for PCF are preoperative (chemo)radiation, the extent of resection, type of reconstruction, a hypopharynx tumor, poor nutritional status, and comorbidities such as hypothyroidism and diabetes.[14,15] Though early oral intake is traditionally thought to lead to increased PCF, several studies have demonstrated that oral intake within 5 days is safe and does not increase the rate of fistulas.[16,17] Initial management can in general be conservative if the fistula is limited; placing the patient on nothing by mouth, a cuffed cannula, and nasogastric feeding tube. If these measures are unsuccessful, operative closure should be considered using, for example, a pedicled muscle flap.

21.2.2 Vocal Rehabilitation

Vocal rehabilitation remains one of the major challenges after TL. In most western countries, tracheoesophageal speech is the method of choice. The placement of a VP in a surgically created fistula between trachea and esophagus allows pulmonary air to be diverted through the VP, causing vibrations of the pharyngoesophageal segment, producing sound. Other options are the use of an electrolarynx or esophageal speech, though not all patients are able to master this technique. A recent meta-analysis on the vocal outcome after TL indicated that tracheoesophageal speech is the preferred rehabilitation method based on acoustic and perceptual outcomes.[18]

Since the first publication on the use of a prosthetic device by Mozolewski et al in 1973, several prosthetic devices have been developed.[19] We have recently analyzed our results in prosthetic vocal rehabilitation in a consecutive cohort of all patients treated by TL between 2000 and 2012 and in follow-up in our hospital with a Provox VP. Median device lifetime was 64 and 68 days for the Provox2 and Provox Vega, respectively, and 143 and 191 days for the problem-solving ActiValve Light and ActiValve Strong.[20] When compared to historical cohorts, the lifetime of the device seems to be decreasing though the main indication for

replacement remains transprosthetic leakage.[21] Lewin et al[22] found similar results in the MD Anderson Cancer Center with a median device lifetime of 61 days, where also the ActiValve had the longest device lifetime of 161 days. In their cohort, previous RT was significantly associated with a lower device lifetime (59 vs. 66 days).[22] In our cohort, a salvage TL or TL for a dysfunctional larynx was significantly associated with a shorter device lifetime. Interestingly, we were also able to demonstrate a significant relation between device lifetime and driving distance to the hospital. Although median driving time was only 26 minutes in our cohort, every 15-minute increase in driving time resulted in a hazard ratio of 0.92 (0.90–0.94, $p < 0.001$) where a hazard ratio of less than 1 means longer device lifetime. It would be very interesting to validate these results in countries where driving distances are longer.

21.3 Tips

- A TL is still associated with the highest overall survival rates for T4 tumors of the larynx, though chemoradiation is a valuable alternative.
- Counsel the patients adequately about the expected overall survival rates and quality of life after the different treatment options for advanced cancer of the larynx.
- Primary insertion of a VP allows for early vocal rehabilitation and optimal social reintegration.
- During TL, attention should be paid to obtain a wide enough stoma, as flat as possible, to allow easy use of HMEs, automatic speaking valves, and adhesives.

21.4 Traps

- Compared to a primary TL, fistula rates are higher following a salvage TL, or a TL for a dysfunctional larynx.
- Conservative treatment is the method of choice in initial management of a PCF. If this treatment is unsuccessful, surgical management with a pedicled flap is advised.

References

[1] EuroQol Group. EuroQol: a new facility for the measurement of health-related quality of life. Health Policy. 1990; 16(3):199–208

[2] Rosen CA, Lee AS, Osborne J, Zullo T, Murry T. Development and validation of the voice handicap index-10. Laryngoscope. 2004; 114(9):1549–1556

[3] Belafsky PC, Mouadeb DA, Rees CJ, et al. Validity and reliability of the Eating Assessment Tool (EAT-10). Ann Otol Rhinol Laryngol. 2008; 117(12):919–924

[4] Wolf GT, Fisher SG, Hong WK, et al; Department of Veterans Affairs Laryngeal Cancer Study Group. Induction chemotherapy plus radiation compared with surgery plus radiation in patients with advanced laryngeal cancer. N Engl J Med. 1991; 324(24):1685–1690

[5] Hoffman HT, Porter K, Karnell LH, et al. Laryngeal cancer in the United States: changes in demographics, patterns of care, and survival. Laryngoscope. 2006; 116(9, pt 2, suppl 111):1–13

[6] Olsen KD. Reexamining the treatment of advanced laryngeal cancer. Head Neck. 2010; 32(1):1–7

[7] Timmermans AJ, van Dijk BA, Overbeek LI, et al. Trends in treatment and survival for advanced laryngeal cancer: a 20-year population-based study in The Netherlands. Head Neck. 2016; 38(suppl 1):E1247–E1255

[8] Petersen JF, Timmermans AJ, van Dijk BAC, et al. Trends in treatment, incidence and survival of hypopharynx cancer: a 20-year population-based study in the Netherlands. Eur Arch Otorhinolaryngol. 2018; 275(1):181–189

[9] McNeil BJ, Weichselbaum R, Pauker SG. Speech and survival: tradeoffs between quality and quantity of life in laryngeal cancer. N Engl J Med. 1981; 305(17):982–987

[10] Hamilton DW, Bins JE, McMeekin P, et al. Quality compared to quantity of life in laryngeal cancer: a time trade-off study. Head Neck. 2015

[11] Hamilton DW, Pedersen A, Blanchford H, et al. A comparison of attitudes to laryngeal cancer treatment outcomes: a time trade-off study. Clin Otolaryngol. 2018; 43(1):117–123

[12] Stacey D, Légaré F, Col NF, et al. Decision aids for people facing health treatment or screening decisions. Cochrane Database Syst Rev. 2014; 1(1):CD001431

[13] Paydarfar JA, Birkmeyer NJ. Complications in head and neck surgery: a meta-analysis of postlaryngectomy pharyngocutaneous fistula. Arch Otolaryngol Head Neck Surg. 2006; 132(1):67–72

[14] Timmermans AJ, Lansaat L, Theunissen EA, Hamming-Vrieze O, Hilgers FJ, van den Brekel MW. Predictive factors for pharyngocutaneous fistulization after total laryngectomy. Ann Otol Rhinol Laryngol. 2014; 123(3):153–161

[15] Patel UA, Moore BA, Wax M, et al. Impact of pharyngeal closure technique on fistula after salvage laryngectomy. JAMA Otolaryngol Head Neck Surg. 2013; 139(11):1156–1162

[16] Medina JE, Khafif A. Early oral feeding following total laryngectomy. Laryngoscope. 2001; 111(3):368–372

[17] Aires FT, Dedivitis RA, Petrarolha SM, Bernardo WM, Cernea CR, Brandão LG. Early oral feeding after total laryngectomy: a systematic review. Head Neck. 2015; 37(10):1532–1535

[18] van Sluis KE, van der Molen L, van Son RJJH, Hilgers FJM, Bhairosing PA, van den Brekel MWM. Objective and subjective voice outcomes after total laryngectomy: a systematic review. Eur Arch Otorhinolaryngol. 2018; 275(1):11–26

[19] Mozolewski E, Zietek E, Jach K. Surgical rehabilitation of voice and speech after laryngectomy. Pol Med Sci Hist Bull. 1973; 15(4):373–377

[20] Petersen JF, Lansaat L, Timmermans AJ, Van der Noort V, Hilgers FJM, van den Brekel MWM. Postlaryngectomy prosthetic voice rehabilitation outcomes in a consecutive cohort of 232 patients over a 13-year period. Head Neck 2018

[21] Op de Coul BM, Hilgers FJ, Balm AJ, Tan IB, van den Hoogen FJ, van Tinteren H. A decade of postlaryngectomy vocal rehabilitation in 318 patients: a single Institution's experience with consistent application of provox indwelling voice prostheses. Arch Otolaryngol Head Neck Surg. 2000; 126(11):1320–1328

[22] Lewin JS, Baumgart LM, Barrow MP, Hutcheson KA. Device life of the tracheoesophageal voice prosthesis revisited. JAMA Otolaryngol Head Neck Surg. 2017; 143:65–71

22 Transoral Robotic Surgical Total Laryngectomy: The Technique Step by Step

Georges Lawson, Abie Mendelsohn, Sebastien Van der Vorst, Marc Remacle, Gilles Delahaut

Abstract

The aim of our study is to demonstrate our technique in performing transoral robotic surgery total laryngectomy (TORS-TL) with the use of the da Vinci robotic system. We provide a comprehensive description of the TORS-TL operative techniques. Two fresh frozen human cadavers were selected after ethical approval to describe the appropriate step-by-step surgical resection. We adopted a five-step procedure that was later applied on two of our patients. The first patient presented initially with a squamous cell carcinoma (SCC) in the laryngeal glottis area. A lack of clinical response to initial treatment by chemoradiotherapy led to the decision of performing salvage total laryngectomy surgery. The second patient had a previous history of head and neck SCC; he had no recurrence of his primary tumor but significantly suffered postoperatively of breathing and swallowing difficulties due to severe laryngeal incompetence. TORS-TL was successfully performed on all cases. The operative time on the two cadavers was approximately 65 and 55 minutes. It was significantly longer on our patients, 210 minutes and 235 minutes, respectively, despite the fact that exactly the same steps were followed throughout all procedures. There were no intraoperative and postoperative complications or surgical morbidity related to the use of the da Vinci robotic system. TORS supraglottic laryngectomy (TORS-SL) for SCC was performed in a safe, reliable, and smooth manner and has shown to be successful in treating our patients. We thus believe our described step-by-step technique for TORS-SL is efficient and reproducible.

Keywords: da Vinci robot, total laryngectomy, transoral robotic surgery, technique, procedure

22.1 Introduction

Transoral surgery is nowadays a well-established procedure for the management of laryngeal diseases, benign or early malignancies. Transoral robotic surgery (TORS) using the da Vinci System (Intuitive Surgical, Sunnyvale, CA) is described as a minimally invasive surgery providing with excellent outcomes and shortening hospital stays.[1] Different laryngeal subsite surgeries has been addressed by TORS such as supraglottic laryngectomy[2] and hypopharyngectomy[3] with feasibility trials and promising initial data. A combination of both procedures is now adapted to perform a TORS total laryngectomy (TORS-TL).

22.2 Patients and Methods

We performed a transoral resection of the entire larynx on two different series. We first operated on two fresh frozen human cadavers in the faculty of medicine anatomy laboratory after ethical approval. Both interventions were performed by the senior author following a predesigned five-step technique. We then operated on live patients in our operative room hospital setting. Both surgeries were also performed by the same surgeon. The da Vinci robotic system was mounted and prepared in the operating room in our usual standard fashion, and we followed exactly the same five-step procedure used during the cadaveric dissection.

Subject selection: The selection of our cadavers was based on the fact that they had to be freshly frozen in order to simulate as closely as possible a real-life situation. A mouth-opening retractor was used to allow exposure and access to the larynx transorally.

The selection of our patients was based on the following criteria: first, both patients should have no general surgical contraindications as confirmed during the preoperative anesthesia consultation. Second, a proper mouth-opening range was required in order to appropriately access the larynges to perform transoral laryngeal resections with a safe margin in case of a tumor.

The first case was a T3N0 glottic cancer that had previously failed an organ preservation strategy based on concomitant chemoradiation therapy. The second case was a patient presenting with a previous history of T3N1 glottic cancer successfully treated by concomitant chemoradiation therapy. A year after treatment, the patient presented to us with a severe laryngeal incompetency, impairing both his breathing and swallowing patterns.

Thus, we decided to perform a functional total laryngectomy.

Operative instruments used were found in our regular open neck tracheotomy surgical case.

Regarding the transoral robotic approach, we recommend (according to GL's learning curve) the use of specific instruments adapted to the da Vinci robot, as well as standard cordectomy instruments and a mouth gag adapted to the surgery: Remacle and Lawson–LARS (Fentex Medical, Neuhausen, Germany) or the FK-WO (Gyrus ACMI, Tuttlingen, Germany).

The five-step procedure is summarized as follows (▶Table 22.1):

1. *Cervical exposure:* The procedure begins with a standard tracheostomy skin incision, approximately 4 cm in length, at the midpoint between the cricoid cartilage and the sternal notch. After superior subplatysmal skin flap is raised, the strap muscles are divided along the midline raphe to expose the trachea and cricoid cartilages. A thyroid isthmusectomy is performed, and the lateral lobes are dissected off of the lateral tracheal walls. A complete transection of the trachea is placed at the third tracheal space with rising posterior tracheal mucosal cuts. Inferior stomal stitches are used to secure the thoracic trachea. The skin incision gives ample visualization to dissect around the remaining rostral trachea and cricoid cartilage, which includes sectioning bilateral recurrent laryngeal nerves. At this point, two 2–0 Vicryl sutures are placed around the lateral walls of the rostral trachea and are threaded through glottis for intraoral

Table 22.1 The five steps of transoral robotic surgery total laryngectomy

1. Cervical exposure, with tracheostomy and laryngeal dissection (▶Fig. 22.1)

2. Intraoral resection with clipping of the laryngeal artery (▶Fig. 22.2)

3. Larynx delivery through the mouth (▶Fig. 22.3)

4. Intraoral reconstruction by suturing the hypopharyngeal mucosa to the base of tongue (▶Fig. 22.4)

5. Cervical closure by suturing cervical skin to the tracheostomy site (▶Fig. 22.5)

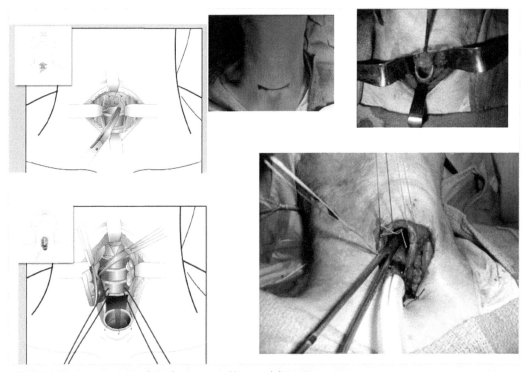

Fig. 22.1 Cervical exposure with tracheostomy and laryngeal dissection.

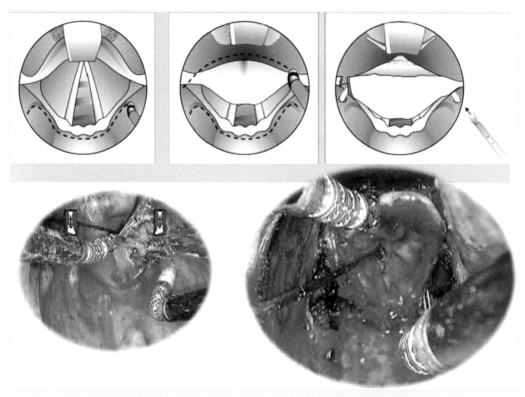

Fig. 22.2 Intraoral resection with clipping of the laryngeal artery.

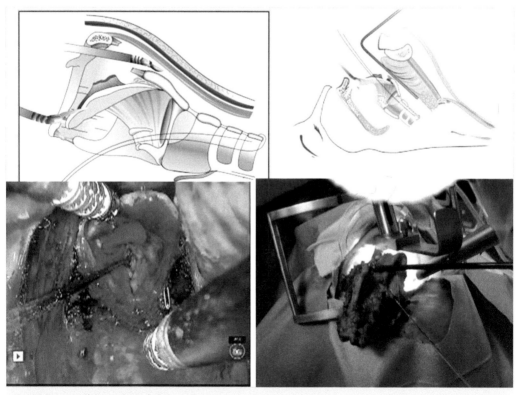

Fig. 22.3 Larynx delivery through the mouth.

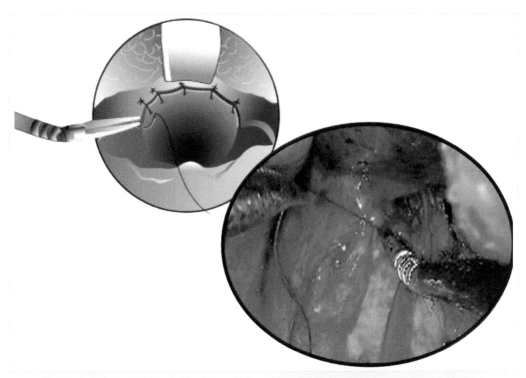

Fig. 22.4 Intraoral reconstruction by suturing the hypopharyngeal mucosa to the base of tongue.

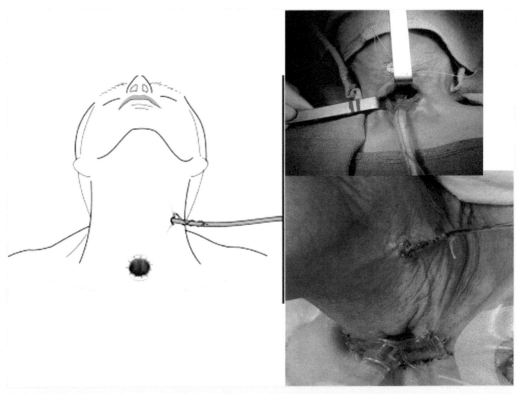

Fig. 22.5 Cervical closure by suturing cervical skin to the tracheostomy site.

retraction. The stoma site is covered with sterile drapes.

2. *Intraoral resection:* The procedure is started with the initial placement of the intraoral retractor with the epiglottis retracted out of view of the glottis. A 0-degree endoscope is used along with 5-mm Maryland dissector and 5-mm spatula Bovie. With optimal retraction and visualization, the initial intraoral incision is placed along the superior aspect of the arytenoid mucosa. With the dissector retracting the mucosa, the Bovie separates the postcricoid mucosa and the medial pyriform sinus wall from the cricoid cartilage. Subsequently, the epiglottis is then released from retraction and the vallecula incision is made along the lingual surface of the epiglottis in a direction toward the superior border of the thyroid cartilage. Extending the vallecular incision laterally and posteriorly, the superior laryngeal vessels are encountered as they course through the thyrohyoid membrane. Multiple clips are placed on the vessels and divided. Dissection is continued caudally until the thyroid cartilage is encountered, keeping the hyoid bone retracted underneath the intraoral retractor blade. The instruments are directed along the external thyroid cartilage perichondrium. As we resume inferiorly, tension will be required on the previously placed inferior tracheal retraction sutures. These sutures will give a rostral pull to the inferior portion of the thyroid cartilage as well as allowing for lateral retraction to improve visualization. Dissection continues caudally and laterally until the larynx is freed from its attachments.

3. *Laryngeal delivery through the mouth:* At the end of the dissection, the larynx is delivered orally.

4. *Intraoral reconstruction:* The mucosa is reapproximated to the base of tongue with 3–0 braided absorbable sutures placed with the use of the 5-mm needle holder arm. In our experience, given the extensive mucosal preservation, the pharyngotomy can be closed in a horizontal orientation. Following the watertight closure, fibrin glue is placed over the incision. At this point, steps of salivary bypass tube placement and primary tracheoesophageal prosthesis placement may be performed in a typical manner depending on surgeon preference. Intraoral retraction is released.

5. *Cervical closure:* With superiorly directed skin retraction, the pharyngotomy may be bolstered with externally placed sutures along the tongue base musculature. The strap muscles are reapproximated over the pharyngotomy site. A small suction drain is placed superior to the stoma site. Superior skin flap is released and the superior stomaplasty is performed using braided absorbable suture. At the end of the procedure, the endotracheal tube is replaced with a laryngectomy tube.

22.3 Discussion

As was discussed in our previous publication,[4] an intraoral approach for total laryngectomy offers a number of benefits over the traditional approach. First, the direct view allows for maximal mucosa sparing, creating a horizontal pharyngotomy closure. Ideal pharyngotomy closure has been subject to debate. In order to reduce the development of pharyngeal shelf and associated neopharyngeal diverticula,[5] Davis et al advocated the T-shaped pharyngotomy closure to improve postlaryngectomy swallowing function.[6] Presently, however, pharyngotomy closure is routinely performed in a vertical linear fashion to minimize technical error as well as to reduce blood supply at the corners of the T-shaped suture line, as postulated. Yet common-day practice leaves the concerns of Davis et al[6] unresolved. The mucosal-sparing TORS incision allows for a substantial improvement in pharyngeal defect size. This results in a linear horizontal closure mitigating the concerns for ischemia while reducing the possibility of pharyngeal shelf and neopharyngeal diverticula formation.

The TORS approach also obviates the need for carotid sheath dissection. As pharyngocutaneous fistula is the most prevalent postlaryngectomy complication,[7] lateral extrusion of the fistula is the most concerning as the infectious contents weakens the carotid arterial wall with subsequent risk for carotid blowout.[8] Avoiding the creation of tissue planes between the pharynx and carotid artery may avert a natural lateral tract for fistula formation. While such high-risk factors as postradiation therapy[9] may continue to lead to pharyngocutaneous fistulas irrespective of surgical approach, TORS-TL may in fact improve the treatment and outcome of this frequent complication by limiting associated morbidity. However, carotid artery protection is removed if concurrent neck dissection is performed.

As demonstrated in the TORS experience, minimally invasive head and neck surgical approaches decrease patient hospital stays and hastens recuperation.[1]

22.4 Conclusion

TORS-SL for SCC was performed in a safe, reliable, and smooth manner and has shown to be successful in treating our patients. We thus believe that the described step-by-step technique for TORS-SL that we developed is efficient and reproducible. The application of TORS to total laryngectomy is expected to follow demonstrated patterns in order to have an effect on the patient and health care strain and costs. To demonstrate the potential benefits of TORS-TL, substantial clinical experience must be collected. Apart from demonstration of feasibility, our initial institutional TORS-TL experience is limited from statistical analysis. To date, we have performed TORS-TL for both oncologic and functional indications. The goal of the present report is to share the surgical protocol successfully utilized in order to encourage the advancement of this surgical technique and shared clinical experiences so conclusive data may be gathered.

References

[1] O'Malley BW, Jr, Weinstein GS, Snyder W, Hockstein NG. Transoral robotic surgery (TORS) for base of tongue neoplasms. Laryngoscope. 2006; 116(8):1465–1472

[2] Alon EE, Kasperbauer JL, Olsen KD, Moore EJ. Feasibility of transoral robotic-assisted supraglottic laryngectomy. Head Neck. 2012; 34(2):225–229

[3] Park YM, Kim WS, Byeon HK, De Virgilio A, Jung JS, Kim SH. Feasibility of transoral robotic hypopharyngectomy for early-stage hypopharyngeal carcinoma. Oral Oncol. 2010; 46(8):597–602

[4] Lawson G, Mendelsohn AH, Van Der Vorst S, Bachy V, Remacle M. Transoral robotic surgery total laryngectomy. Laryngoscope. 2013; 123(1):193–196

[5] Deschler DG, Blevins NH, Ellison DE. Postlaryngectomy dysphagia caused by an anterior neopharyngeal diverticulum. Otolaryngol Head Neck Surg. 1996; 115(1):167–169

[6] Davis RK, Vincent ME, Shapshay SM, Strong MS. The anatomy and complications of "T" versus vertical closure of the hypopharynx after laryngectomy. Laryngoscope. 1982; 92(1):16–22

[7] Paydarfar JA, Birkmeyer NJ. Complications in head and neck surgery: a meta-analysis of postlaryngectomy pharyngocutaneous fistula. Arch Otolaryngol Head Neck Surg. 2006; 132(1):67–72

[8] Boscolo-Rizzo P, De Cillis G, Marchiori C, Carpenè S, Da Mosto MC. Multivariate analysis of risk factors for pharyngocutaneous fistula after total laryngectomy. Eur Arch Otorhinolaryngol. 2008; 265(8):929–936

[9] Remacle M, Matar N, Lawson G, Bachy V. Laryngeal advanced retractor system: a new retractor for transoral robotic surgery. Otolaryngol Head Neck Surg. 2011; 145(4):694–696

23 Locally Advanced Supraglottic Cancer: Organ-Preservation Protocol

Roberta Granata, Lisa Licitra

Abstract

We describe a case of a man with a supraglottic laryngeal carcinoma stage T2N1 (stage III) treated with induction chemotherapy (cisplatin + paclitaxel), followed by radiation (RT) alone. Treatment goals of patients with limited-stage cancer of the larynx are: curing the cancer, preserving laryngeal functions, and maximizing the patient's quality of life. Traditionally, primary treatment approaches, with equivalent outcome results, includes primary larynx-preserving surgery, when feasible, followed by RT or chemoradiation in high-risk cases or as an alternative option a combination of chemoradiation and radiation therapy. Treatment choice aim at maximizing in the patient organ function, quality of life, and overall. In this situation, the optimal decision-making requires an experienced multidisciplinary team for initial evaluation, response assessment as well as supportive care, and rehabilitation during and after treatment. In addition to the extent of the tumor, pretreatment laryngeal function, coexisting chronic disease, and patient expectations are critical factors in selecting surgical or nonsurgical primary treatment.

Keywords: supraglottic cancer, organ preservation, multidisciplinary team, induction chemotherapy, chemoradiation

23.1 Case Report

A 67-year-old Caucasian male presented in another hospital with left laterocervical adenopathy where he was followed by hematologists for monoclonal gammopathy of undetermined significance (MGUS) immunoglobulin Mκ (IgMκ). An excisional biopsy of the lymph node was performed. The pathological report described a squamous cell carcinoma (G2). He stated that he was a 45 pack year cigarette smoker, and had a history of alcohol abuse with chronic liver disease (steatosis grade 1).

At the time of our consultation, the patient was healthy; he had a transverse scar on the left neck and a new lymph node of 3cm in the left neck. A direct laryngoscopy revealed a vegetant lesion of the lingual surface of the epiglottis that also involved the left glossoepiglottic vallecula. The lesion reached to and infiltrated the right pharyngeal epiglottic fold without vocal cord fixation.

We performed an MRI scan that showed a lesion occupying the left glossoepiglottic vallecula, the lingual surface of the epiglottis without infiltration of the base of tongue, aryepiglottic fold, or piriform sinus. There was a left submandibular lymph node of 23 × 19 mm.

Due to the past smoking history and presence of comorbidities possibly associated with occurrence of secondary primaries, we completed the staging with a PET scan that confirmed the locoregional extension of the tumor and no distinct metastatic disease. We concluded that the tumor was cT2N1M0, stage III, according to the seventh edition of the American Joint Committee on Cancer (AJCC; ▶ Fig. 23.1).

We examined the patient in our multidisciplinary clinic. A surgical conservation approach was excluded due to the extent of the cancer. An organ-preservation protocol was offered to the patient. The patient started chemotherapy with paclitaxel plus cisplatin 3 weekly treatment for three cycles. The treatment well tolerated except for a grade 2 neutropenia after the first cycle and no other side effects.

We repeated the MRI scan after two cycles of chemotherapy and with a 70% reduction in the size of the cancer according to Response Evaluation

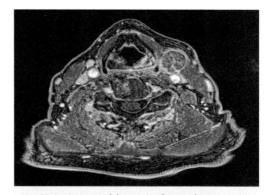

Fig. 23.1 MRI scan of diagnosis of supraglottic carcinoma with metastasis to the left neck.

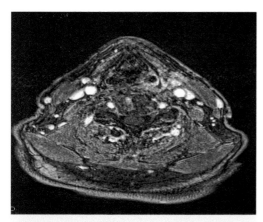

Fig. 23.2 MRI scan after two cycles of induction chemotherapy.

Criteria In Solid Tumors (RECIST) criteria.[1] Vocal cord mobility was maintained. In larynx preservation (LP) trials, a response to induction chemotherapy of more than 50%, along with cord remobilization, was the standardized criterion used for selecting patients for radiation, thus allowing for organ preservation (▶ Fig. 23.2).

After the third cycle of chemotherapy, the patient started radiotherapy alone; he received intensity-modulated radiotherapy (IMRT) to a total dose of 69.96 Gy in 33 fractions on tumor and adenopathy (left level II); in particular, supraglottic larynx and left II to III neck level received 61.05 Gy in 33 fractions; larynx plus bilateral neck received 54.45 Gy in 33 fractions.

Radiotherapy was well tolerated. He had grade 2 mucositis and grade 1 dysphagia. The treatment ended in September 2015. After three years, the patient is alive and free of cancer with no report of any late symptoms such as dysphagia and dysphonia. In January 2018, he developed a postradiation hypothyroidism and replacement therapy was started.

23.2 Discussion

The first study on the role of chemotherapy for organ preservation in larynx cancer was published in 1991.[2] In that study, induction chemotherapy followed by radiation therapy proved to be an effective strategy total laryngectomy, with a high rate of LP, local control, and long-term survival in patients with advanced cancer of the larynx.[2] Total response rate was 77% with complete response in 26% and partial response in 51%.[2] In this study, surgery and induction chemotherapy followed by radiation has the same survival. In this context, a response to induction chemotherapy serves as a selection procedure of radioresponsive cases, which allows for LP without adding any benefit in survival.

The following study on LP compared induction chemotherapy versus chemoradiation versus radiotherapy alone. In Radiation Therapy Oncology Group (RTOG) 91–11, the patients with stage III or IV glottic or supraglottic squamous cell cancer were randomly assigned to induction cisplatin/5-fluorouracil (PF) followed by RT (control arm), concomitant cisplatin/RT, or RT alone. The composite endpoint of laryngectomy-free survival (LFS) was the primary endpoint.[3]

The study concluded that induction PF followed by RT and concomitant cisplatin/RT show similar efficacy for the composite endpoint of LFS. Locoregional control and LP were significantly improved with concomitant cisplatin/RT compared with the induction arm or RT alone.

The results of a subsequent study supported that docetaxel, cisplatin, and 5-fluorouracil (TPF) is the best induction chemotherapy treatment compared to PF.[4]

Another phase III study comparing induction PF versus induction TPF, enrolling patients with cancer of the larynx and hypopharynx, confirmed a significantly higher response rate with induction TPF (80 vs. 59%), thereby selecting more patients to undergo definitive RT, which translated into a significantly higher LP rate (3-year estimates, 70 vs. 57.5%).[4] No other outcome was improved with TPF; the rates of local recurrence, late salvage surgery, metastases, and overall survival were the same in both groups. The small sample size precluded analysis by primary site.

The TREMPLIN (Radiotherapy with Cisplatin versus Radiotherapy with Cetuximab after Induction Chemotherapy for Larynx Preservation) randomized phase II trial evaluated the feasibility of a sequential approach for LP seeking for solutions to reduce toxicity of chemoradiation.[5] A total of 153 operable patients with cancer of the larynx or hypopharynx (T2–T3 and N0–N3) received three cycles of induction TPF. Responders would then be randomly assigned to either cetuximab or cisplatin concurrent with RT. The primary endpoint was LP 3 months after treatment, with an expected rate of 80%. The TREMPLIN study did not meet the prespecified LP endpoint because of a high dropout rate (24%) before random assignment that was related to both substantial toxicity from TPF and insufficient tumor response. Also, cetuximab/RT proved as toxic as cisplatin/RT, causing the same rate of grade 3 to 4 acute mucositis but worse in-field skin toxicity. More local failures among patients treated with cetuximab raised the possibility that for larynx cancer, epidermal growth factor receptor inhibition/RT may be inferior to cisplatin/RT for achieving local control. This feasibility trial demonstrated that both cetuximab/RT and cisplatin/RT were difficult to administer after induction TPF. Moreover, the LP rate was no better than that observed with TPF, followed by RT alone in GORTEC 2000–2001.[5]

In 2009, a consensus panel met to review all the clinical trial results. The experts proposed the adoption of a new composite study endpoint in organ-preservation clinical trials: laryngoesophageal dysfunction-free survival; moreover, they underlined the importance of a multidisciplinary team for the selection of therapy for the individual patient.[6]

In the light of the challenges posed by the interpretation of organ preservation study results, we reanalyzed the updated results of RTOG 91–11 study. We used the numbers provided in the RTOG 91–11 paper's Table 1[3] and we noticed that the proportion of patients alive at 10 years is always *numerically* higher with induction over concomitant chemoradiation: overall survival is 38.8 versus 27.5%, survival with larynx is 28.9 versus 23.5%, and survival without larynx is 9.9 versus 4% with induction and concomitant, respectively.[7]

In summary, the results of RTOG 91–11 fail to provide any support to the superiority of concomitant chemoradiation, suggesting that sequential treatment may actually be more effective, with a comparable increase in the proportion of long-term survivors with and without larynx.[7]

In accordance with these data, we adopted our favorite organ-preservation approach. We personalized the choice of induction chemotherapy schedule with paclitaxel and cisplatin, due to the presence of comorbidity that would have precluded full dose of TPF.

References

[1] Eisenhauer EA, Therasse P, Bogaerts J, et al. New response evaluation criteria in solid tumours: revised RECIST guideline (version 1.1). Eur J Cancer. 2009; 45(2):228–247

[2] Karp DD, Vaughan CW, Carter R, et al. Larynx preservation using induction chemotherapy plus radiation therapy as an alternative to laryngectomy in advanced head and neck cancer. A long-term follow-up report. Am J Clin Oncol. 1991; 14(4):273–279

[3] Forastiere AA, Zhang Q, Weber RS, et al. Long-term results of RTOG 91–11: a comparison of three nonsurgical treatment strategies to preserve the larynx in patients with locally advanced larynx cancer. J Clin Oncol. 2013; 31(7):845–852

[4] Pointreau Y, Garaud P, Chapet S, et al. Randomized trial of induction chemotherapy with cisplatin and 5-fluorouracil with or without docetaxel for larynx preservation. J Natl Cancer Inst. 2009; 101(7):498–506

[5] Lefebvre JL, Pointreau Y, Rolland F, et al. Induction chemotherapy followed by either chemoradiotherapy or bioradiotherapy for larynx preservation: the TREMPLIN randomized phase II study. J Clin Oncol. 2013; 31(7):853–859

[6] Lefebvre JL, Ang KK; Larynx Preservation Consensus Panel. Larynx preservation clinical trial design: key issues and recommendations—a consensus panel summary. Head Neck. 2009; 31(4):429–441

[7] Licitra L, Bonomo P, Sanguineti G, et al. A different view on larynx preservation evidence-based treatment recommendations. J Clin Oncol. 2018; 36(13):1376–1377

24 Salvage Surgery after Primary Radiotherapy: Transoral Laser Microsurgery

Mohssen Ansarin, Augusto Cattaneo, Francesco Chu

Abstract

Radiotherapy (RT) is widely used as primary treatment for early-stage cancer of the larynx. In the case of persistent/recurrent cancer of the larynx after RT, different salvage treatments are to be considered: total laryngectomy, open partial laryngectomy, and transoral laser microsurgery (TLM). TLM is the first-line treatment for early and intermediate laryngeal cancer, but it can also be considered as salvage surgery after RT in selected cases. Candidates for salvage surgery should be chosen on the basis of careful clinical and radiological examination. Clinical examination should include detailed laryngoscopy, combined with MRI or CT scan of the larynx, even in the case of a superficial suspicious lesion. The selection criteria for TLM in recurrent cancer of the larynx are very strict. It is important to achieve a good exposure of the larynx with full visualization of the anterior commissure. Minimal cordectomies (e.g., I, II, or III) are not recommended. Hemilaryngectomy (types IV and V) is generally suggested, even for apparently superficial lesions because after RT it is not easy to detect the real boundaries of the tumor. Here we present two clinical cases in which the patients underwent TLM as salvage surgery after RT failure for cancer of the larynx.

Keywords: transoral laser microsurgery, salvage surgery, microlaryngoscopy, radiation failure

24.1 Case Reports

24.1.1 Patient 1

A 77-year-old male patient presented to our clinic because of persistent dysphonia. He is a non-smoker and complains of "rough voice." Eight months previously, he underwent radiation (66 Gy) for "cT1a" squamous cell carcinoma (SCC) of the larynx. Clinical records reveal type II diabetes, severe renal failure, and hypertension. Videolaryngoscopy shows a leukoerythroblastic lesion of the left vocal fold extending to the laryngeal ventricle; laryngeal mobility is mildly reduced. No lymph nodes are detected on the palpation of the neck.

A biopsy of the lesion was taken and the final histopathological examination was SCC.

A neck and chest CT scan was performed, demonstrating enhanced areas at the level of the left vocal fold and anterior commissure (AC). The lesion extends to the left ventricle, without infiltration of the left paraglottic space (PGS). No cervical lymphadenopathy was detected. No suspicious pulmonary lesions were noted. The lesion was classified as yT2, N0M0 (▶ Fig. 24.1a).

The patient is intubated with a laser-safe tubing (Laser-Flex Tracheal Tube; Mallinckrodt Inc., St Louis, MO); a direct laryngoscopy evaluation with 30- and 70-degree rigid endoscopes revealed a lesion involving the left vocal fold, extending to the AC and the contralateral vocal fold. The tumor extended superiorly to involve the anterior one-third of the left false vocal fold (▶ Fig. 24.1b).

The exposure of the larynx was achieved by using a large bore laryngoscope. A type V left hemilaryngectomy was performed using a CO_2 laser. "En bloc" resection of the cancer includes the left vocal fold, the false vocal fold, the anterior commissure, and the anterior two-thirds of the right vocal fold. The inner perichondrium of the thyroid cartilage was exposed in order to remove completely the PGS. Both arytenoids were preserved. For the procedure, a 25-W carbon dioxide laser (Martin,

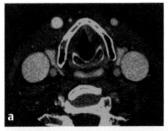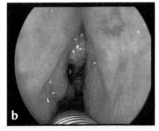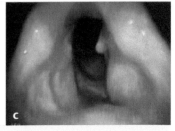

Fig. 24.1 (a) CT scan. (b) Intraoperative evaluation. (c) Postoperative evaluation.

Tuttlingen, Germany) with an output power of 0.8 to 3.4 W in superpulse mode and with a beam width of 150 μm was used. Specimens are orientated, fixed in 10% buffered formalin for 24 hours, and paraffin embedded. Five-micrometer sections stained with hematoxylin and eosin. Resection margins stained with Indian ink. The final pathological results showed poorly differentiated SCC of the larynx, infiltrating the subepithelial connective tissue near the thyroid cartilage with a "close" (<1 mm) margin at the level of the deep plane. All margins are free from neoplastic infiltration. After multidisciplinary discussion, the patient was referred to close follow-up and he is currently cancer free after 41 months of follow-up (▶ Fig. 24.1c).

24.1.2 Patient 2

A 72-year-old male patient was referred to our clinic because of persistent mild dysphonia. He is not a smoker and takes no medications. In 1994, he underwent radiation therapy (66 Gy) for a "cT1a" SCC of the right vocal fold. Three years later, he underwent type I cordectomy because of carcinoma in situ of the right vocal fold. Outpatient laryngoscopy reveals mild edema of the larynx. I-scan examination reveals a 4-mm submucosal lesion at the level of the right ventricle. No lymph nodes are detectable on palpation of the neck (▶ Fig. 24.2a).

CT scan demonstrates mild asymmetry of the supraglottic region and a 4-mm submucosal lesion of the right ventricle. The PGS is unaltered, and there are no enlarged signs of infiltration of the laryngeal cartilages and lymph nodes were detected (▶ Fig. 24.2b).

The patient underwent microlaryngoscopy under general anesthesia. He was intubated with a laser-safe tubing (Laser-Flex Tracheal Tube; Mallinckrodt Inc.) and a direct laryngoscopy evaluation with 30- and 70-degree rigid endoscopes

revealed a small submucosal lesion between the upper surface of the right vocal fold and the floor of the ventricle. Frozen sections on intraoperative biopsy confirms SCC (▶ Fig. 24.2c).

The exposure of the vocal folds and the AC is obtained with a large bore laryngoscope. A type IV right hemilaryngectomy was performed; "en bloc" resection of the cancer includes the right vocal fold and the false vocal fold. The inner perichondrium of thyroid cartilage is exposed in order to remove completely the PGS. Specimens are harvested as previously described in patient one. The final pathological results revealed an in situ SCC with all margins free of cancer. The patient is referred to follow-up and he is currently free from disease.

24.2 Discussion

Radiotherapy (RT) is widely used as primary treatment for early-stage laryngeal cancer. The reported 5-year rate of local control (LC) after primary radiation ranges from 84 to 95% for T1 and from 50 to 85% for T2; for early-stage supraglottic cancers, LC rates up to 100% for T1 and up to 86% for T2 tumors.[1,2,3]

In case of persistent/recurrent cancer of the larynx after RT, different salvage treatments are to be considered. Total laryngectomy (TL) remains the gold standard and the most widely used for advanced-stage recurrences not amenable to conservation laryngeal surgery (CLS). Open partial laryngectomy (OPHLs) can provide high LC although they are not recommended for unfit patients due to the risk of postoperative complications (salivary fistula and aspiration pneumonia), unpredictable functional recovery, and long hospitalization time.[4]

TLM is a standard surgical treatment for the early and intermediate cancer of the larynx.[5] The role of TLM as a salvage surgery after RT in selected cases is also widely reported in the literature.[6,7,8,9,10] Shah et al reported that, in case of recurrences,

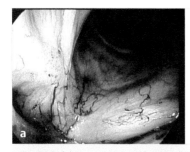 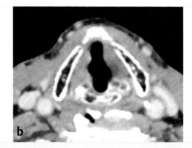 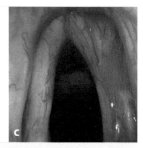

Fig. 24.2 (a) Preoperative evaluation. (b) CT scan. (c) Intraoperative evaluation.

if the T-stage is higher than primary tumor, CLS should be avoided.[11] It is also well known that recurrences after RT are allegedly related to an initial tumor understaging since diagnosis is based on clinical imaging, without the support of pathological examination of tumor margins. At the time of recurrence, tissue inflammation (edema or erythema) and fibrotic laryngeal changes negatively affect the evaluation of tumor extension.[12] Candidates for salvage surgery should be selected on the basis of a careful clinical and radiological examination. The first step is flexible video fiberoptic laryngoscopy (with white light, I-scan systems or with narrowband imaging) to evaluate local extension of the tumor, arytenoid/vocal fold motility, and the affected laryngeal subsites.

Preoperative imaging of the larynx (CT scan or MRI with surface coils) is mandatory in order to exclude involvement of the PGS and/or pre-epiglottic space (PES), infiltration of the laryngeal framework (AC and at the cricoarytenoid region) and to assess the nodal status.[13] It is to be highlighted that endoscopic examination and radiological imaging for laryngeal recurrences have a diagnostic accuracy of 38%, with 10% of the tumors being overstaged and 52% understaged.[12] Due to this limit, authors report a lower LC rate for advanced rT3–rT4 stage recurrences when compared to early rT1–rT2 stages.[14]

The selection criteria for TLM in recurrent laryngeal cancer are very restricted. It is important to achieve a good exposure of the larynx with full visualization of the AC. Only 20% of laryngeal recurrences demonstrate a single concentric pattern of growth; more commonly, multifocal nests of cancer (dissociated cancer cells and perineural foci of infiltration) are encountered, not easily detectable at the out-patient-clinic laryngoscopy.[7] Intraoperative rigid endoscopy, under general anesthesia, with angled telescopes provides a more detailed evaluation of the cancer. TLM is potentially feasible for rT1 and rT2. On the contrary, massive involvement of the PGS/PES, arytenoid fixation, and infiltration of the laryngeal framework are absolute contraindications to TLM.

24.3 Tips

- Outpatient laryngoscopy with white light and narrowband imaging/I-scan permits a better visualization of the mucosal changes after RT.
- A CT scan or MRI with surface coils is mandatory, even in the case of a superficial suspicious lesion: the AC, paralaryngeal spaces, subglottic area, and laryngeal cartilages should be specifically evaluated.
- A good intraoperative exposure of all the laryngeal subsites is an indispensable prerequisite for TLM. If the lesion reaches the AC and the AC cannot be visualized, TLM should not be performed because of the risk of a nonradical surgery.
- Minimal cordectomies (e.g., I, II, or III) are not recommended. Hemilaryngectomy (types IV and V) is generally suggested, even for apparently superficial lesions because after RT it is difficult to detect the true boundaries of the tumor.

24.4 Traps

- Vocal fold or arytenoid hypomotility should never be underestimated because of the risk of insidious submucosal growth of the cancer.
- Lesions involving the AC are potentially ycT4: be careful with staging of the cancer.

References

[1] Hartl DM, Ferlito A, Brasnu DF, et al. Evidence-based review of treatment options for patients with glottic cancer. Head Neck. 2011; 33(11):1638–1648

[2] Mendenhall WM, Parsons JT, Mancuso AA, Stringer SP, Cassisi NJ. Radiotherapy for squamous cell carcinoma of the supraglottic larynx: an alternative to surgery. Head Neck. 1996; 18(1):24–35

[3] Hinerman RW, Mendenhall WM, Amdur RJ, Stringer SP, Villaret DB, Robbins KT. Carcinoma of the supraglottic larynx: treatment results with radiotherapy alone or with planned neck dissection. Head Neck. 2002; 24(5):456–467

[4] Laccourreye O, Weinstein G, Naudo P, Cauchois R, Laccourreye H, Brasnu D. Supracricoid partial laryngectomy after failed laryngeal radiation therapy. Laryngoscope. 1996; 106(4):495–498

[5] Forastiere AA, Ismaila N, Lewin JS, et al. Use of larynx-preservation strategies in the treatment of laryngeal cancer: American Society of Clinical Oncology Clinical Practice Guideline Update. J Clin Oncol. 201 8; 36(11):1143–1169

[6] Fink DS, Sibley H, Kunduk M, et al. Functional outcomes after salvage transoral laser microsurgery for laryngeal squamous cell carcinoma. Otolaryngol Head Neck Surg. 2016; 155(4):606–611

[7] Chen MM, Holsinger FC, Laccourreye O. Salvage conservation laryngeal surgery after radiation therapy failure. Otolaryngol Clin North Am. 2015; 48(4):667–675

[8] Steiner W, Vogt P, Ambrosch P, Kron M. Transoral carbon dioxide laser microsurgery for recurrent glottic carcinoma after radiotherapy. Head Neck. 2004; 26(6):477–484

[9] Del Bon F, Piazza C, Mangili S, Redaelli De Zinis LO, Nicolai P, Peretti G. Transoral laser surgery for recurrent glottic cancer after radiotherapy: oncologic and functional outcomes. Acta Otorhinolaryngol Ital. 2012; 32(4):229–237

[10] Ansarin M, Planicka M, Rotundo S, et al. Endoscopic carbon dioxide laser surgery for glottic cancer recurrence after

radiotherapy: oncological results. Arch Otolaryngol Head Neck Surg. 2007; 133(12):1193–1197

[11] Shah JP, Loree TR, Kowalski L. Conservation surgery for radiation-failure carcinoma of the glottic larynx. Head Neck. 1990; 12(4):326–331

[12] Zbären P, Nuyens M, Curschmann J, Stauffer E. Histologic characteristics and tumor spread of recurrent glottic carcinoma: analysis on whole-organ sections and comparison with tumor spread of primary glottic carcinomas. Head Neck. 2007; 29(1):26–32

[13] Preda L, Conte G, Bonello L, et al. Diagnostic accuracy of surface coil MRI in assessing cartilaginous invasion in laryngeal tumours: do we need contrast-agent administration? Eur Radiol. 2017; 27(11):4690–4698

[14] Meulemans J, Delaere P, Nuyts S, Clement PM, Hermans R, Vander Poorten V. Salvage transoral laser microsurgery for radiorecurrent laryngeal cancer: indications, limits, and outcomes. Curr Otorhinolaryngol Rep. 2017; 5(1):83–91

25 Salvage Surgery after Radiotherapy: Supracricoid Laryngectomy

Sandro J. Stoeckli

Abstract

Conservation surgery in the form of transoral laser microsurgery and open partial laryngectomy is increasingly used for salvage of recurrent cancer of the larynx following radiation therapy in order to avoid the sequelae of total laryngectomy. Supracricoid partial laryngectomy with cricohyoidoepiglottopexy or cricohyoidopexy has been proven to be oncologically sound and to provide satisfactory voice and swallowing function in this setting. Keys to success are correct selection of patients and cancer, experience with this technically demanding surgery, and swallowing rehabilitation with a team of dedicated speech and swallowing therapists. Review of the literature reveals good oncological outcome of supracricoid partial laryngectomy as salvage procedure after failure of radiation in very well selected patient cohorts. Conversion to total laryngectomy either during surgery due to unexpected tumor extension or postoperatively due to failed swallowing rehabilitation has to be discussed with the patient.

Keywords: supracricoid partial laryngectomy, CHEP, laryngeal cancer, recurrence, salvage surgery, partial laryngectomy

25.1 Case Report

A 71-year-old Caucasian male presented with progressive hoarseness over a period of 3 months. The patient denied any pain, swallowing was normal without clinical signs for aspiration, and there was no dyspnea. He stated having stopped smoking cigarettes 10 years ago with an estimated cumulative consumption of 40 pack-years. The patient experienced a myocardial infarction 2 years ago and has been under medication with aspirin since that time.

At consultation, the patient presented in good general health, but with a severely hoarse voice. Laryngoscopy revealed an exophytic lesion of the anterior part of both vocal folds with extension to the anterior commissure (▶ Fig. 25.1). There was no supraglottic or subglottic extension of the tumor. On videostroboscopy, there was an impaired motility of the right vocal cord. Vocal fold vibration was totally absent.

High-resolution computed tomography (CT) of the larynx demonstrated a tumor involving both vocal ligaments anteriorly with invasion of the anterior commissure (▶ Fig. 25.2).

The tumor was staged cT2 cN0. Because of bilateral vocal fold invasion, the patient underwent primary radiation of the larynx. Unfortunately, the tumor recurred within the first year after completion of radiotherapy. The recurrent cancer had

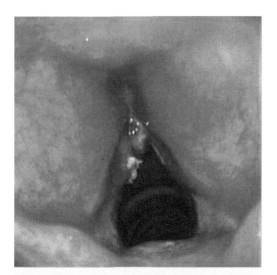

Fig. 25.1 Laryngoscopic view of the larynx.

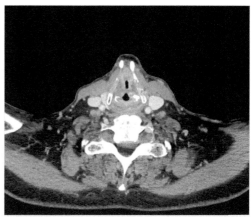

Fig. 25.2 Axial CT of the larynx.

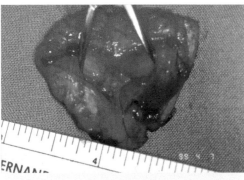
Fig. 25.3 Laryngeal resection specimen.

almost exactly the same extension as prior to therapy. No subglottic extension was noted on endoscopy. CT revealed no extralaryngeal spread. The cancer was staged rT2 rN0. Due to deep invasion of the anterior commissure and inadequate exposure on endoscopy TLM was judged as not feasible. The patient was in good general health with normal pulmonary function. After thorough discussion with the patient and his family and Multidisciplinary Tumor Board decision, the patient was offered supracricoid partial laryngectomy (SCPL). The patient was also consented for total laryngectomy in case unexpected extension of the cancer was discovered intraoperatively. A percutaneous endoscopic gastrostomy (PEG) tube was placed at the beginning of surgery. The SCPL with cricohyoidoepiglottopexy (CHEP) was uneventful and frozen sections of the margins at the cricoid showed clear resection margins (▶ Fig. 25.3). There were no complications during the postoperative course, and the patient was decannulated 4 weeks after surgery. Swallowing rehabilitation was prolonged with PEG removal after 5 months. The patient had a good but hoarse voice. Currently, he is doing well with no evidence of cancer after 3 years.

25.2 Discussion

In the last decades, organ-preservation strategies have been increasingly used in the treatment of cancer of the larynx. The number of total laryngectomies as initial treatment has dramatically decreased in most parts of the world. Progress in radiation technology and the introduction of chemotherapy as an adjunct to radiation has led to the increased use of nonsurgical therapy strategies in laryngeal oncology. The widespread use

of transoral laser microsurgery (TLM) and the advances in open partial laryngectomies have diminished the number of total laryngectomies. The ultimate goal of all these achievements was to equal the excellent tumor control provided by total laryngectomy, but to preserve the organ's function.

Treatment options for residual or recurrent cancer after primary radiation or chemoradiation include total laryngectomy, open partial laryngectomy, and TLM.[1] The primary treatment choice in the radiorecurrent setting in most centers even nowadays is total laryngectomy. In contrast to other head and neck subsites, the larynx yields a favorable outcome after salvage surgery with overall survival rates above 60%.[2] Diagnosis and management of recurrent cancer of the larynx remains challenging due to postradiation chronic inflammation, edema, and fibrosis. Tumor extension is difficult to visualize and even getting a reliable biopsy often proves to be difficult. Larynx sparing surgical procedures for a radiorecurrent cancer have been recently reported with encouraging results. Conservation surgery has been compared to total laryngectomy in a series of 726 salvage patients from the National Cancer Database in the United States.[3] All patients presented with initial T1 or T2 lesions prior to radiation. Slightly more than 7% of patients required salvage surgery, 24% receiving total laryngectomy, 35.1% open partial laryngectomy, and 40.9% TLM. In this selected cohort, conservation surgery by either open partial laryngectomy or TLM yielded comparable outcome to total laryngectomy. In a series from Italy of 71 patients, 31% of patients with recurrence after primary radiation underwent TLM, 21% open partial laryngectomy, and 48% total laryngectomy.[4] There was no statistically significant difference in terms of disease-free survival between the three groups. In a systematic review and meta-analysis evaluating the outcome of TLM for radiorecurrent laryngeal carcinoma, the pooled mean estimates for local control at 24 months were 56.9% after first TLM and 63.8% after repeat TLM and the pooled mean laryngeal preservation 72.3%.[5] The authors conclude that TLM for recurrent laryngeal cancer is an oncologically sound procedure in very well selected patients with earlier stage (rT1/2) lesions. In summary, early-stage recurrences of cancer of the larynx are suitable for conservation surgery in a subset of very well selected patients, either by TLM in case of well-circumscribed lesions with adequate laryngeal exposure or by open partial laryngectomy.

SCPL is an open partial laryngectomy procedure that involves the resection of the entire larynx and impaction of the hyoid bone with the cricoid ring. In case of preservation of the suprahyoid part of the epiglottis, the reconstruction is a CHEP, and in case of total resection of the epiglottis a cricohyoidopexy (CHP). Initially described by Majer and Rieder in 1959 and further developed in France and other European countries, the SCPL was mainly used for initial treatment of glottic and supraglottic cancer avoiding the permanent tracheostoma of a total laryngectomy.[6] The technique proved to be oncologically sound even for advanced (T3) cancer and provided good function with regard to swallowing and voice.[7,8,9]

SCPL has also been advocated in recent years for the management of recurrent laryngeal cancer after primary radiation. The advantages of SCPL over total laryngectomy are the avoidance of a permanent stoma and the preservation of voice. As in the primary setting, SCPL is only suited for a select group of cancers. Subglottic extension to the level of the cricoid, invasion of the hyoid bone, fixation of the arytenoids, and extralaryngeal spread are contraindications. From the patient side, inability to adhere to postoperative rehabilitation of swallowing and speech and compromised respiratory function are factors against a SCPL. In a report by Sperry et al, 96 patients undergoing SCPL for primary laryngeal cancer in 54, and recurrent laryngeal cancer in 42 cases, have been evaluated.[10] Out of the 42 recurrent cases, 23 were staged rT1, 12 rT2, 6 rT3, and 1 rT4. The 5-year local control rate with larynx preservation was 89%, while the ultimate 5-year local control rate with total laryngectomy in case of recurrence 100%. A recent systematic review and meta-analysis of SCPL for radiorecurrent laryngeal cancer revealed promising results.[11] Only patients with tumors staged rT2 and rT3 were included. The pooled local control rate, disease-free survival, and overall survival for all 251 patients out of 11 studies achieved 92, 80, and 79%, respectively. The mean pooled larynx preservation rate was 85.2%, the mean pooled decannulation rate was 92.1%, the pooled mean rate of efficient swallowing was 96.5%, the pooled mean PEG dependence rate was 3.5%, and the pooled mean aspiration pneumonia rate was 6.4%. Total laryngectomy due to chronic aspiration was necessary in only two cases. The authors concluded that SCPL is a valid option in radiorecurrent cancer of the larynx with excellent oncological and functional outcome. Indications include rT1 and rT2 lesions with limited endoscopic exposure and/or invasion of the anterior commissure, rT2 lesions with impaired vocal cord mobility, and rT3 lesions with limited invasion of the paraglottic and pre-epiglottic space and no extralaryngeal extension.

The major concern in SCPL is functional outcome, in particular swallowing function. Swallowing is a fundamental function heavily impacting the patient's quality of life. Aspiration pneumonia is a potentially life-threatening complication. The reluctance in performing SCPL is even higher in the radiorecurrent setting because of functional concerns and fear from complications. In a comparison of 82 SCPL for radiation failures versus untreated cases, there were no statistical differences with regard to postoperative complications and functional outcomes as assessed for decannulation rate, swallowing, and phonation.[12] A similar comparison in another study in 27 patients confirmed these good results.[13] In contrast to these favorable results, there are also studies in the literature that report on high rates of surgical complications, prolonged swallowing rehabilitation, and frequent aspiration pneumonias.[14,15,16,17,18,19] In summary, most authors agree on SCPL to be an oncologically sound and also with regard to complications and functional outcome valid option in the setting of a radiorecurrent laryngeal cancer. To select the right patient with the right cancer seems to be the key for success.

25.3 Tips

- Choose the right patient: Sufficient pulmonary function, good performance status, and sufficient cognitive function for prolonged swallowing rehabilitation. Otherwise, opt for total laryngectomy
- Choose the right cancer: Indications include rT1 and rT2 lesions not suited for TLM with or without invasion of the anterior commissure, rT2 lesions with impaired vocal cord mobility, and rT3 lesions with limited invasion of the paraglottic and pre-epiglottic space. Fixation of the arytenoids, extralaryngeal spread, and extended subglottic invasion are contraindications.
- Swallowing rehabilitation after SCPL requires a dedicated and experienced team of speech and swallowing therapists.

- Consider upfront PEG instead of nasogastric tube insertion.
- Always consent the patient for total laryngectomy in case of unexpected tumor extension detected during surgery. Use frozen sections to assure resection with free margins, in particular at the cricoid margin.
- Perfect alignment of hyoid and cricoid is crucial for wound closure and function.

25.4 Traps

- Be careful with preoperative imaging. Imaging might underestimate extension of the cancer because of postradiation alterations.
- Failure of postoperative swallowing rehabilitation may lead to completion laryngectomy. The patient should be made aware of this.
- Failure of anterior fixation of arytenoids to the cricoid ring can be the cause for poor voice quality and aspiration.

References

[1] Fried M, Ferlito A, eds. Part V. Neoplasms of the larynx. In: The Management of Recurrent Laryngeal Cancer. The Larynx. 3rd ed. San Diego, CA: Plural Publishing Inc.; 2009

[2] Goodwin WJ, Jr. Salvage surgery for patients with recurrent squamous cell carcinoma of the upper aerodigestive tract: when do the ends justify the means? Laryngoscope. 2000; 110(3, pt 2, suppl 93):1–18

[3] Cheraghlou S, Kuo P, Mehra S, Yarbrough WG, Judson BL. Salvage surgery after radiation failure in T1/T2 larynx cancer: outcomes following total versus conservation surgery. Otolaryngol Head Neck Surg. 2018; 158(3):497–504

[4] Piazza C, Peretti G, Cattaneo A, Garrubba F, De Zinis LO, Nicolai P. Salvage surgery after radiotherapy for laryngeal cancer: from endoscopic resections to open-neck partial and total laryngectomies. Arch Otolaryngol Head Neck Surg. 2007; 133(10):1037–1043

[5] Ramakrishnan Y, Drinnan M, Kwong FN, et al. Oncologic outcomes of transoral laser microsurgery for radiorecurrent laryngeal carcinoma: a systematic review and meta-analysis of English-language literature. Head Neck. 2014; 36(2):280–285

[6] Majer EH, Rieder W. Technique de laryngectomie permettant de conserver la perméabilité respiratoire:la crico-hyoido-pexie. Ann Otolaryngol Chir Cervicofac. 1959; 76:677–683

[7] Mannelli G, Lazio MS, Luparello P, Gallo O. Conservative treatment for advanced T3–T4 laryngeal cancer: meta-analysis of key oncological outcomes. Eur Arch Otorhinolaryngol. 2018; 275(1):27–38

[8] Gallo A, Manciocco V, Simonelli M, Pagliuca G, D'Arcangelo E, de Vincentiis M. Supracricoid partial laryngectomy in the treatment of laryngeal cancer: univariate and multivariate analysis of prognostic factors. Arch Otolaryngol Head Neck Surg. 2005; 131(7):620–625

[9] Dufour X, Hans S, De Mones E, Brasnu D, Ménard M, Laccourreye O. Local control after supracricoid partial laryngectomy for "advanced" endolaryngeal squamous cell carcinoma classified as T3. Arch Otolaryngol Head Neck Surg. 2004; 130(9):1092–1099

[10] Sperry SM, Rassekh CH, Laccourreye O, Weinstein GS. Supracricoid partial laryngectomy for primary and recurrent laryngeal cancer. JAMA Otolaryngol Head Neck Surg. 2013; 139(11):1226–1235

[11] De Virgilio A, Pellini R, Mercante G, et al. Supracricoid partial laryngectomy for radiorecurrent laryngeal cancer: a systematic review of the literature and meta-analysis. Eur Arch Otorhinolaryngol. 2018

[12] Pellini R, Manciocco V, Spriano G. Functional outcome of supracricoid partial laryngectomy with cricohyoidopexy: radiation failure vs previously untreated cases. Arch Otolaryngol Head Neck Surg. 2006; 132(11):1221–1225

[13] Bussu F, Galli J, Valenza V, et al. Evaluation of swallowing function after supracricoid laryngectomy as a primary or salvage procedure. Dysphagia. 2015; 30(6):686–694

[14] Pellini R, Pichi B, Ruscito P, et al. Supracricoid partial laryngectomies after radiation failure: a multi-institutional series. Head Neck. 2008; 30(3):372–379

[15] León X, López M, García J, Viza I, Orús C, Quer M. Supracricoid laryngectomy as salvage surgery after failure of radiation therapy. Eur Arch Otorhinolaryngol. 2007; 264(7):809–814

[16] Laccourreye O, Weinstein G, Naudo P, Cauchois R, Laccourreye H, Brasnu D. Supracricoid partial laryngectomy after failed laryngeal radiation therapy. Laryngoscope. 1996; 106(4):495–498

[17] Marchese-Ragona R, Marioni G, Chiarello G, Staffieri A, Pastore A. Supracricoid laryngectomy with cricohyoidopexy for recurrence of early-stage glottic carcinoma after irradiation. Long-term oncological and functional results. Acta Otolaryngol. 2005; 125(1):91–95

[18] Sewnaik A, Hakkesteegt MM, Meeuwis CA, de Gier HH, Kerrebijn JD. Supracricoid partial laryngectomy with cricohyoidoepiglottopexy for recurrent laryngeal cancer. Ann Otol Rhinol Laryngol. 2006; 115(6):419–424

[19] Makeieff M, Venegoni D, Mercante G, Crampette L, Guerrier B. Supracricoid partial laryngectomies after failure of radiation therapy. Laryngoscope. 2005; 115(2):353–357

26 Salvage Surgery after Radiotherapy: Total Laryngectomy

Fabio Ferreli, Giuseppe Mercante, Giuseppe Spriano

Abstract

Radiotherapy for cT1 and cT2 and selected cases of cT3 laryngeal carcinoma is widely used. The recurrence of laryngeal cancer following (chemo) radiotherapy offers ample possibilities for surgical salvage options, if compared to other sites of the head and neck, but various factors must be considered. The diagnosis and staging of laryngeal relapses remains a challenging task. Differentiating between radiation reaction such as edema, fibrosis, and soft-tissue and cartilage necrosis, and recurrent cancer is a difficult clinical and radiological issue. Laryngeal cancer recurs more frequently in the primary site (T) than in cervical lymph nodes (N) or at distance (M). Radiorecurrent cancer is more aggressive due to its high propensity to infiltrate surrounding tissue, are less differentiated lesions, and have typical histological growth pattern with multifocal, lymphovascular and perineural infiltration. For these reasons, in the majority of cases, salvage total laryngectomy (STL) is the only choice in case of persistent/recurrent advanced cancer of the larynx after organ preservation protocols. STL is technically more difficult than primary laryngectomy and is associated with a higher number of complications such as hematoma, edema, suture dehiscence, subcutaneous abscess, and tissue necrosis with consequent pharyngocutaneous fistula (PCF). A second surgical procedure for closing the PCF may be necessary if wound dressing and spontaneous healing are not adequate. Surgical pearls and suggestions have been proposed for preventing PCF; nonetheless, pedicle or free flap harvesting from nonirradiated areas is one of the most commonly used techniques.

Keywords: salvage total laryngectomy, radiotherapy failure, recurrent laryngeal cancer, pharyngocutaneous fistula

26.1 Case Report

A 66-year-old male ex-cigarette smoker was affected by squamous cell carcinoma of the larynx involving the right vocal cord and the homolateral supraglottic regions, extending to the posterior commissure and the right arytenoid. An MRI scan was performed, confirming posterior extension of the cancer, involving the posterior commissure and the right arytenoid, in conjunction with osteosclerotic aspects of the same arytenoid. The paraglottic space was involved as the anterior commissure, without erosion of the perichondrium of the thyroid cartilage. The lesion was in close contact with the cricoarytenoid joint and the thyroarytenoid space was obliterated. No subglottic extension of the cancer was identified (▶ Fig. 26.1). The cancer was staged as cT3N0-G2. Following a multidisciplinary team assessment, radiotherapy (RT) was delivered. Two weeks before starting RT, the patient presented severe acute dyspnea and an emergency tracheostomy was carried out. The patient was treated with intensity-modulated radiation therapy (IMRT) with a total dose of 70 Gy to the tumor, 63 Gy to the peristomal region and 58 Gy to the bilateral neck (levels II–V). Four months following RT, the MRI showed a recurrent/persistent lesion involving the right glottic and supraglottic region, with infiltration of the paraglottic space but without erosion of the thyroid cartilage. The posterior commissure was involved by the cancer with contralateral extension to the left posterior paraglottic space. The lesion extended also inferiorly into the subglottic region, both anteriorly and posteriorly (▶ Fig. 26.2a,b). The tumor was

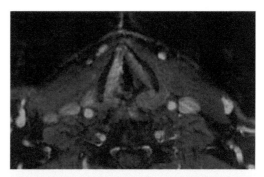

Fig. 26.1 The axial MRI showed a right vocal cord tumor with involvement of the homolateral paraglottic space, the right arytenoid, and the posterior commissure.

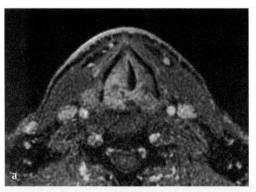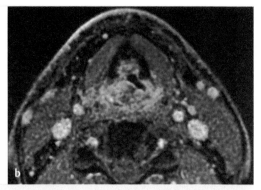

Fig. 26.2 The axial plane of the MRI performed after 4 months from the end of radiotherapy showed a persistent lesion in the right glottic plane with infiltration of the paraglottic space (a). The lesion involved the posterior commissure. The right arytenoid was not identifiable because it was completely subverted by the tumor. The lesion extended inferiorly in the anterior and posterior hypoglottic space (b).

restaged as yrcT4aN0. Biopsies in microlaryngoscopy confirmed recurrence; therefore, salvage total laryngectomy (STL) was planned. Bilateral neck dissections, total laryngectomy, and prophylactic temporoparietal myofascial free flap was harvested to reinforce the pharyngeal closure in order to prevent complications such as pharyngocutaneous fistula (PCF).

26.2 Surgical Technique

The patient was placed in the head extended position. The surgical procedure was performed under general anaesthesia, with intubation through the previous tracheostomy. A nasogastric feeding tube (NGFT) was inserted.

A traditional "apron" incision was performed, which consisted of a bilateral curvilinear midneck incision incorporated with the planned skin excision of the previous tracheotomy. This incision allows to adequately expose the contents of the lateral neck for bilateral selective neck dissection (levels II–IV). After completing the neck dissection, the thyroid gland was released from the trachea on both sides, completely sectioning the isthmus. In this case, there was no suspicion of anterior spread of the tumor; otherwise, the hemithyroid with tumor involvement is left attached to the larynx and is removed along with it. The superior laryngeal artery and vein were identified at the level of the thyrohyoid membrane and sectioned bilaterally. Inferior constrictor muscles were exposed and incised at the insertion on the posterior border of the thyroid cartilage; thus, the superior cornu was skeletonized, thereby releasing the larynx. The hyoid bone was cranially identified and preserved.

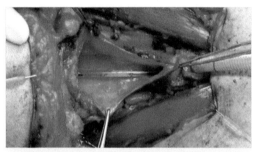

Fig. 26.3 The pharyngeal defect after total laryngectomy and before the primary closure.

The hyothyroepiglottic space was dissected and the thyrohyoid membrane was incised at the inferior border of the hyoid bone, in order to access the valleculae. The inferior limit of the resection was performed at the level of the third tracheal ring as needed considering the previous tracheostomy and the subglottic extension of the cancer. The posterior portion of the cricoid was dissected out of the overlying mucosa. The laryngeal frame was finally detached from the anterior esophageal wall through a pharyngotomy (▶Fig. 26.3). A T-shaped closure of the pharynx was carried out. A second layer closure was performed using the inferior constrictor muscles. Finally, the tracheostomy was harvested. The temporoparietal fascia free flap was harvested and insert directly over the pharyngeal closure (▶Fig. 26.4a, b).

Bilateral cervical and right temporal drains were inserted. The postoperative period was uneventful and the drains were removed within 3 days. Oral intake of liquids started 3 weeks after surgery. The period of hospitalization was 30 days.

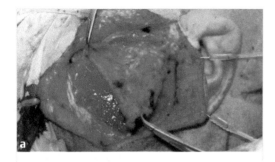

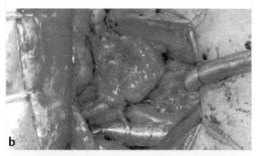

Fig. 26.4 Harvesting technique of the temporoparietal fascia free flap and closure of the pharyngeal defect. Based on the superficial temporal artery and vein, the temporoparietal fascia is elevated (**a**). Temporoparietal fascia is used as a patch and is positioned over the pharyngeal suture to support it (**b**).

The final pathology report showed yrpT4aN0 squamous cell laryngeal carcinoma (G1) with free margins.

No local complications were observed nor any other comorbidities occured. The patient did not have any symptoms of pharyngeal stenosis.

26.3 Discussion

Since publishing the study by the Veterans Affairs Laryngeal Cancer Study Group[1] and the Radiation Therapy Oncology Group Trial 91–11,[2] there has been a shift from primary surgery to an increase in (chemo)radiotherapy as the primary treatment of advanced cancer of the larynx. Concurrent treatment regimens using cisplatin-based chemoradiotherapy have emerged as the preferred treatment choice for organ preservation in case of advanced laryngeal cancer, with adequate healing rates and improved quality of life for many patients.[3] Despite the development of organ-preservation strategies, there still are patients who require surgical salvage due to treatment failure. In fact, persistent or local recurrence of the cancer primary occurs in approximately 30% of patients with advanced cancer of the

larynx submitted to nonsurgical organ-preservation treatments.[1] As a result, STL is now most often performed in cases of recurrent cancer or incomplete cancer response to nonsurgical treatment. Conservation surgery (open partial laryngectomies or endoscopic procedures) with preservation of voice and deglutition has been the treatment option of choice for initial recurrences or cancer of the larynx that present in stages rT1 and rT2, although selected cases of rT3 cancer may also be eligible for these procedures and have been included in the published series.[4,5,6] Radio-recurrent tumors are more aggressive due to the high propensity for infiltrating surrounding tissue, moreover are less differentiated lesions and have typical histological growth pattern aspects with multifocal foci and lymphovascular and perineural infiltration.[7] For these reasons STL remains the standard treatment for advanced recurrent/residual local cancer of the larynx after (chemo) radiotherapy. Regarding the oncological outcomes, Sandulache et al demonstrated that only nodal status at the time of STL and the time between completion of initial nonsurgical treatment and STL (disease-free interval) correlated with overall survival (OS) and time to recurrence via univariate and multivariate analyses.[8]

The role of elective neck dissection during STL remains unclear. Although some authors have illustrated improved survival outcomes with elective neck dissection,[8,10,11] others have demonstrated no benefits.[8,12,13] In the Sandulache study of a subset of 201 patients without preoperative evidence of neck disease, 13 patients developed regional recurrence after STL and neck dissection (13 of 95; 14%) compared with 15 patients who developed regional recurrence after STL without neck dissection (15 of 106; 14%; p = NS). Therefore, the authors have not found any demonstrable benefits of the elective neck dissection.[9]

Salvage surgery is technically more difficult than primary surgery and is associated with a higher number of complications such as hematoma, edema, suture dehiscence, subcutaneous abscess, and tissue necrosis with consequent PCF. A recent review demonstrated an overall complication rate of 67.5% and the PCF was the most frequently reported complication of STL with a pooled incidence of 28.9%.[14]

Salivary fistulas may occur in patients undergoing salvage surgery for laryngohypopharyngeal cancer after (chemo)radiotherapy. RT and chemotherapy target cancer cells, but, in spite of modern techniques, the surrounding healthy tissue is irradiated as well. Tissue damaged by radiation must undergo repair. During the repair process, the injured tissue may be replaced by normal functioning tissue. On the other hand, tissue repair mechanisms may cause replacement of normal tissue with fibrotic tissue. Tissues become noncompliant, contracted, and atrophic, resulting in altered function and significant symptom burden. Surgery is a further insult and previously irradiated tissue may not heal. After chemoradiotherapy, there is a time window (usually from 4 to 6 weeks after the end of treatment until 4–5 months into follow-up) in which salvage surgery may be undertaken with limited or no additional morbidity. In the postoperative period, hypoxic and avascular irradiated normal tissues may not be able to heal after further surgical damage. This aspect leads to complications, such as suture dehiscence and subsequent fistulas. Basheeth et al demonstrated that performance of STL within 1 year after completion of RT and performing concomitant bilateral neck dissection were significant risk factors for the development of salivary fistulas.[15] Other surgeons reported complications which include wound infections, pharyngeal stenosis/stricture, stomal stenosis, and tracheoesophageal fistula.[14] Given the increased patient morbidity, prolonged hospitalization, knowledge of the incidence of these type of complications is crucial for pretreatment counseling.

The most commonly used reconstruction modalities are pedicled pectoralis major muscle flaps (PMMFs) and fasciocutaneous free flaps (FFF) such as radial forearm flap and anterolateral thigh flap.

Guimarães et al in a recent review analyzed the efficacy of prophylactic use of PMMF to reduce the PCF rate, including data from 12 observational retrospective studies (742 patients; 253 in the PMMF group and 489 in the control group). The incidence of PCF was 30.9%. The practical use of PMMF decreases the risk of the incidence of fistula of approximately 22%, proving the rationale for the elective use of the PMMF as well-vascularized, nonirradiated tissue for safer closure of the pharynx.[16] The muscle flap is generally harvested while the pharynx is being closed, thus adding minimal operative time. Being a regional pedicle flap, the PMMF does not require a separate reconstructive team or microvascular experience. Other advantages include reduced operative time and hospital costs and resources, low failure rate, and abundance of tissue. However, there are disadvantages: reduced neck mobility, the need to rotate the vascular pedicle when using the skin paddle, and the thickness of the flap, possibly leading to

a reduction in swallowing function. In a recent study, Nguyen and Thuot demonstrated that FFF reconstruction led to better functional outcomes than PMMF reconstruction regarding swallowing function, with similar rates of postoperative complications.[17] There is also the potential donor site morbidity after harvesting the PMMF, such as shoulder dysfunction, impaired postlaryngectomy speech due to the presence of muscle over the neopharynx, and excessive muscle bulk, which may be cosmetically less acceptable and may result in the inability to close the neck incisions. In contrast, the FFF presents a higher relative freedom of movement due to a higher versatility of inset. In this case, we performed a temporoparietal fascia flap, which was described by Higgins et al in 12 patients.[18] This is an interesting free flap, which has some advantages. This flap is thin and pliable and adequate in size, but with limited pedicle length. The inherent thin and pliable nature brings this very robust vascular network in close proximity to the neopharyngeal suture line in order to promote neovascularization. Finally, harvesting of this flap is associated with no significant donor site morbidity, in comparison to the PMMF or the radial forearm flap. Classic STL using transcervical approach requires wide surgical exposure in order to stage the neck dissection. The common skin flap is a superior base "apron-shaped" flap including the skin, the subcutaneous adipose tissue, and the platysma muscle that are detached from the cervical fascia. Recently, our group proposed a minimally invasive lateral cervical approach in order to reduce the surgical trauma on the neck harvesting an anterior myocutaneous (AMC) flap.[19,20,21] This lateral cervical approach is feasible for salvage STL as well as for most challenging cases, which needed a circular pharyngolaryngectomy.[21] In a recent study, the pectoralis major myocutaneous pedicle flap was harvested to complete the circumference of the digestive tube because the pharyngeal mucosa was not sufficient for direct closure. In spite of this, all the surgical steps (neck dissection, laryngopharyngeal resection, reconstruction) were performed through a single 8-cm lateral cervical incision. The AMC flap has the advantage of sparing healthy tissue. The preservation of the hyoid bone and its muscle insertions contribute to respecting tissue for covering the suture line. Another advantage could be represented by a better cosmetic profile of the lateral neck avoiding the posterior retraction of the classic TL. This surgical procedure seems to be indicated in laryngeal and hypopharyngeal tumors without anterior spread outside the external perichondrium and/or invasion of the hyoid bone or its inserted muscles, as both upfront and/or salvage surgery. Further studies are needed to confirm the advantages in terms of reduction of PCF compared to other techniques.

26.4 Tips

- When planning salvage surgical treatment, it is mandatory to consider the initial extent of the cancer.
- After open conservative surgery on the larynx, such as vertical or horizontal laryngectomies (types I, II, or III of the European Laryngological Society classification), it is reasonable to perform an aggressive surgery such as total laryngectomy due to the modification of the anatomical boundaries for the spread of the cancer.
- In case of STL after (chemo)radiotherapy, it is necessary to use a nonirradiated vascularized flap (pedicled or free flaps) to prevent local complications, such as PCF.

26.5 Traps

- Clinico-radiological evaluation of the larynx after (chemo)radiotherapy remains challenging despite the use of endoscopies and modern imaging; therefore, it is difficult to define the tumor stage of the cancer.
- Recurrent/persistent cancer of the larynx after (chemo)radiotherapy has a pattern of features of local invasion less predictable than cancer arising de novo.
- STL has been associated with high rates of postoperative local complications, especially after chemoradiotherapy, such as PCF, operative wound infection, and bleeding.

References

[1] Wolf GT, Fisher SG, Hong WK, et al; Department of Veterans Affairs Laryngeal Cancer Study Group. Induction chemotherapy plus radiation compared with surgery plus radiation in patients with advanced laryngeal cancer. N Engl J Med. 1991; 324(24):1685–1690

[2] Weber RS, Berkey BA, Forastiere A, et al. Outcome of salvage total laryngectomy following organ preservation therapy: the Radiation Therapy Oncology Group trial 91–11. Arch Otolaryngol Head Neck Surg. 2003; 129(1):44–49

[3] Forastiere AA, Goepfert H, Maor M, et al. Concurrent chemotherapy and radiotherapy for organ preservation in advanced laryngeal cancer. N Engl J Med. 2003; 349(22):2091–2098

[4] Spriano G, Piantanida R, Maffioli M. Salvage surgery after unsuccessful radiotherapy of cancer of the larynx Acta Otorhinolaryngol Ital. 1989; 9(2):161–168

[5] Spriano G, Pellini R, Romano G, Muscatello L, Roselli R. Supracricoid partial laryngectomy as salvage surgery after radiation failure. Head Neck. 2002; 24(8):759–765

[6] Pellini R, Pichi B, Ruscito P, et al. Supracricoid partial laryngectomies after radiation failure: a multi-institutional series. Head Neck. 2008; 30(3):372–379

[7] Zbären P, Nuyens M, Curschmann J, Stauffer E. Histologic characteristics and tumor spread of recurrent glottic carcinoma: analysis on whole-organ sections and comparison with tumor spread of primary glottic carcinomas Head Neck. 2007; 29:26–32

[8] Sandulache VC, Vandelaar LJ, Skinner HD, et al. Salvage total laryngectomy after external-beam radiotherapy: a 20-year experience. Head Neck. 2016; 38(suppl 1):E1962–E1968

[9] Hilly O, Gil Z, Goldhaber D, et al. Elective neck dissection during salvage total laryngectomy: a beneficial prognostic effect in locally advanced recurrent tumours. Clin Otolaryngol. 2015; 40(1):9–15

[10] Hilly O, Stern S, Horowitz E, Leshno M, Feinmesser R. Is there a role for elective neck dissection with salvage laryngectomy? A decision-analysis model. Laryngoscope. 2013; 123(11):2706–2711

[11] Koss SL, Russell MD, Leem TH, Schiff BA, Smith RV. Occult nodal disease in patients with failed laryngeal preservation undergoing surgical salvage. Laryngoscope. 2014; 124(2):421–428

[12] Basheeth N. Elective neck dissection for N0 neck during salvage total laryngectomy. JAMA Otolaryngol Head Neck Surg. 2013; 139(8):790–796

[13] Pezier TF, Nixon IJ, Scotton W, et al; Should elective neck dissection be routinely performed in patients undergoing salvage total laryngectomy? J Laryngol Otol. 2014; 128(3):279–283

[14] Hasan Z, Dwivedi RC, Gunaratne DA, Virk SA, Palme CE, Riffat F. Systematic review and meta-analysis of the complications of salvage total laryngectomy Eur J Surg Oncol. 2017; 43(1):42–51

[15] Basheeth N, O'Leary G, Sheahan P. Pharyngocutaneous fistula after salvage laryngectomy: impact of interval between radiotherapy and surgery, and performance of bilateral neck dissection. Head Neck. 2014; 36(4):580–584

[16] Guimarães AV, Aires FT, Dedivitis RA, et al. Efficacy of pectoralis major muscle flap for pharyngocutaneous fistula prevention in salvage total laryngectomy: a systematic review. Head Neck. 2016; 38(suppl 1):E2317–E2321

[17] Nguyen S, Thuot F. Functional outcomes of fasciocutaneous free flap and pectoralis major flap for salvage total laryngectomy. Head Neck. 2017; 39(9):1797–1805

[18] Higgins KM, Ashford B, Erovic BM, Yoo J, Enepekides DJ. Temporoparietal fascia free flap for pharyngeal coverage after salvage total laryngectomy. Laryngoscope. 2012; 122(3):523–527

[19] Spriano G, Mercante G, Pellini R, Ferreli F. Total laryngectomy: a new lateral cervical approach. Clin Otolaryngol. 2017; 43(2):784–785

[20] Spriano G, Mercante G, Cristalli G, Pellini R, Ferreli F. Lateral cervical approach for supracricoid partial laryngectomy. Am J Otolaryngol. 2017; 38(5):598–602

[21] Spriano G, Mercante G, Manciocco V, Cristalli G, Sanguineti G, Ferreli F. A new lateral cervical approach for salvage total laryngo-pharyngectomy. Acta Otorhinolaryngol Ital. 2017

27 Strategy for Avoiding Pharyngocutaneous Fistula: Pectoralis Muscle Flap for Salvage Total Laryngectomy

Pankaj Chaturvedi, Manish Mair

Abstracts

There has been a paradigm shift in the primary management of cancer of the larynx since the results of the Veterans Affairs and Radiation Therapy Oncology Group trials were published. This has led to an increase in the use of organ-preservation protocol (OPP) over laryngeal surgery. Subsequent failure after OPP requires salvage total laryngectomy. The complication rate following salvage total laryngectomy is higher than primary surgery, most probably, due to tissue fibrosis and obliterative endarteritis. The incidence of major and minor complications is reported between 52 and 59%. Pharyngocutaneous fistula (PCF) is the most common component of these complications. These complications increase hospitalization time, cost of treatment, and future incidence of pharyngeal stenosis, significantly impacting the quality of life of patients. There is robust evidence supporting the use of vascularized tissue in the closure of defects following salvage laryngectomy to decrease complications. The vascularized tissue can be a local flap, pedicle flap, or free flap. However, local flap based on sternocleidomastoid or infrahyoid musculature, being located in the radiation field, precludes their use in the salvage setting. These flaps can be used as an overlay or an interpositional flap. Overlay flaps are placed over the primary closure and interpositional flaps are primarily used to augment inadequate pharyngeal mucosa. Using options other than vascularized flaps such as good nutritional support, a salivary bypass tube, timing of starting oral feeds, and avoiding unnecessary neck dissections helps in decreasing the complication rates. In this chapter, we discuss the various strategies for avoiding PCF with a special emphasis on reconstruction using the pectoralis muscle flap in salvage laryngectomy.

Keywords: organ-preservation protocol, salvage laryngectomy, complications, vascularized flap, pharyngocutaneous fistula

27.1 Case Report

A 63-year-old retired farmer with no comorbidities, and euthyroid, retired farmer, presented with progressive hoarseness for the last 4 months. He had no history of aspiration or difficulty in breathing. He was a beedi smoker, smoking through one pack a day for 20 years as well as drinking socially. At the time of consultation, the patient had good Eastern Cooperative Oncology Group (ECOG) status and presented with a change in voice, having narrow vocal range. No abnormality was detected in the examination of oral cavity and cervical palpation. Examination with a Hopkins rod revealed an ulcero-infiltrative lesion in the entire left true and false vocal cord, which extended to the anterior commissure and reaching the ipsilateral arytenoids without involvement of infraglottis larynx. The mobility of the left vocal fold was restricted. For a better deeper evaluation, a CT scan was performed, which revealed an infiltrative, irregular lesion at the left vocal fold having heterogeneous contrast enhancement. It was seen that the lesion infiltrated the anterior commissure and posteriorly was reaching the ipsilateral arytenoid. There were no signs of extension to the right vocal fold, paraglottic space, and pre-epiglottis space. All the cartilages were intact. Microlaryngoscopy was performed and it was seen that the lesion was involving the anterior commissure, making its complete exposure difficult. Histology was confirmed as squamous cell carcinoma. The patient was diagnosed with cancer of the glottis staged as T2N0. In view of inadequate microlaryngoscopy exposure, the patient was not considered suitable for laser excision and he underwent radical radiation, which consisted of 70 Gy in 35 fractions. However, after a disease- and symptom-free interval of 1.5 year, he presented again with a progressive increase in hoarseness. He did not have any signs of aspiration or difficulty breathing. On Hopkins rod examination, the lesion was seen on the left vocal fold. It had similar extension as seen prior to the radiation. On direct laryngoscopy, the extent of the lesion was confirmed and it was found to have an infraglottic extension (▶ Fig. 27.1). The left cord was fixed and the right cord was edematous as a sequel to radiation. Biopsy confirmed recurrent cancer with PET contrast-enhanced CT (CECT) demonstrating fluorodeoxyglucose (FDG) avid lesion in the anterior commissure with erosion of the left lamina of the thyroid and exolaryngeal extension (▶Fig. 27.2). In view of its infraglottic extension, any form of conservative laryngeal surgery was not possible. The patient underwent total laryngectomy with primary closure of the remnant mucosa. Essentially, the steps of salvage total laryngectomy are similar to a routine total laryngectomy. However, in this case, an overlay pectoralis myofascial flap was used to cover the mucosal closure (▶Fig. 27.3). The patient had an uneventful satisfactory postoperative period. He was started on liquid diet on the 10th postoperative day. The nasogastric tube was removed on the 12th day after surgery. The final histopathological report is shown in ▶Fig. 27.4.

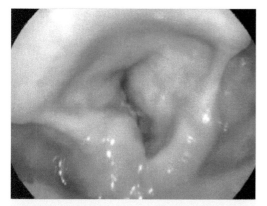

Fig. 27.1 Fiberoptic laryngoscopy finding post radical radiation.

27.2 Discussion

There has been a major shift in the management of laryngeal cancer from surgery to OPP. This paradigm shift occurred following publication of the results of Veterans Affairs (VA) Laryngeal Cancer Study Group[1] and Radiation Therapy Oncology Group (RTOG) 91–11[2] trials. They demonstrated that OPP had similar survival outcomes as compared to surgery and considering the morbidity associated with total laryngectomy, there was an obvious increase in the use of OPP. Subsequently, with the failure of OPP, there was an understandable rise in the rate of salvage laryngectomy. Stankovic et al[3] have shown poor survival with salvage laryngectomy as compared to primary laryngectomy. Apart from recurrence, salvage laryngectomy is also occasionally considered in cases of stage IV chondronecrosis (Chandler's classification)[4] with patients having debilitating symptoms. The reported major and minor complications associated with salvage laryngectomy ranged from 52 to 59% in view of previously irradiated tissue.[5] In the same study, the incidence of pharyngocutaneous fistula (PCF) was 15% after radiation only and 30% after chemoradiation. In a meta-analysis by Hasan et al, consisting of 50 studies and 3,292 patients, the overall complication rate was 67.5% and PCF was seen in 28.9% cases.[6] These complications lead to prolonged hospitalization, increased treatment costs, and potential need for reoperations. Therefore, it is

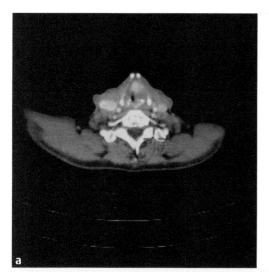
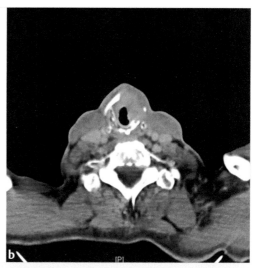

Fig. 27.2 (a, b) Axial images of PET-CECT scans after radical radiation treatment.

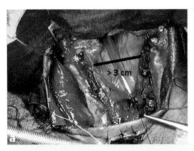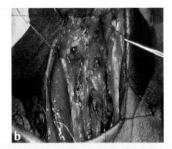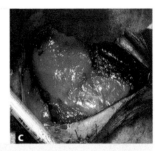

Fig. 27.3 **(a)** Adequate remnant pharyngeal mucosa for primary closure. **(b)** Primary closure of pharyngeal mucosa. **(c)** Overlay PMMF over primary closure of remnant pharyngeal mucosa.

Histopathology report

Poorly differentiated squamous cell carcinoma

Tumor size: 3 cm × 2 cm

Uni-focal tumor

Thyroid cartilage is involved

Thyroid gland is free

Closest cut margin is anterior soft tissue: 0.7 cm

No perineural invasion or lymphovascular emboli

Bilateral cervical lymph nodes: all reactive

Fig. 27.4 Histopathological report of the laryngectomy specimen.

crucial to discuss various preventive methods that can reduce these complication rates.

There are several predisposing factors to fistula formation such as preexisting comorbidities, pre- and postoperative low hemoglobin and albumin levels, tumor site and stage, concurrent neck dissection, hypothyroidism, etc. As per the VA trial,[1] the rate of salvage laryngectomy was higher in glottic cancer, fixed cords, cartilage erosion, T4, and stage IV cancers. The incidence of salvage laryngectomy in the VA trial was 36%. It was 28, 16, and 31% in patients who received neoadjuvant chemotherapy (NACT) followed by radiotherapy (RT), concurrent chemoradiotherapy (CCRT), and only RT, respectively, in RTOG-9111 trial.[2] Salvage laryngectomy was required within 2 years of completion of treatment in 80% of the cases. In a post hoc analysis of the laryngopharyngeal cancers in the TAX 324 trial, there was no significant difference in the incidence of salvage laryngectomy between two-drug (docetaxel and cisplatin [TP]) and three-drug (docetaxel, cisplatin, and fluorouracil [TPF]) groups (20 vs. 11%).[7]

27.2.1 Reduction in Leak Rate

Tissue fibrosis and obliterative endarteritis following radiation are major contributory factors increasing the incidence and severity of complications associated with salvage laryngectomy.[8] Pharyngeal stenosis is a long-term sequel that further impacts swallowing and voice of these patients. The use of a vascularized tissue flap has been studied extensively for reducing the rate of PCF. The flap can be interpositional or overlay. Overlay flap is used when adequate remnant pharyngeal mucosa is available for primary closure. A study by Hui et al in 1996 has shown that 1.5 cm relaxed and 2.5 cm stretch pharyngeal remnant mucosa are adequate for primary closure.[9] The interpositional flap is mainly used to augment inadequate pharyngeal remnant mucosa. However, it is preferred by a few institutes over onlay flap even when adequate pharyngeal remnant mucosa is available. The markings used for an interpositional flap is shown in ▶ Fig. 27.5.

Paleri et al[10] in a systemic review consisting of 591 patients suggested that there is a definite advantage in using vascularized tissue from outside the radiation field after salvage laryngectomy. Thus, local flaps based on sternocleidomastoid or infrahyoid musculature preclude their use in salvage setting[11,12] as they are within the radiation field. Another meta-analysis by Sayles and Grant[13] similarly showed that the rate of PCF after primary closure was 27.6%, which reduced significantly with a flap-reinforced closure (10.3%). A multi- institutional retrospective study[14] consisting of 359 patients from eight institutions also showed that the use of nonirradiated, vascularized flaps reduced the incidence and duration of fistula. The PCF rate was lowest with pectoralis

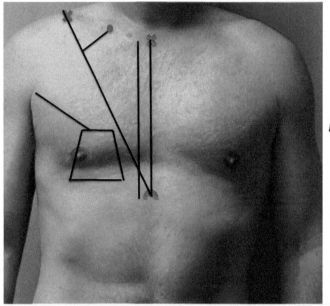

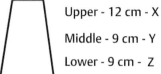

Upper - 12 cm - X

Middle - 9 cm - Y

Lower - 9 cm - Z

X = Mucosal width at BOT

Y = Mucosal width in middle part

Z = Mucosal width in lower part

Fig. 27.5 Marking of interpositional pectoralis myocutaneous flap.

onlay flap (15%) as compared to interposed free flap (25%) or primary closure (35%).

The vascularized flap can be a pectoralis major myofascial flap (PMMF) or a free flap. Comparing them, Chao et al reviewed 36 studies, with 301 patients reconstructed with PMMF and 605 patients with free flaps. Pooled-data analysis revealed that PMMF had higher reported rates of fistula (24.7 vs. 8.9%), requirement for second surgery (11.3 vs. 5.5%), and fewer PMMF patients produced tracheoesophageal speech (17.5 vs. 52.1%). They found no difference in stricture rates or swallowing outcomes.[15] However, the use of free flaps requires surgical expertise, infrastructure, and longer duration of surgery, and also carries a higher risk of flap failure. PMMF has the advantage of a simpler flap harvest and can be performed simultaneously with primary closure of the pharynx, thus reducing overall duration of surgery. Moreover, the bulk of the muscle will cover the great vessels of the neck preventing any major blowout. Coming on to the long-term functional outcomes comparing PMMF and free flap when used for reconstruction specifically after salvage laryngectomy, it was seen that the requirement for esophageal dilatation was higher after PMMF (25 vs. 9%) and 38.7% had a limited oral intake compared to

15.2% of patients who received free flaps. However, the complication rates were similar in both the groups. Subgroup analyses showed a smaller amount of PCFs as well as wound dehiscence in patients where onlay PMMF was used, compared to inset pectoralis myocutaneous flap (pectoralis major myocutaneous [PMMC]).[16] In our case, there was adequate remnant mucosa of more than 3 cm and primary closure was performed along with an overlay PMMF.

Another consideration is the timing of starting oral feeds in the postoperative period. A meta-analysis incorporating four randomized controlled trials and three nonrandomized controlled trials by Hay et al[17] compared patients who had early or late postoperative feeds. This meta-analysis showed there was no difference in complication rate when early feeding was started. However, the population under analysis was heterogeneous, where some studies included postirradiated patients, while others exclude them. Moreover, the method of randomization is not mentioned in three out of four studies. Thus, timing of oral feeds impacting PCF still remains a matter of debate.

It has been postulated that leak rate can decrease further by the use of salivary bypass tube. It helps funnel saliva into the esophagus bypassing the anastomosis; however, a few surgeons believe them to be propagators of fistulas due to constant pressure and irritation along the suture line. It was seen that the rate of PCF was less in patients in whom salivary bypass tube was used (24.6 vs. 8.3%)[18]; however, it was not significant on multivariate analysis. Bondi et al[19] and Punthakee et al[20] also showed lower fistula rates; however, the sample size was small and multivariate analysis was not done. Thus, the use of a salivary bypass tube to decrease the rate of fistula needs further research.

27.2.2 Impact of Neck Dissection on Rates of PCF

The main aim of any surgery is to achieve good control rate and have least complications. A meta-analysis by Paydarfar and Birkmeyer[21] has shown that performing neck dissection is an important factor that increases the rate of PCF. Few other authors have also shown that there is a decrease in complication rates when neck dissection is not performed without compromising a the oncologic outcomes of the patients.[22,23] As far as control is concerned, recent PETNECK trial[24] has shown that PET-CT–guided surveillance has similar survival outcomes as planned neck dissection with considerably fewer operations and better cost-effectiveness. However, the majority of patients in this trial had a primary cancer in the oropharynx and were human papillomavirus (HPV) positive. Thus, its implication in the management of laryngeal cancer during salvage setting needs further confirmation through a randomized control trial. Apart from these interventions, it is important to provide adequate nutritional support to the patients and correct any thyroid hormone imbalance by giving thyroxine supplements whenever required.

27.3 Tips

- Older age, smoking cigarette, chronic obstructive pulmonary disease (COPD), hypopharyngeal more than laryngeal cancer, and increasing T-stage have higher complication rates.
- Along with PCF, other complications include wound infection, pharyngeal stenosis, bleeding, and dysphagia.
- Putting an overlay vascularized flap tissue has been shown to reduce leak rates, but it needs to be proven in a randomized control trial.

- Respectful handling of prior irradiated tissue is important in salvage laryngectomy cases.
- Keeping a cuff of pharyngeal constrictors around the remnant mucosa is essential as it can be used as a second closure layer over the mucosal closure.
- The width of the remnant mucosa is important in order to decide whether a vascularized flap will be used for augmentation or an overlay flap.

27.4 Traps

- PET-CECT is essential in cases of salvage laryngectomy as it gives us an idea about deeper extension of the cancer and also rules out distant metastasis.
- Timing of PET-CECT is important, as it may show false-positive results in the first 8 to 12 weeks after OPP.
- Various methods may help in reducing the complication rate, but one must be well equipped to handle them.

References

[1] Wolf GT, Fisher SG, Hong WK, et al; Department of Veterans Affairs Laryngeal Cancer Study Group. Induction chemotherapy plus radiation compared with surgery plus radiation in patients with advanced laryngeal cancer. N Engl J Med. 1991; 324(24):1685–1690

[2] Forastiere AA, Zhang Q, Weber RS, et al. Long-term results of RTOG 91-11: a comparison of three nonsurgical treatment strategies to preserve the larynx in patients with locally advanced larynx cancer. J Clin Oncol. 2013; 31(7):845–852

[3] Stankovic M, Milisavljevic D, Zivic M, Stojanov D, Stankovic P. Primary and salvage total laryngectomy. Influential factors, complications, and survival. J BUON. 2015; 20(2):527–539

[4] Chandler JR. Radiation fibrosis and necrosis of the larynx. Ann Otol Rhinol Laryngol. 1979; 88(4, pt 1):509–514

[5] Weber RS, Berkey BA, Forastiere A, et al. Outcome of salvage total laryngectomy following organ preservation therapy: the Radiation Therapy Oncology Group trial 91-11. Arch Otolaryngol Head Neck Surg. 2003; 129(1):44–49

[6] Hasan Z, Dwivedi RC, Gunaratne DA, Virk SA, Palme CE, Riffat F. Systematic review and meta-analysis of the complications of salvage total laryngectomy. Eur J Surg Oncol. 2017; 43(1):42–51

[7] Posner MR, Norris CM, Wirth LJ, et al; TAX 324 Study Group. Sequential therapy for the locally advanced larynx and hypopharynx cancer subgroup in TAX 324: survival, surgery, and organ preservation. Ann Oncol. 2009; 20(5):921–927

[8] Teknos TN, Myers LL. Surgical reconstruction after chemotherapy or radiation. Problems and solutions. Hematol Oncol Clin North Am. 1999; 13(4):679–687

[9] Hui Y, Wei WI, Yuen PW, Lam LK, Ho WK. Primary closure of pharyngeal remnant after total laryngectomy and partial pharyngectomy: how much residual mucosa is sufficient? Laryngoscope. 1996; 106(4):490–494

[10] Paleri V, Drinnan M, van den Brekel MWM, et al. Vascularized tissue to reduce fistula following salvage total laryngectomy: a systematic review. Laryngoscope. 2014; 124(8):1848–1853

[11] Albirmawy OA. Prevention of postlaryngectomy pharyngocutaneous fistula using a sternocleidomastoid muscle collar flap. J Laryngol Otol. 2007; 121(3):253–257

[12] Kadota H, Fukushima J, Kamizono K, et al. A minimally invasive method to prevent postlaryngectomy major pharyngocutaneous fistula using infrahyoid myofascial flap. J Plast Reconstr Aesthet Surg. 2013; 66(7):906–911

[13] Sayles M, Grant DG. Preventing pharyngo-cutaneous fistula in total laryngectomy: a systematic review and meta-analysis. Laryngoscope. 2014; 124(5):1150–1163

[14] Patel UA, Moore BA, Wax M, et al. Impact of pharyngeal closure technique on fistula after salvage laryngectomy. JAMA Otolaryngol Head Neck Surg. 2013; 139(11):1156–1162

[15] Chao JW, Spector JA, Taylor EM, et al. Pectoralis major myocutaneous flap versus free fasciocutaneous flap for reconstruction of partial hypopharyngeal defects: what should we be doing? J Reconstr Microsurg. 2015; 31(3):198–204

[16] Nguyen S, Thuot F. Functional outcomes of fasciocutaneous free flap and pectoralis major flap for salvage total laryngectomy. Head Neck. 2017; 39(9):1797–1805

[17] Hay A, Pitkin L, Gurusamy K. Early versus delayed oral feeding in patients following total laryngectomy. Adv Otolaryngol. 2014; 2014

[18] Hone RWA, Rahman E, Wong G, et al. Do salivary bypass tubes lower the incidence of pharyngocutaneous fistula following total laryngectomy? A retrospective analysis of predictive factors using multivariate analysis. Eur Arch Otorhinolaryngol. 2017; 274(4):1983–1991

[19] Bondi S, Giordano L, Limardo P, Bussi M. Role of Montgomery salivary stent placement during pharyngolaryngectomy, to prevent pharyngocutaneous fistula in high-risk patients. J Laryngol Otol. 2013; 127(1):54–57

[20] Punthakee X, Zaghi S, Nabili V, Knott PD, Blackwell KE. Effects of salivary bypass tubes on fistula and stricture formation. JAMA Facial Plast Surg. 2013; 15(3):219–225

[21] Paydarfar JA, Birkmeyer NJ. Complications in head and neck surgery: a meta-analysis of postlaryngectomy pharyngocutaneous fistula. Arch Otolaryngol Head Neck Surg. 2006; 132(1):67–72

[22] Basheeth N, O'Leary G, Sheahan P. Elective neck dissection for no neck during salvage total laryngectomy: findings, complications, and oncological outcome. JAMA Otolaryngol Head Neck Surg. 2013; 139(8):790–796

[23] Dagan R, Morris CG, Kirwan JM, et al. Elective neck dissection during salvage surgery for locally recurrent head and neck squamous cell carcinoma after radiotherapy with elective nodal irradiation. Laryngoscope. 2010; 120(5):945–952

[24] Mehanna H, Wong WL, McConkey CC, et al. PET-CT surveillance versus neck dissection in advanced head and neck cancer N Engl J Med. 2016; 374(15):1444–1454

28 Reconstruction for Advanced Cancer: Pectoralis Major Myocutaneous Flap

Genival B. de Carvalho, José G. Vartanian, Luiz P. Kowalski

Abstract

In many head and neck surgery services, the pectoralis major myocutaneous flap remains the mainstay reconstructive method because of the lack of availability of a specialized reconstructive surgical team and the costly instrumentation required to perform free flaps. Even in head and neck surgery services in which free flaps are used routinely, pectoralis major fasciocutaneous or myocutaneous flaps can be performed in combination with free flaps to reconstruct larger tridimensional surgical defects, to protect critical vessels at risk for rupture, and to manage or prevent salivary fistulas. Therefore, pectoralis major flaps must be part of the armamentarium of every head and neck surgeon who provides major surgical procedures.

Keywords: head and neck reconstruction, pectoralis major myocutaneous flap, pedicled flap, complications, salvage surgery

28.1 Introduction

Since Ariyan's first report in 1979,[1] the pectoralis major myocutaneous flap (PMMF) has been one of the most widely used methods for reconstruction of major defects in head and neck cancer surgery because of its technical ease, versatility, proximity to the head and neck region, and the possibility of carrying well-vascularized tissue to irradiated areas.[2] Even in head and neck centers where free flaps are available, PMMF can be used in association with free flaps for major defect repair, for protection of critical vessels at risk of exposure and rupture, and to avoid or to minimize the occurrence and severity of pharyngocutaneous fistula, especially in patients undergoing salvage surgery after radiotherapy or radiochemotherapy.[3]

28.2 Surgical Technique

In our institution, we delimit the island of skin according to the defect to be reconstructed. In most cases, we perform an island flap, partially preserving the upper part of the pectoralis major muscle with a low skin incision , decreasing the functional impairment of the arm, while allowing a possible future use of a Bakamijan deltopectoral flap if necessary. After incision of the skin, the cutaneous flap is elevated laterally to preserve the muscular fascia to reduce bleeding; the section of the muscular fibers of the major pectoralis is performed at the lower border of the flap to facilitate identification of the vascular pedicle, which passes between the fibers of the pectoralis major and pectoralis minor. Rotation of the PMMF to the cervical region can be done through a tunnel on or below the clavicle, which has the advantage of increasing the upper limit of reach of the flap by approximately 2 to 3 cm. We recommend sectioning part of the subclavian muscle in the topography of the passage of the vascular pedicle, to reduce the risk of compression.[4] In obese patients and patients with a bulky pectoralis major, passage of the flap through the subclavicle route may not be feasible.

28.3 Primary Indications in the Treatment of Advanced Laryngeal Tumors

PMMF is widely used for reconstruction in patients undergoing surgical treatment of advanced laryngeal tumors. PMMF can be used for reconstruction of the partial or total defect of the pharynx, for reconstruction of the skin, for protection of the great vessels in patients at high risk for dehiscence and exposure, as well as for the prevention of pharyngocutaneous fistulas in cases of primary closure of the pharynx in salvage surgery, primarily after radiotherapy (with or without associated chemotherapy).

28.3.1 Reconstruction of Pharyngeal Defects

Regarding the reconstruction of defects after total pharyngolaryngectomies, PMMF has been the second option in centers where free flaps are available, and its use is indicated primarily for patients with poor clinical performance.[5] In the study by Chan et al, 202 patients underwent total reconstruction of the pharynx after resection of advanced laryngeal or hypopharyngeal cancer: 92 patients underwent reconstruction with PMMF; 24 patients underwent reconstruction with free anterolateral thigh (ALT) flap; and 24 patients underwent reconstruction with free jejunal flap. The fistula rate in the PMMF group was 23.9%; it was 12.5% in the free ALT group, and just 2.3% in the jejunum flap group. With regard to late stenosis, it was 27.2% in the PMMF group, 12.5% in the ALT group, and 2.3% in the jejunal flap group. Reconstruction of mucosal defects with myocutaneous or fasciocutaneous flaps presents a higher rate of pharyngocutaneous fistulas and late stenosis. Conversely, in total pharyngolaryngectomies extended to the base of the tongue, reconstruction with jejunum may not be feasible.[6]

In situations in which reconstruction with the jejunal free flap is impossible, PMMF should be sutured to the prevertebral fascia in the reconstructions after total pharyngolaryngectomy, since it presents a lower complication rate compared with the use of PMMF as a tunnel. Carvalho et al, evaluated the results of 69 patients undergoing total pharyngeal reconstruction, 45 patients underwent reconstruction with PMMF, of which 29 were made with the muscle sutured the prevertebral fascia and 16 were made as a tunnel with PMMF to reconstruct the pharynx. In this subgroup of patients, a general rate of immediate postoperative complications of 51.7% was observed in the group sutured to the prevertebral fascia, and a rate of 62.5% in the muscle in the tunnel. The most common immediate complication in the group of patients with muscle sutured to the fascia was infection of the surgical site (37.9%), whereas in the muscle group with tunnel, the most immediate complication was fistula formation (50%). The most common late complication in the group with muscle sutured to in the fascia was stenosis (21.4%), whereas in the muscle group with tunnel, 37.5% of patients had stenosis.[7]

28.3.2 Prevention of Pharyngocutaneous Fistula

One of the most common complications after total laryngectomy or pharyngolaryngectomy is pharyngocutaneous fistula, especially in salvage surgery after failed radiotherapy or radiochemotherapy. Rates of pharyngocutaneous fistula found in the literature range from 14 to 57%.[8,9] In an initial (unpublished) study from our service that analyzed the treatment of 69 patients with advanced laryngeal or hypopharyngeal cancer with complications in radiochemical surgeries, the rate of pharyngocutaneous fistula was 55% in a subgroup of 18 patients with treatment failure at the primary site. The rotation of the myocutaneous flap of the pectoralis major to cover and reinforce the primary closure of the mucosa is related to a significant decrease in the fistula rate, even when only the fasciomuscular flap was performed.[10] In the systematic review, the use of PMMF reduced the risk of pharyngocutaneous fistula by 22% in patients undergoing salvage pharyngolaryngectomy.[11] Conversely, a small retrospective series with 64 patients did not show a significant decrease in the fistula rate with the use of pectoralis major flaps (17.6 vs. 13.3%, $p = 0.74$).[12]

The use of a salivary bypass tube has also been described as a strategy for the prevention of salivary fistulas and stenosis. In a study of a prospective cohort with 105 patients who underwent anterolateral arm cutaneous flap reconstruction or antebrachial flap associated with salivary bypass, the authors compared the group with a retrospective cohort of patients who underwent PMMF, anterolateral arm, or antebrachial without the routine use of salivary bypass. In this study, the authors observed a significant reduction in the fistula and stenosis rates in the salivary bypass group: 26 versus 7% ($p < 0.001$) and 18 versus 3% ($p = 0.001$), respectively.[13]

28.4 Complications

PMMF is a safe, technically easy flap to perform. In a study with a retrospective cohort of 437 patients, PMMF below the clavicle did not present a higher complication rate than PMMF over the clavicle: 33.8 versus 38.2% ($p = 0.796$), respectively. In this study, a review of the literature demonstrated that rates of partial necrosis of the flap range from 4 to 29%, those of total necrosis range from 0 to 5.9%, and fistulas range from 5 to 29%.[3] In addition to these complications, another study with 211 patients undergoing PMPF reconstruction described that 24% of the patients had surgical site infection and 7% had a hematoma.[14] Other possible complications are a reduction in shoulder flexion and a decrease in flexural strength.[15]

28.5 Functional Results

In a retrospective series of 126 patients who underwent reconstruction following salvage total laryngectomy, 93 had PMMF and 33 had microsurgical fasciocutaneous flaps. A better functional outcome occurred ($p < 0.05$) in patients who had microsurgical fascicular cutaneous flaps, with a return of normal feeding in 85 compared to 61% in the PMMF group.[16] A systematic review by Mahalingam et al evaluated quality of life and functional outcomes in patients undergoing pharyngolaryngectomy. A better functional outcome for swallowing was found in patients who had reconstruction with jejunal microsurgical flap and better outcome with a tracheoesophageal prosthesis.[17] Moreover, the incidence rates of voice failure and shoulder disability were significantly higher in the PMMF group.[12]

28.6 Clinical Cases

28.6.1 Use of Myocutaneous Flap of the Pectoralis Major for Complete Post Total Pharyngolaryngectomy Reconstruction

Case 1

A 68-year-old man, Eastern Cooperative Oncology Group (ECOG) stage 3, with transglottic squamous cell carcinoma of the larynx, cT4aN2bM0, with extension to the tongue base and the lateral wall of the pharynx on the left side. The patient had a tracheostomy performed 4 months previously. The patient underwent total pharyngolaryngectomy extending to the base of the tongue, lateral pharyngeal wall, cervical skin, and the previous tracheostomy tract with bilateral neck dissection of levels II to V and VI and total thyroidectomy. Due to the extension of the resection to the base of the tongue and lateral wall of the pharynx, a decision was made to reconstruct the defect with a PMMF in to better close the resection area at the base of the tongue and the lateral wall of the pharynx. The surgical team planned to perform

an extension of the island of skin below the mammary areola to facilitate the closure of the defect (▶Fig. 28.1). ▶Fig. 28.2 shows the PMMF suture to the prevertebral fascia.

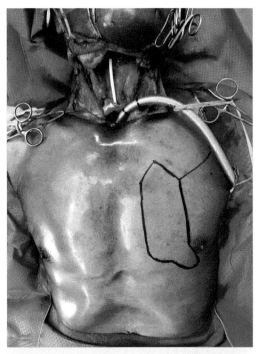

Fig. 28.1 The surgical team planned to perform an extension of the island of skin below the mammary areola to facilitate the closure of the defect.

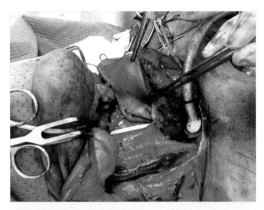

Fig. 28.2 The pectoralis major myocutaneous flap sutured to the prevertebral fascia.

28.6.2 Use of PMMF for Pharyngocutaneous Fistula Protection and Reconstruction of the Cervical Skin Defect

Case 2

A 56-year-old man, ECOG stage 2, had been diagnosed with transglottic squamous cell cancer of the larynx, cT4aN0M0, with invasion of the cervical skin and tracheostoma, for 3 months. The patient underwent total laryngectomy and partial pharyngectomy extended to include cervical skin and tracheostoma with bilateral neck dissection of levels II to IV and VI and total thyroidectomy. The pharyngeal remnant closure was done primarily, and PMMF was performed to reduce the risk of a fistula and closure of the cervical skin. ▸ Fig. 28.3 shows the planning of the incision with resection of the cervical skin and the tracheostoma trajectory, whereas ▸ Fig. 28.4 shows the postresection defect. ▸ Fig. 28.5 shows the final result of the reconstruction with PMMF.

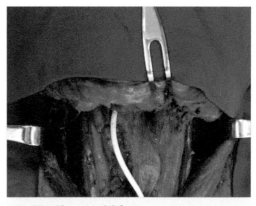

Fig. 28.4 The surgical defect.

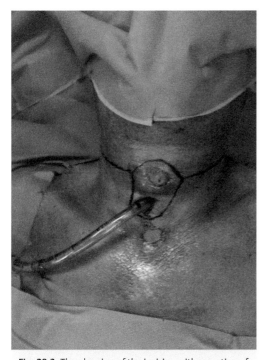

Fig. 28.3 The planning of the incision with resection of the cervical skin and the tracheostoma trajectory.

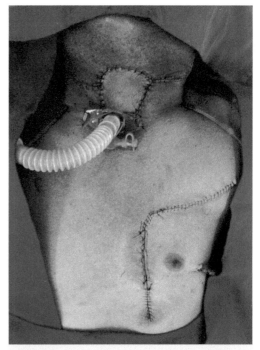

Fig. 28.5 The reconstruction with pectoralis major myocutaneous flap.

References

[1] Ariyan S. The pectoralis major myocutaneous flap. A versatile flap for reconstruction in the head and neck. Plast Reconstr Surg. 1979; 63(1):73–81

[2] Zhang X, Li MJ, Fang QG, Sun CF. A comparison between the pectoralis major myocutaneous flap and the free anterolateral thigh perforator flap for reconstruction in head and neck cancer patients: assessment of the quality of life. J Craniofac Surg. 2014; 25(3):868–871

[3] Vartanian JG, Carvalho AL, Carvalho SM, Mizobe L, Magrin J, Kowalski LP. Pectoralis major and other myofascial/myocutaneous flaps in head and neck cancer reconstruction: experience with 437 cases at a single institution. Head Neck. 2004; 26(12):1018–1023

[4] de Azevedo JF. Modified pectoralis major myocutaneous flap with partial preservation of the muscle: a study of 55 cases. Head Neck Surg. 1986; 8(5):327–331

[5] You YS, Chung CH, Chang YJ, Kim KH, Jung SW, Rho YS. Analysis of 120 pectoralis major flaps for head and neck reconstruction. Arch Plast Surg. 2012; 39(5):522–527

[6] Chan YW, Ng RW, Liu LH, Chung HP, Wei WI. Reconstruction of circumferential pharyngeal defects after tumour resection: reference or preference. J Plast Reconstr Aesthet Surg. 2011; 64(8):1022–1028

[7] Carvalho AL, Miguel VER, Santos CR, Magrin J, Filho JG, Kowalski LP. Total pharyngeal reconstruction: review of 69 cases. Rev Col Bras Cir. 1999; 26(2):85–89

[8] Stoeckli SJ, Pawlik AB, Lipp M, Huber A, Schmid S. Salvage surgery after failure of nonsurgical therapy for carcinoma of the larynx and hypopharynx. Arch Otolaryngol Head Neck Surg. 2000; 126(12):1473–1477

[9] Schwartz SR, Yueh B, Maynard C, Daley J, Henderson W, Khuri SF. Predictors of wound complications after laryngectomy: a study of over 2000 patients. Otolaryngol Head Neck Surg. 2004; 131(1):61–68

[10] Gilbert MR, Sturm JJ, Gooding WE, Johnson JT, Kim S. Pectoralis major myofascial onlay and myocutaneous flaps and pharyngocutaneous fistula in salvage laryngectomy. Laryngoscope. 2014; 124(12):2680–2686

[11] Guimarães AV, Aires FT, Dedivitis RA, et al. Efficacy of pectoralis major muscle flap for pharyngocutaneous fistula prevention in salvage total laryngectomy: A systematic review. Head Neck. 2016; 38(suppl 1):E2317–E2321

[12] Sittitrai P, Srivanitchapoom C, Reunmakkaew D. Prevention of pharyngocutaneous fistula in salvage total laryngectomy: role of the pectoralis major flap and peri-operative management. J Laryngol Otol. 2018; 132(3):246–251

[13] Piazza C, Bon FD, Paderno A, et al. Fasciocutaneous free flaps for reconstruction of hypopharyngeal defects. Laryngoscope. 2017; 127(12):2731–2737

[14] Shah JP, Haribhakti V, Loree TR, Sutaria P. Complications of the pectoralis major myocutaneous flap in head and neck reconstruction. Am J Surg. 1990; 160(4):352–355

[15] Moukarbel RV, Fung K, Franklin JH, et al. Neck and shoulder disability following reconstruction with the pectoralis major pedicled flap. Laryngoscope. 2010; 120(6):1129–1134

[16] Nguyen S, Thuot F. Functional outcomes of fasciocutaneous free flap and pectoralis major flap for salvage total laryngectomy. Head Neck. 2017; 39(9):1797–1805

[17] Mahalingam S, Srinivasan R, Spielmann P. Quality-of-life and functional outcomes following pharyngolaryngectomy: a systematic review of literature. Clin Otolaryngol. 2016; 41(1):25–43

29 Reconstruction for Advanced Cancer: Supraclavicular Island Flap

Leandro L. de Matos, Helio R. Nogueira Alves, Claudio R. Cernea

Abstract

The supraclavicular island flap (SCIF) is very versatile option for the reconstruction of defects in the head and neck and are used in the reconstruction of skin defects (mainly the lower third of the face, such as the malar, parotid, auricular, and cervical regions), the mucosa (oral cavity, oropharynx, and hypopharynx), and lateral defects, and for skull base repair (especially in the lateral and posterior regions). In this chapter we describe a case of a patient with a recurrent squamous cell carcinoma of the neopharynx following a salvage total laryngectomy that was resected and the circular defect was reconstructed with a SCIF with a very good result. The tips and traps about the flap's operative technique are described. The SCIF may be harvested rapidly, and it may be used in a single reconstruction procedure with no need to change the patient's position. The literature also reports that the supraclavicular flap presents similar success rates compared to other flaps and can still be safely used in patients with various comorbidities. The results of our group demonstrate that the average time for flap harvesting was approximately 50 minutes. There were 14.9% of partial flap necrosis (7 of 47 cases). Four cases required surgical debridement and primary closure, and there were three cases of fistula, all of which occurred in the four cases of hypopharyngeal reconstruction that had complete resolution with conservative treatment. All patients exhibited an adequate functional response at the end of 6 months of follow-up after reconstruction.

Keywords: laryngeal neoplasms, pharyngeal neoplasms, salvage therapy, surgical flaps, reconstructive surgical procedures

29.1 Case Report

The patient was a 64-year-old Caucasian male patient previously treated with chemoradiotherapy (3 years prior) as an organ preservation protocol for a stage III (T3N0M0) transglottic squamous cell carcinoma (SCC). Two years after this treatment, he presented with a local recurrence and underwent salvage total laryngectomy with primary closure. The histopathological examination revealed a 1.9-cm grade 2 rpT4a (stage IVa) SCC of the left vocal cord with extension to the supraglottis, both piriform sinuses and the thyroid cartilage, with free margins. No adjuvant treatment was performed at that time. The patient presented with another recurrence at the neopharynx (▸Fig. 29.1) and circumferential resection of the pharynx, including two tracheal rings (▸Fig. 29.2) that demonstrated a 7.0-cm grade 2 rpT4a rpN0 (stage IVa) SCC including the pharyngeal mucosa and involving the thyroid gland skin of the anterior neck, esophageal mucosa, and left common carotid artery. A supraclavicular island flap (SCIF) of 8 × 24 cm was used to reconstruct the pharyngeal defect (▸Fig. 29.3 and ▸Fig. 29.4). The patient stayed in the hospital for 30 days due to complications at the donor site. A cervical hematoma was drained on postoperative day 6, and two resutures were performed to treat donor area dehiscences.

The patient was started on a liquid diet and gradually advanced to a normal diet 45 days after the operation. The feeding tube was removed on the 70th postoperative day. He then received re-irradiation treatment and one cisplatin cycle (the chemotherapy was withdrawn due to nephrotoxicity). The neopharyngeal aspect and the videodeglutogram 6 months after the surgery are displayed in ▸Fig. 29.5. Unfortunately, 8 months after the surgery and only 3 months after the end of re-irradiation therapy, a new recurrence was discovered and the patient died 3 months later.

29.2 Discussion

A SCIF is very versatile option for the reconstruction of defects of the head and neck. Initially described for the treatment of burn scar retractions, it is now widely used in reconstruction following the reconstruction of oncologic defects. In this context, SCIFs are used in the reconstruction of skin defects (mainly the lower third of the face, such as the malar, parotid, auricular, and cervical regions), the mucosa (oral cavity, oropharynx, and hypopharynx), and lateral defects, and for skull base repair (especially in the lateral

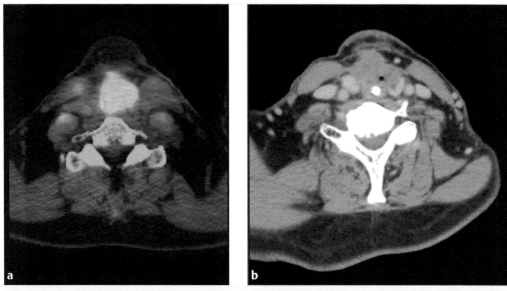

Fig. 29.1 Clinical appearance of the pharyngeal recurrence. **(a)** 18-fluorodeoxyglucose-PET-CT demonstrating intense metabolic activity. **(b)** CT scan identifying a circumferential mass invading the neopharynx and cervical esophagus.

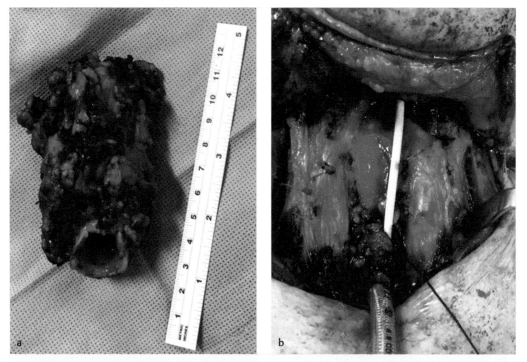

Fig. 29.2 Aspect of the surgical specimen and defect. **(a)** Surgical specimen with circumferential resection of the neopharynx and two tracheal rings. **(b)** Circumferential defect of the pharynx (the cervical esophagus is repaired just behind the trachea).

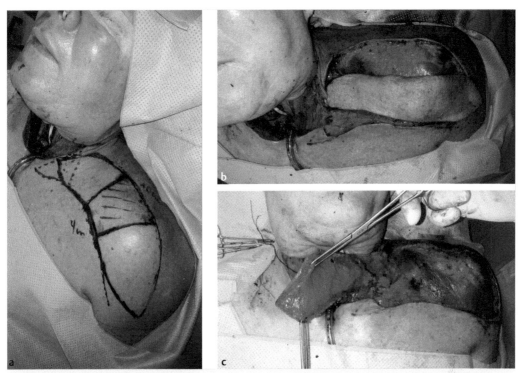

Fig. 29.3 Supraclavicular flap harvesting. **(a)** The flap is planned based on the triangle delimited for the posterior border of the sternocleidomastoid muscle, the medial superior border of the clavicle, and the external jugular vein. The flap is then drawn in a fusiform island between the anterior border of the trapezius muscle and an anterior parallel line up to the deltoid muscle, enough to reach the upper limit of the defect. As a modification of the technique, if necessary, the omohyoid muscle can be sectioned to increase the reach of the flap. In the same way, the external jugular vein can also be ligated and sectioned, as it contributes in a secondary way to the drainage of the supraclavicular veins. **(b)** The flap is elevated in the subfascial plane from lateral to medial, until the supraclavicular fossa. Some perforators from the deltoid muscle are cauterized during this process without compromising the vascularization of the flap. **(c)** Usually, the dissection ends after dividing the superficial cervical fascia (in cases where extra length is needed, the omohyoid muscle can be divided).

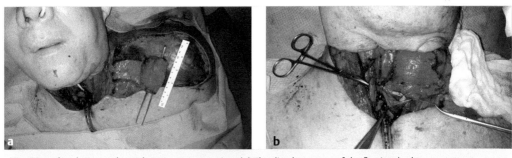

Fig. 29.4 Flap design and neopharynx reconstruction. **(a)** The distal segment of the flap is tubed to reconstruct the circumferential defect of the pharynx, and the remaining proximal segment is deepithelialized to be tunneled. **(b)** Suture between the remaining esophagus and the supraclavicular island flap.

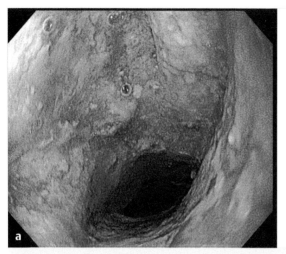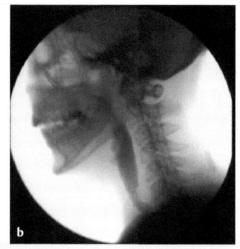

Fig. 29.5 Final aspect of the reconstruction, 6 months after the operation. **(a)** Endoscopic view of the neopharynx. **(b)** Videodeglutogram demonstrating the good caliber of the neopharynx, without stenosis, during the swallowing of solid food.

and posterior regions). This usage, in the authors' opinion, is because the flap accommodates better in these positions, as it is a thin flap that is inadequate for reconstructing areas that require a large volume of tissue. It is important to note that this statement is the opinion of the authors of this chapter and is based on their personal experiences. The literature clearly supports the use of the flap in other situations.[1]

The SCIF is also fast and easy to harvest, and it may be used in a single reconstruction procedure with no need for change in the patient's position. The flap has a glabrous skin area. The donor area usually can be primarily closed, and no functional sequelae have been observed.[2]

The literature[3] also reports that the supraclavicular flap presents similar success rates compared to other flaps and can still be safely used in patients with various comorbidities such as obesity, malnutrition, diabetes, radiotherapy, and smoking. The SCIF can also be used in reconstruction following salvage surgery reconstructions, but the integrity of the vascular pedicle must be ensured before beginning the flap harvesting, which can be identified by angiotomography or angioresonance.[4]

The study carried out at our hospital published in 2012[5] describes 47 consecutive cases of head and neck reconstructions (4 hypopharyngeal, 19 intraoral, and 24 cutaneous defects). The average time for flap harvesting was 50 minutes, and there was no damage to the vascular pedicle during

resection. The treatment of the donor area was primary closure in all cases, with five cases of conservative treatment for dehiscence. There were seven cases of partial flap necrosis (14.9%): four (three intraoral and one cutaneous defect) were submitted to surgical debridement and primary closure, and there were three cases of fistula, all of which occurred in the four cases of hypopharyngeal reconstruction that had complete resolution with conservative treatment. All patients exhibited a functional response at the end of 6 months of follow-up after reconstruction. These rates are similar to other studies,[3,6,7,8,9] and the description of total flap losses are punctual and often associated with technical issues.[3]

29.3 Tips

When the dissection reaches the supraclavicular fossa, caution must be exercised in dividing the superficial cervical fascia to avoid damaging the supraclavicular pedicle. Usually, the dissection can be finished at this point; if more length is required, the omohyoid muscle can be divided. Rarely, the pedicle is skeletonized.

The tunnel must be adequate to avoid compression of the flap; moreover, care should be taken not to compress the flap in the weeks after to surgery (especially the first 21 days) to avoid compromising its vascularization. It is recommended that the tracheostomy tube be fixed with sutures rather than with a shoelace and that no cervical bandage be placed, for example. The patient is also maintained in a neutral position postoperatively, without the use of pillows.

Special care should be taken in the suturing of the base of the flap; commonly, leftover skin must be accommodated in the cervical region. To better accommodate the base of the pedicle, it is possible to join the posterior and anterior lines in the flap next to the skin triangle, but one should always be careful to avoid compromising the vascularization of the flap.

29.4 Traps

Special care must be taken when using this flap in neck dissection of levels IV and V, which are precisely the territories of the transverse cervical artery and its branches. This procedure, as well as previous radiotherapy treatment, is not a contraindication to the use of the flap,[10] but it is recommended to preserve the pedicle that emerges from the transverse cervical branch to the SCIF. In 2012, Alves[5] described nine cases of supraclavicular flap use in patients submitted to modified radical cervical dissection without loss of the flap or relevant complications. Some authors[3,8,11,12] also recommend that the fascia along the supraclavicular vessels be preserved as a form of protection for the flap's vascularization.

References

[1] Chen WL, Zhang DM, Yang ZH, et al. Extended supraclavicular fasciocutaneous island flap based on the transverse cervical artery for head and neck reconstruction after cancer ablation. J Oral Maxillofac Surg. 2010; 68(10):2422–2430

[2] Herr MW, Bonanno A, Montalbano LA, Deschler DG, Emerick KS. Shoulder function following reconstruction with the supraclavicular artery island flap. Laryngoscope. 2014; 124(11):2478–2483

[3] Chiu ES, Liu PH, Friedlander PL. Supraclavicular artery island flap for head and neck oncologic reconstruction: indications, complications, and outcomes. Plast Reconstr Surg. 2009; 124(1):115–123

[4] Adams AS, Wright MJ, Johnston S, et al. The use of multislice CT angiography preoperative study for supraclavicular artery island flap harvesting. Ann Plast Surg. 2012; 69(3):312–315

[5] Alves HR, Ishida LC, Ishida LH, et al. A clinical experience of the supraclavicular flap used to reconstruct head and neck defects in late-stage cancer patients. J Plast Reconstr Aesthet Surg. 2012; 65(10):1350–1356

[6] Wu H, Chen WL, Yang ZH. Functional reconstruction with an extended supraclavicular fasciocutaneous island flap following ablation of advanced oropharyngeal cancer. J Craniofac Surg. 2012; 23(6):1668–1671

[7] Chiu ES, Liu PH, Baratelli R, Lee MY, Chaffin AE, Friedlander PL. Circumferential pharyngoesophageal reconstruction with a supraclavicular artery island flap. Plast Reconstr Surg. 2010; 125(1):161–166

[8] Sandu K, Monnier P, Pasche P. Supraclavicular flap in head and neck reconstruction: experience in 50 consecutive patients. Eur Arch Otorhinolaryngol. 2012; 269(4):1261–1267

[9] Nthumba PM. The supraclavicular artery flap: a versatile flap for neck and orofacial reconstruction. J Oral Maxillofac Surg. 2012; 70(8):1997–2004

[10] Razdan SN, Albornoz CR, Ro T, et al. Safety of the supraclavicular artery island flap in the setting of neck dissection and radiation therapy. J Reconstr Microsurg. 2015; 31(5):378–383

[11] Di Benedetto G, Aquinati A, Pierangeli M, Scalise A, Bertani A. From the "charretera" to the supraclavicular fascial island flap: revisitation and further evolution of a controversial flap. Plast Reconstr Surg. 2005; 115(1):70–76

[12] Vinh VQ, Van Anh T, Ogawa R, Hyakusoku H. Anatomical and clinical studies of the supraclavicular flap: analysis of 103 flaps used to reconstruct neck scar contractures. Plast Reconstr Surg. 2009; 123(5):1471–1480

30 Reconstruction for Advanced Cancer: Latissimus Dorsi Myocutaneous Flap

S. van Weert, C. René Leemans

Abstract

The pedicled myocutaneous latissimus dorsi flap is a versatile flap that is suitable in reconstruction of the head and neck due to its thinness, wide arc of rotation, and possible (large) dimensions. The surgical technique is straightforward and reported complication rates are relatively low. The flap can be used in pharyngeal reconstruction as an alternative to free tissue transfer when primary closure is not feasible. A case is reported of advanced laryngeal cancer reconstructed with a latissimus dorsi flap. The history, background, and possible (contra)indications are mentioned. The surgical technique is meticulously described. Specific subjects are addressed such as the necessity of awareness of the angiosomes and the trajectory and branching of the pedicle. The position of the skin paddle should not be designed too caudal in relation to the muscle to allow proper perfusion of the paddle. It is necessary to ligate the branches to the underlying serratus muscle to achieve adequate mobilization to the head and neck area. Finally, the most important tips and traps are described in order to achieve an optimal result in performing the latissimus dorsi flap in pharyngeal reconstruction.

Keywords: pharyngectomy, latissimus dorsi, anatomy, surgical technique, angiosomes

30.1 Case Report

A 70-year-old male presented with progressive hoarseness and dysphagia over the past 5 months. He had a history of recurrent airway infections and coughing during deglutition suggesting aspiration. His medical history noted a transient ischemic attack and hypercholesterolemia for which he used anticoagulants and statins. The patient was a current cigarette smoker and had a smoking history of 55 pack-years. He never used alcohol.

On physical examination, the patient had a hoarse voice and frequent coughing. Direct laryngoscopy revealed a large ulcerating lesion originating from the left supraglottic area and extending to the left hypopharynx. The left vocal cord was immobile. There was evidence of saliva, penetrating the glottis. There were no palpable lymph nodes in the neck.

An MR of the larynx was performed showing a left supraglottic cancer with growth to the piriform sinus on the left. There was obvious cartilage invasion (▶ Fig. 30.1).

Enlarged ipsilateral cervical nodes in levels II and III were identified for which an ultrasound with fine-needle aspiration cytology was performed.

An examination under general anesthesia was performed for biopsy and to evaluate the exact extent of the cancer. The cancer extended from the left false vocal cord to the laryngeal aspect of the epiglottis and the glottis. There was extension of the lesion to the medial wall of the left hypopharynx without invading the posterior pharyngeal wall. Biopsies were taken.

Histopathology showed a moderately differentiated squamous cell carcinoma. Cytology showed two cancer-positive nodes in the ipsilateral neck in levels II and III. The was staged as a pT4aN2b carcinoma of the supraglottic larynx.

Due to the extent of disease and poor functionality of the larynx, a total laryngectomy with partial pharyngectomy and a left selective neck

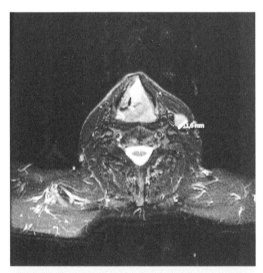

Fig. 30.1 T2-weighted axial MR image of the lesion showing the extent from the larynx to the left hypopharynx.

dissection of levels II to IV was advised by the multidisciplinary head and neck team. A latissimus dorsi (LD) myocutaneous flap was suggested for pharyngeal reconstruction.

The patient underwent the above-mentioned surgery including a hemithyroidectomy on the left. Cricopharyngeal myotomy was performed as well as placement of a voice prosthesis. Pharyngeal closure was achieved using a myocutaneous LD flap from the left.

For harvesting of the flap, the patient was placed in the right lateral decubitus position. The shoulder was abducted for exposure of the axillary area by suspension of the forearm. The patient was placed on special cushioning to avoid excessive pressure specifically on the iliac crest. The flap was outlined by measuring the distance from the surgical defect to the pectoral–humeral junction and by assessing the length needed to reach the recipient site. The lateral border of the muscle was outlined running from the midpoint of the axilla to the posterior iliac crest as depicted by the white dotted line in ▶ Fig. 30.2.

The skin paddle was designed over the second angiosome to ensure proper perfusion (▶ Fig. 30.3).

The dimensions of the skin island were determined based on the dimensions of the surgical defect. Incision commenced from the midpoint of the axilla down to the lateral border of the skin paddle. While incising anteriorly of the paddle, the lateral border of the muscle was identified.

Once proper attachment of muscle and skin was identified, the muscle was mobilized from the underlying structures by dissecting it in the posterior direction. The serratus anterior muscle was exposed and dissection proceeded in the plane between these muscles. After detaching the distal tip of the skin paddle and transection of the muscle caudally, dissection was started at the medial insertion of the LD muscle for further cranial mobilization. In this area, multiple intercostal arteries were identified and ligated. Mobilizing the muscle upward, the thoracodorsal vessels that constitute the pedicle were carefully identified. Branches to the serratus anterior muscle were ligated and divided as well as the thoracodorsal nerve for adequate mobilization. When the muscle was fully mobilized and only attached to its vascular pedicle, it was delivered to the recipient site via transfer through the axillary fossa and tunneled subcutaneously (▶ Fig. 30.4).

Care was taken to make the tunnel wide enough to avoid compression of the pedicle. The skin paddle was trimmed to the correct size to fit the pharyngeal defect. The skin paddle was sutured into the defect using continuous semipermanent sutures ensuring a watertight closure of the neopharynx. The donor site was closed primarily after leaving two suction drain catheters after some undermining and without undue tension. The skin was closed using staples.

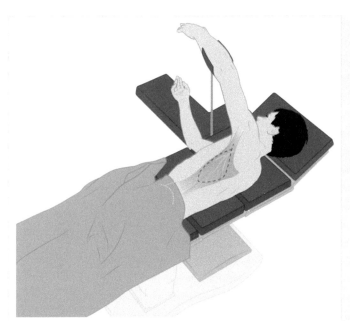

Fig. 30.2 Intraoperative positioning of the patient. The lateral decubitus position with the ipsilateral arm raised in abduction and fixed at the level of the forearm. Note the white dotted line delineating the lateral border of the muscle as well as the iliac crest. The black dotted line marks the skin paddle design.

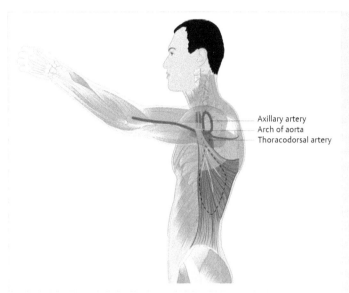

Axillary artery
Arch of aorta
Thoracodorsal artery

Fig. 30.3 Latissimus dorsi muscle with its blood supply and landmarks. The thoracodorsal artery supplies the skin paddle (*dotted line*). Note that ligation of the branches toward the serratus muscle constitutes a wider arc of rotation. The angiosomes (*yellow-green-blue*) designate the levels of perforator density (from good in yellow and green to poor in blue). The skin paddle overlaps the first and second angiosomes.

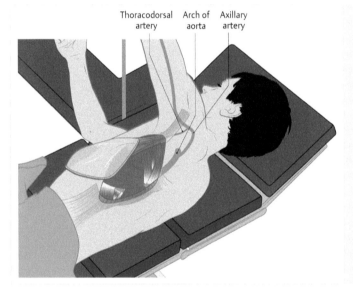

Thoracodorsal artery   Arch of aorta   Axillary artery

Fig. 30.4 The myocutaneous flap has been mobilized and is ready to be transferred to the recipient site through the axillary fossa. Transfer can be done both intrapectoral and subcutaneous.

The patient remained on a nothing by mouth for 7 days, after which a barium swallow examination was performed. There were no signs of fistula and the patient started uneventful oral intake. He immediately had a clear prosthetic voice. He was discharged from the hospital 12 days after surgery.

30.2 Discussion

In the case of advanced cancer of the larynx with poor functionality prior to treatment, general consensus exists that total laryngectomy is superior to organ-preservation strategies.[1,2] Once the decision is made for total laryngectomy, one should evaluate whether primary pharyngeal closure is possible with acceptable functional outcome.

Several reconstructive techniques after partial pharyngectomy have been described, each with its pros and cons.

In the case described here, partial pharyngectomy was necessary, leaving enough pharyngeal mucosa to be used in combination with tissue transfer. According to Hui et al, a 2.5-cm-wide remnant of pharyngeal mucosa is considered sufficient for primary closure and after resecting one-third to three-fourths, partial reconstruction is necessary.[3,4] A choice should be made to use a pedicled or a free flap. For free tissue transfer, the surgical teams need to be experienced in microvascular surgery and operating time is usually longer. The functional outcome with regard to strictures, however, seems to be superior in the case of free flap reconstruction.[5] Free tissue transfers mostly used in pharyngeal reconstruction are the radial forearm flap (RFFF), anterolateral thigh flap (ALT), and the jejunal graft. The latter method has the drawbacks of additional abdominal surgery, relatively high complication rate, and often less than optimal outcome with regard to swallowing and prosthetic speech in comparison to skin-covered reconstruction.[4]

Once the choice is made for a pedicled flap, one should consider the bulk needed, the geometry, and the donor site morbidity as well as cosmesis. Relative contraindications for the LD flap are a history of surgery or radiation in the axilla—although successful LD flap reconstruction after axillary node dissection has been reported[6]—or a cardiac implant device for a pectoralis major (PM) flap. The disadvantage of a PM flap is its relative large bulk—in comparison to an LD flap—and the possible breast deformity that would make it less favorable in female patients. Another pedicled (fasciocutaneous) flap reported for pharyngeal reconstruction is the supraclavicular artery island flap (SCAIF).[7]

Although Iginio Tansini was credited for first describing the LD flap for mammary reconstruction in 1906, a later review of his work suggests that this flap was in fact a compound scapular flap.[8] Moore and Harkins were the first to describe the "true" pedicled LD reconstruction for breast reconstruction in 1953.[9] In 1978, Quillen et al reported on the first case of a pedicled LD flap in head and neck surgery. They described an "island flap" with the advantage of a long pedicle and a large skin paddle, which makes it suitable for large defects in the head and neck area.[10]

The vascular pedicle is constituted by the thoracodorsal artery and vein, which branch from the subscapular artery, which in turn branches from the axillary artery (▶Fig. 30.3). The thoracodorsal nerve runs along the vascular pedicle and needs to be divided for appropriate mobilization. There are some known varieties specifically in the number of branches supplying the serratus anterior muscle.[11]

To assess the reliability of the overlying skin paddle, it is important to take notice of the three angiosomes or territories of the LD muscle; the further caudal of the scapula, the less reliable the viability of the paddle. Preferably, the paddle is designed over the second angiosome to ensure good perfusion and a wide arc of rotation to reach the head and neck area. The paddle can have maximum dimensions of 10 cm in width and 15 cm in length to allow primary closure.[11]

To avoid seroma formation, two suction drain catheters need to be placed, and quilted suturing of the donor site should be considered.[12,13]

The LD flap is very reliable and has few complications. Watson et al, for example, described total loss of a flap due to a narrow tunnel underneath the PM, which compromised the pedicle. To reach the level of the pharynx, a subcutaneous tunnel should suffice and minimizes possible damage to the thoracodorsal and thoracoacromial pedicle. Another avoidable error is designing the skin paddle too distal, resulting in inadequate perfusion of the skin paddle.[14,15] Otherwise, the excellent arc of rotation, considerable dimensions, ease of harvest, and thinness of the muscle make it one of the most suitable pedicled flaps in head and neck reconstruction.

30.3 Tips

- Consider a pedicled LD flap for pharyngeal reconstruction when patients seem unfit for free tissue transfer.
- The pedicled LD flap has large dimensions, is easy to harvest, thin, and has a relative low complication rate.
- Be aware of the angiosomes of the LD muscle to guarantee proper perfusion of the skin paddle.
- Divide the arterial branches to the serratus anterior muscle in order to provide tension-free mobilization of the thoracodorsal pedicle.
- Generous drainage of the donor site using multiple suction drain catheters should be used to prevent seroma formation. Quilted suturing may aid in this.

30.4 Traps

- Previous surgery or radiation in the axillary area should be considered a relative contraindication for a pedicled LD flap.
- Do not forget the added operating time needed and briefing with the anesthesiology team due to positioning and repositioning of the patient from supine to lateral decubitus and back.

- Do not make a too narrow tunnel for transfer to the recipient site in order to not compromise the pedicle.

References

[1] Lefebvre JL. Larynx preservation. Curr Opin Oncol. 2012; 24(3):218–222

[2] Forastiere AA, Ismaila N, Lewin JS, et al. Use of larynx-preservation strategies in the treatment of laryngeal cancer: American Society of Clinical Oncology Clinical Practice Guideline Update. J Clin Oncol. 2018; 36(11):1143–1169

[3] Hui Y, Wei WI, Yuen PW, Lam LK, Ho WK. Primary closure of pharyngeal remnant after total laryngectomy and partial pharyngectomy: how much residual mucosa is sufficient? Laryngoscope. 1996; 106(4):490–494

[4] de Bree R, Rinaldo A, Genden EM, et al. Modern reconstruction techniques for oral and pharyngeal defects after tumor resection. Eur Arch Otorhinolaryngol. 2008; 265(1):1–9

[5] Piazza C, Bon FD, Paderno A, et al. Fasciocutaneous free flaps for reconstruction of hypopharyngeal defects. Laryngoscope. 2017; 127(12):2731–2737

[6] Hartmann CE, Branford OA, Malhotra A, Chana JS. Survival of a pedicled latissimus dorsi flap in breast reconstruction without a thoracodorsal pedicle. J Plast Reconstr Aesthet Surg. 2013; 66(7):996–998

[7] Giordano L, Di Santo D, Occhini A, et al. Supraclavicular artery island flap (SCAIF): a rising opportunity for head and neck reconstruction. Eur Arch Otorhinolaryngol. 2016; 273(12):4403–4412

[8] Ribuffo D, Cigna E, Gerald GL, et al. Iginio Tansini revisited. Eur Rev Med Pharmacol Sci. 2015; 19(13):2477–2481

[9] Moore HG, Jr, Harkins HN. The use of a latissimus dorsi pedicle flap graft in radical mastectomy. Surg Gynecol Obstet. 1953; 96(4):430–432

[10] Quillen CG, Shearin JC, Jr, Georgiade NG. Use of the latissimus dorsi myocutaneous island flap for reconstruction in the head and neck area: case report. Plast Reconstr Surg. 1978; 62(1):113–117

[11] Godat DM, Sanger JR, Lifchez SD, et al. Detailed neurovascular anatomy of the serratus anterior muscle: implications for a functional muscle flap with multiple independent force vectors. Plast Reconstr Surg. 2004; 114(1):21–29, discussion 30–31

[12] Lee J, Bae Y, Jung JH, et al. Effects of quilting suture interval on donor site seromas after breast reconstruction with latissimus dorsi muscle flap: a randomized trial. Clin Breast Cancer. 2016; 16(6):e159–e164

[13] Daltrey I, Thomson H, Hussien M, Krishna K, Rayter Z, Winters ZE. Randomized clinical trial of the effect of quilting latissimus dorsi flap donor site on seroma formation. Br J Surg. 2006; 93(7):825–830

[14] Urken ML, Cheney ML, Blackwell KE, Harris JR, Hadlock TA, Futra N. Atlas of Regional and Free Flaps for Head and Neck Reconstruction. 2nd ed. Baltimore, MD: Lippincott Williams & Wilkins; 2012:336

[15] Watson JS, Robertson GA, Lendrum J, Stranc MF, Pohl MJ. Pharyngeal reconstruction using the latissimus dorsi myocutaneous flap. Br J Plast Surg. 1982; 35(4):401–407

31 Gastric Pull-Up

Sundeep Alapati, Jatin P. Shah

Abstract

The gastric pull-up procedure for reconstruction of circumferential pharyngoesophageal defects was introduced in the 1960s. The procedure was popularized and refined in the 1970s and 1980s. It was during this period that large case series demonstrating the procedure as safe and reliable were published. Classic indications for the procedure are for reconstruction of circumferential pharyngeal defects after total laryngopharyngectomy and/or cervical esophagectomy. The procedure is completed in three steps. First, the larynx and the pharyngoesophageal region and upper thoracic esophagus are mobilized through the neck. Second, the stomach and lower esophagus are mobilized in and through the abdominal cavity. The last step involves transposition of the stomach into the neck, followed by pharyngogastric anastomosis to restore continuity of the alimentary tract. The advantage of this procedure is the immediate reconstruction of a mucosal lined alimentary tract with only a single anastomosis required. The major disadvantage is the morbidity of operating in three separate visceral spaces. Recently, the popularity of gastric pull-up has decreased with the advent of microvascular free flap reconstruction. However, for reconstruction after total laryngopharyngoesophagectomy and upper thoracic esophagectomy, gastric pull-up remains a good option.

Keywords: gastric pull-up, laryngopharyngectomy, cervical esophagectomy

31.1 History

Reconstruction of the upper alimentary tract following circumferential resection of cancer of the hypopharynx and cervical esophagus has long been a challenge. In the first half of the 20th century, reconstruction was mainly performed by using local flaps as described by Trotter (1912) and Wookey (1940).[1] Multistaged reconstruction with tubed pedicled flaps was the next advancement in pharyngeal reconstruction, which took up to 6 to 8 months to complete the reconstruction. Some patients already had recurrence by the time reconstruction was complete. The multiple stages required prolonged hospitalization, and during which time, the patient was dependent upon nasogastric tube feedings. The deltopectoral flap, popularized by Bakamjian et al, was a major advancement and took only two procedures to complete the reconstruction.[2] In 1960, Ong and Lee reported their experience with pharyngogastric anastomosis following pharyngolaryngoesophagectomy.[3] Le Quesne and Ranger, and later Harrison and Thompson, refined the technique in favor of trans-hiatal pull-through, without opening the chest, and thus the gastric transposition or gastric pull-up operation was born.[4,5,6,7] This operation accomplished reconstruction of the alimentary tract in a single stage, reducing the prolonged morbidity of multistage procedures. Patients are able to swallow a normal diet in less than 2 weeks postoperatively (▶Fig. 31.1). In 1981, Spiro and his colleagues at the Memorial Hospital

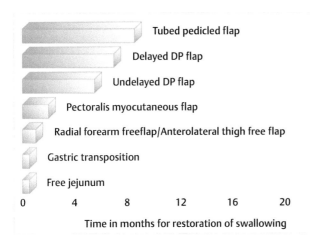

Fig. 31.1 Time required for restoration of normal swallowing after pharyngeal reconstruction by various surgical methods. (Reproduced with permission from Shah JP, Patel SG, Singh B. Head and Neck Surgery and Oncology. Philadelphia, PA: Elsevier; 2012.)

Tubed pedicled flap

Delayed DP flap

Undelayed DP flap

Pectoralis myocutaneous flap

Radial forearm freeflap/Anterolateral thigh free flap

Gastric transposition

Free jejunum

0   4   8   12   16   20   24

Time in months for restoration of swallowing

published a series of 120 patients who were reconstructed with the gastric transposition following cervical esophagectomy or circumferential pharyngectomy.[8,9] This series established that the procedure was safe and highly reliable in carefully selected patients. However, the postoperative morbidity for this procedure was high. Refinements in surgical techniques using laparoscopic and thoracoscopic esophagogastric approaches to mobilize the stomach and esophagus have not reduced the morbidity.[10]

31.2 Indications

The classic indications for the gastric pull-up procedure are for reconstruction of circumferential pharyngeal defects after total laryngopharyngectomy and/or cervical esophagectomy.[11,12] However, the usefulness of this procedure has been further modified to reconstruct the hypopharynx and cervical esophagus in non-oncologic disease processes in both adults and children. These indications include severe stricture or fistula after caustic ingestion, infection, and in the treatment of esophageal atresia. The advantage of the gastric pull-up is the immediate restoration of a mucosal lined alimentary tract with tissue from elsewhere in the alimentary tract with only a single mucosal anastomosis required. In recent years, however, the gastric pull-up procedure has fallen out of favor because of significant morbidity of dissection in three separate visceral spaces and the availability and reliability of free tissue transfer for reconstruction.[13,14,15] However, for reconstruction after total laryngopharyngoesophagectomy and upper thoracic esophagectomy, gastric pull-up remains the best option.[11,12]

31.3 Contraindications

Cancers involving the upper thoracic esophagus and perforating through the membranous trachea are not suitable for the gastric pull-up procedure. Similarly, radiologically demonstrated mediastinal lymph nodes are a contraindication. Previous surgery on the stomach, such as partial gastrectomy or the presence of other pathology in the stomach or esophagus such as esophageal varices, a peptic ulcer, or gastric tumor makes the stomach unsuitable for transposition. Patients with previous mediastinal surgery are not ideal candidates for safe dissection and mobilization of upper thoracic esophagus.

31.4 Preoperative Preparation

The preoperative evaluation should include imaging of the head, neck, and mediastinum using CT scan with contrast or MRI. In addition, an upper gastrointestinal (GI) series with barium esophagogram should be included to evaluate the suitability of the stomach for transposition. Any abnormalities should be further investigated, and alternative methods of reconstruction should be pursued if the stomach is not suitable for transposition. Esophagoscopy, tracheobronchoscopy, and upper GI endoscopy are essential, and a biopsy is required for confirmation of tissue diagnosis. Preoperative consultation with a thoracic surgeon is required for participation in the surgery.

A thorough bowel preparation prior to the operation and admission to the hospital a day prior to surgery is desirable for IV hydration. A detailed informed consent from the patient must be obtained after discussing risk, benefits, alternatives, and possible complications and sequela of the operation. These include complications of surgery and anesthesia, including the risk of fistula, mediastinitis, and pneumothorax. The patient should be informed of the postoperative sequela of dumping syndrome, gastric outlet obstruction, and gastric reflux. The likelihood of postoperative hypothyroidism and hypoparathyroidism should be discussed, and the patient should be made aware of the need for thyroid and calcium replacement. In the past, the risk of intraoperative and postoperative mortality was high, and the patient should be advised of the small but finite risk of death.

31.5 Operative Steps

The patient is positioned on the operating table in the supine position with the neck extended. The procedure is started with both the head and neck and thoracic surgery teams working simultaneously. This allows the procedure to proceed efficiently and can minimize the total operative time. However, if there is any question about the resectability of the primary tumor, that is, involvement of the prevertebral fascia, carotid artery, or invasion of thoracic trachea, then the abdominal and mediastinal components of the procedure should be delayed until the head and neck surgeon can make such a determination. Excessive crowding around the operating table can be avoided by having the two surgeons stand on opposite sides of the table. The head and neck team can use the area around the head of the bed for any assistant surgeons. The skin of the patient is prepped with Betadine solution from the upper lip, to the pubis, and separate drapes are applied to isolate the fields for dissection in the neck and laparotomy.[16,17,18,19,20]

31.5.1 Cervicothoracic Dissection

A transverse incision in the midcervical region is preferred, leaving a distance of at least 3 cm, above the upper border of the permanent tracheostome (▸ Fig. 31.2). Alternatively, a U-shaped curvilinear incision can be employed along the anterior border of the sternocleidomastoid muscles, ending at the lower end with the circular incision for the tracheostome. The permanent tracheostome is ideally placed in the suprasternal notch. If required,

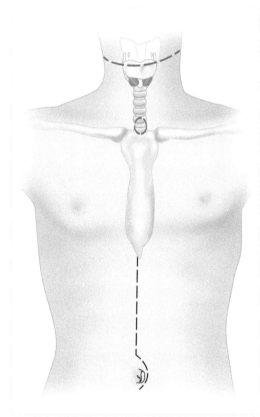

Fig. 31.2 The cervical and abdominal incisions are outlined. (Reproduced with permission from Shah JP, Patel SG, Singh B. Head and Neck Surgery and Oncology. Philadelphia, PA: Elsevier; 2012.)

the incision can be extended below the tracheostome in the midline of the anterior chest wall overlying the manubrium sterni. This extension facilitates excision of the manubrium in patients with distal tracheal invasion requiring substernal tracheal resection. Resection of the manubrium can also be used to facilitate transposition of the stomach through the thoracic inlet in obese patients, in whom the normal thoracic inlet is not sufficient to deliver the stomach in to the neck.

31.5.2 Laryngopharyngectomy and Mobilization of the Upper Thoracic Esophagus

The skin incision is deepened through the platysma, and the upper and lower skin flaps are elevated. The deep cervical fascia at the anterior border of the sternocleidomastoid muscle is incised. This facilitates the beginning of the neck dissections as needed, either unilaterally or bilaterally. In the clinically negative neck, levels II, III, and IV are dissected bilaterally. The extent of neck dissection in patients with documented nodal metastases is dictated by the extent and location of metastatic nodes. Following completion of the neck dissections, attention is focused to the central compartment of the neck. The strap muscles are divided low in the neck, at the suprasternal notch. The middle thyroid vein is ligated permitting access to the tracheoesophageal (TE) groove. The prevertebral plane can be accessed now and a determination of resectability of the cancer can be made.

In patients with lateralized cancers, ipsilateral thyroid lobectomy is performed, largely to enable better clearance of lymph nodes in the TE groove. In circumferential lesions at the level of the thyroid gland, a total thyroidectomy is performed. The thyroid isthmus is exposed, mobilized from the pretracheal plane, and divided if a lobectomy is planned. During this part of the operation, careful search for the parathyroid glands is performed, and as many of the four parathyroids as possible are preserved with their blood supply intact. The parathyroids are retracted laterally.

The permanent tracheostome is then created by excising a circular disc of skin measuring 2 cm in diameter in the suprasternal notch. The trachea is then divided in an oblique beveled fashion. The edges of the distal trachea are sutured to the skin edges of the circular opening to create the permanent tracheostome. A flexible reinforced

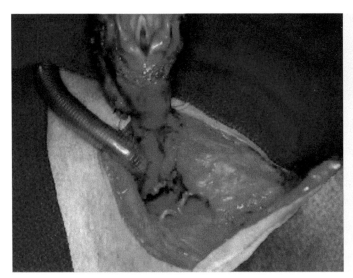

Fig. 31.3 The mobilized larynx permits traction on the cervical esophagus. (Reproduced with permission from Shah JP, Patel SG, Singh B. Head and Neck Surgery and Oncology. Philadelphia, PA: Elsevier; 2012.)

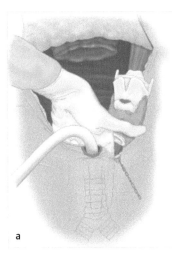
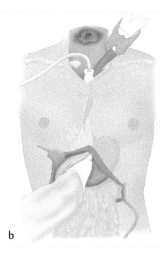

a   b

Fig. 31.4 (a) The upper thoracic esophagus is mobilized using digital dissection via the mediastinum. **(b)** The carina is reached in the posterior mediastinum. (Reproduced with permission from Shah JP, Patel SG, Singh B. Head and Neck Surgery and Oncology. Philadelphia, PA: Elsevier; 2012.)

endotracheal tube is introduced in to the distal trachea, and anesthesia is switched over from the orotracheal tube to this tube. The membranous trachea is gently dissected off of the esophagus posterior to the tracheostome to create a plane of dissection.

Attention is now focused on the superior aspect of the central compartment at the hyoid bone. The suprahyoid muscles are detached from the superior border of the hyoid bone using electrocautery. Attention is paid to the hypoglossal nerves and the lingual arteries, which are often very close to the greater cornua of the hyoid bone. The neurovascular pedicles, containing the superior laryngeal arteries and nerves, at the lateral aspect of the thyrohyoid membrane are carefully isolated, divided,

and ligated. The pharynx is now entered through the vallecula. The remainder of the pharyngeal mucosa and muscular wall are divided circumferentially under direct vision. The superior aspect of the specimen is now completely separated from the oropharynx and can now be used to provide traction on the upper thoracic esophagus (▶ Fig. 31.3).

The upper thoracic esophagus is mobilized circumferentially under direct vision using long instruments and intermittent digital dissection (▶ Fig. 31.4). Meticulous gentle dissection should be undertaken in the TE plane as distal as possible, carefully avoiding inadvertent perforation of the membranous trachea. The anesthesiologist is asked to deflate the balloon of the endotracheal tube to release stretch on the membranous trachea.

Rough digital dissection in the TE plane can easily produce a tear of the membranous trachea, which is difficult to repair. Vascular clips should be used for hemostasis in difficult-to-reach areas. The major blood supply to the upper esophagus is segmental through the branches of the intercostal vessels and prevertebral vessels. These vessels can be clipped and divided as necessary during the dissection.

As the membranous trachea is separated from the esophagus, a Deaver retractor can be used to retract the trachea, providing a direct view of the upper thoracic esophagus. The esophagus can be mobilized laterally and posteriorly at this point in a similar fashion. Blind dissection should absolutely be avoided. By keeping the dissection near the esophagus, entry into the pleural space can be avoided. The surgeon, however, should be on high alert for this potential complication. If the pleural space is entered, the anesthesia team should be alerted and positive pressure respiratory support should be initiated.

31.5.3 Mobilization of the Stomach and Lower Thoracic Esophagus

A midline skin incision in the upper abdomen is made from the xyphoid process up to the umbilicus. The rectus sheath is divided in the midline and the peritoneum is entered and a self-retaining retractor is used to expose the abdominal cavity. The liver and celiac nodes should be palpated for evidence of disease. The triangular ligament of the left lobe of the liver may need to be divided in order to facilitate retraction of the liver and better exposure of the stomach.

The stomach is mobilized by dividing the gastrocolic and gastrosplenic ligaments. The short gastric, left gastric, and left gastroepiploic vessels are sequentially divided and ligated. The blood supply to the mobilized stomach from the right gastric and right gastroepiploic vessels is carefully preserved. The individual branches of the gastroepiploic vessels leading to the gastrocolic ligament must be ligated.

A drainage procedure such as a pyloromyotomy or pyloromyectomy must be performed on the pylorus since the patient will undergo a bilateral vagectomy during the total esophagectomy. A pyloromyectomy is most optimal as it will allow for drainage without constricting the lumen at the gastroduodenal junction. A wedge-shaped segment of the pyloric muscle is removed up to the pyloric mucosa, carefully avoiding mucosal perforation. However, pyloromyotomy or pyloroplasty can be considered as well.

A Penrose drain can now be wrapped around the cardio-esophageal junction allowing for retraction of the cardiac end of the stomach and exposure of the diaphragmatic hiatus. The esophageal hiatus is incised in a semicircular fashion and then dilated manually. This maneuver provides exposure for dissection of the distal esophagus. If there is inadequate space to facilitate dissection, then the diaphragmatic crura can also be divided. The distal esophagus is now circumferentially mobilized using gentle digital dissection and liberal use of vascular clips. Lighting may be difficult in this region and a flexible fiberoptic light source should be utilized. A Harrington retractor may be used to provide gentle anterior retraction of the heart. Retraction of the heart may cause hypotension and intermittent relaxation, and breaks in retraction should be provided. The mobilization is continued until the carina is reached. During these final stages of mobilization, it may be useful to release the esophagus from the stomach toward the neck and vice versa. This "railroading" of the esophagus will allow identification of the last few attachments of the esophagus, permitting its division (▶ Fig. 31.4).

31.5.4 Transposition into the Neck and Anastomosis

Once the thoracic esophagus is completely mobilized, it is ready for transposition into the neck. Traction is applied to specimen in the neck while the stomach, and distal esophagus are fed by the thoracic surgeon from the abdomen through the chest. Forceful retraction of the esophagus must never be performed, because the esophagus can easily tear and the upper end come out through the neck, leaving the lower half and stomach in the abdomen. The thoracic esophagus is gently delivered into the neck, followed by the cardiac end of the stomach. A Babcock clamp can be placed on the cardia to allow delivery of the fundus of the stomach in the neck. It is important to note that enough of the fundus must be delivered to allow a tension-free anastomosis to the pharyngeal mucosa.

The cardioesophageal junction is divided, and the specimen can now be removed (▶ Fig. 31.5).

The transected cardia is closed with either a GI stapler or sharp division and closure in a double-layer fashion. The preferred closure method is to use interrupted inverting chromic suture, while a second layer of serosal sutures is placed using 3–0 silk. A gastrotomy is then made in the upper border of the fundus of the stomach. The incision should be parallel to the serosal vessels and the mucosa should be examined for disease. The gastrotomy should be at least three fingerbreadths in width. Next, the anastomosis between the stomach and pharynx is performed. This can be done in a single-layer fashion using interrupted 2–0 chromic catgut. The posterior anastomotic suture incorporates the prevertebral fascia to hold the stomach in position and avoid traction on the suture line. This pexy maneuver ensures that the stomach is adequately anchored in the neck and allows a tension-free anastomosis (▶ Fig. 31.6). A nasogastric tube is passed through the stomach into the proximal duodenum and its placement is confirmed by palpation. This is best done prior to performing the anterior portion of the anastomosis. The neck and abdomen are then inspected for any signs of bleeding, which should be appropriately controlled. The wounds are copiously irrigated with bacitracin solution. A drain is placed on each side of the neck and sutured securely to the skin. The neck can be closed in a double-layer fashion using 3–0 Vicryl or chromic catgut for platysma and 5–0 Monocryl for skin. The abdomen is closed in the usual fashion.

31.5.5 Postoperative Care

A postoperative chest radiograph must be performed to rule out pneumothorax. In the setting of a postoperative pneumothorax, a chest tube should be placed to drain the pleural cavity. Periodic chest radiographs should be ordered to monitor lung expansion. The chest tubes can be removed once lung expansion is confirmed.

The neck drains should be attached to wall suction units. The drains can be removed once drain output is minimal. A laryngectomy tube can be used to minimize oozing and crusting at the suture line of the tracheostoma. Occasionally, the prolapsing stomach may push the membranous trachea anteriorly, causing functional stomal obstruction.

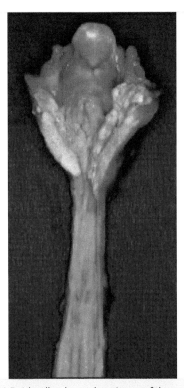

Fig. 31.5 A locally advanced carcinoma of the cervical esophagus extending up to the post cricoid region. (Reproduced with permission from Shah JP, Patel SG, Singh B. Head and Neck Surgery and Oncology. Philadelphia, PA: Elsevier; 2012.)

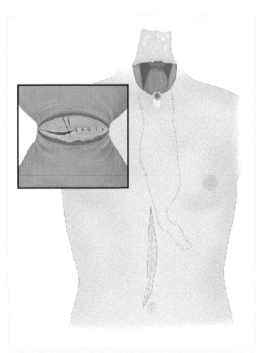

Fig. 31.6 Anastamosis between the stomach and pharynx. (Reproduced with permission from Shah JP, Patel SG, Singh B. Head and Neck Surgery and Oncology. Philadelphia, PA: Elsevier; 2012.)

The nasogastric tube is also attached to suction drainage until peristalsis returns. Tube feeding is initiated once bowel sounds are confirmed. In the setting of good wound healing, oral feeding can start between the 7th and 14th postoperative day. A barium swallow is first performed to rule out anastomotic leak. In patients with a history of radiation, it may be prudent to wait longer than 1 week to initiate feeding. Regurgitation is common in the absence of a cricopharyngeal sphincter. The patient should remain upright while eating to alleviate this. A reflux protocol should also be initiated once the patient begins oral feeding. Some patients may also experience symptoms of dumping, but this is usually transient.

An electrolarynx can be used in the immediate postoperative period for voice restoration.[21] Some patients can learn some degree of "gastric speech", although this is a suboptimal form of voice rehabilitation.[14] Secondary TE puncture has also been shown to be a safe and effective method of voice restoration after gastric pull-up.[21,22,23]

31.6 Complications

A wide range of postoperative mortality (5–20%) is reported in the literature. Complications, such as pharyngogastric fistula is reported in to 22%, and the overall incidence of complications from 26 to 55% are reported.[8] As mentioned previously, in the early years of the procedure, the reported mortality rate was relatively high. A review of a large series of patients in 1981 found a hospital mortality rate of 31%.[13] However, a 1991 review of the experience of 120 patients from Memorial Hospital reported an in-hospital mortality rate of 11%.[8] A similar downward trend has been seen in major and minor complication rates.[13] The largest and most recent series report an anastomotic leak rate of 9 and 13%.[8,13,14] The dreaded complication of circumferential gastric necrosis has been reported in the literature from 0 to 24%, and the rate of death secondary to gastric necrosis is 28%.[24] The surgeon should have a high index of suspicion for anastomotic leak. The mucosa of the stomach is sensitive to photons, and late hemorrhagic complications have occurred in patients who have received radiotherapy with photons after gastric transposition.[8,9]

Overall, the gastric pull-up reconstruction is a safe operation that accomplishes alimentary tract restoration in a single stage, with a single anastomosis, and without the need for microvascular expertise.[16]

References

[1] Wookey H. The surgical treatment of carcinoma of the hypopharynx and the oesophagus. Br J Surg. 1948; 35(139):249–266

[2] Bakamjian VY, Long M, Rigg B. Experience with the medially based deltopectoral flap in reconstructve surgery of the head and neck. Br J Plast Surg. 1971; 24(2):174–183

[3] Ong GB, Lee TC. Pharyngogastric anastomosis after oesophago-pharyngectomy for carcinoma of the hypopharynx and cervical oesophagus. Br J Surg. 1960; 48:193–200

[4] Le Quesne LP, Ranger D. Pharyngolaryngectomy, with immediate pharyngogastric anastomosis. Br J Surg. 1966; 53(2):105–109

[5] Harrison DF. Surgical repair in hypopharyngeal and cervical esophageal cancer. Analysis of 162 patients. Ann Otol Rhinol Laryngol. 1981; 90(4, pt 1):372–375

[6] Harrison DF. Resection of the manubrium. Br J Surg. 1977; 64(5):374–377

[7] Harrison DF, Thompson AE. Pharyngolaryngoesophagectomy with pharyngogastric anastomosis for cancer of the hypopharynx: review of 101 operations. Head Neck Surg. 1986; 8(6):418–428

[8] Spiro RH, Bains MS, Shah JP, Strong EW. Gastric transposition for head and neck cancer: a critical update. Am J Surg. 1991; 162(4):348–352

[9] Spiro RH, Shah JP, Strong EW, Gerold FP, Bains MS. Gastric transposition in head and neck surgery. Indications, complications, and expectations. Am J Surg. 1983; 146(4):483–487

[10] DePaula AL, Macedo AL, Cernea CR, et al. Reconstruction of upper digestive tract: reducing morbidity by laparoscopic pull-up. Otolaryngol Head Neck Surg. 2006; 135(5):710–713

[11] Patel RS, Goldstein DP, Brown D, Irish J, Gullane PJ, Gilbert RW. Circumferential pharyngeal reconstruction: history, critical analysis of techniques, and current therapeutic recommendations. Head Neck. 2010; 32(1):109–120

[12] Chan YW, Ng RW, Liu LH, Chung HP, Wei WI. Reconstruction of circumferential pharyngeal defects after tumour resection: reference or preference. J Plast Reconstr Aesthet Surg. 2011; 64(8):1022–1028

[13] Wei WI, Lam KH, Choi S, Wong J. Late problems after pharyngolaryngoesophagectomy and pharyngogastric anastomosis for cancer of the larynx and hypopharynx. Am J Surg. 1984; 148(4):509–513

[14] Wei WI, Lam LK, Yuen PW, Wong J. Current status of pharyngolaryngo-esophagectomy and pharyngogastric anastomosis. Head Neck. 1998; 20(3):240–244

[15] Disa JJ, Pusic AL, Hidalgo DA, Cordeiro PG. Microvascular reconstruction of the hypopharynx: defect classification, treatment algorithm, and functional outcome based on 165 consecutive cases. Plast Reconstr Surg. 2003; 111(2):652–660, discussion 661–663

[16] Shah JP, Patel SG, Singh B, et al. Jatin Shah's Head and Neck Surgery and Oncology 4th ed. Philadelphia, PA: Elsevier/Mosby; 2012

[17] Bains MS, Spiro RH. Pharyngolaryngectomy, total extrathoracic esophagectomy and gastric transposition. Surg Gynecol Obstet. 1979; 149(5):693–696

[18] Lam KH, Wong J, Lim ST, Ong GB. Surgical treatment of carcinoma of the hypopharynx and cervical oesophagus. Ann Acad Med Singapore. 1980; 9(3):317–322

[19] Lam KH, Choi TK, Wei WI, Lau WF, Wong J. Present status of pharyngogastric anastomosis following

pharyngolaryngo-oesophagectomy. Br J Surg. 1987; 74(2):122–125

[20] Lam KH, Wong J, Lim ST, Ong GB. Pharyngogastric anastomosis following pharyngolaryngoesophagectomy. Analysis of 157 cases. World J Surg. 1981; 5(4):509–516

[21] Medina JE, Nance A, Burns L, Overton R. Voice restoration after total laryngopharyngectomy and cervical esophagectomy using the duckbill prosthesis. Am J Surg. 1987; 154(4):407–410

[22] Singer MI, Blom ED, Hamaker RC. Voice rehabilitation after total laryngectomy. J Otolaryngol. 1983; 12(5):329–334

[23] Noel D, Fink DS, Kunduk M, Schexnaildre MA, DiLeo M, McWhorter AJ. Secondary tracheoesophageal puncture using transnasal esophagoscopy in gastric pull-up reconstruction after total laryngopharyngoesophagectomy. Head Neck. 2016; 38(3):E61–E63

[24] Butskiy O, Anderson DW, Prisman E. Management algorithm for failed gastric pull up reconstruction of laryngopharyngectomy defects: case report and review of the literature. J Otolaryngol Head Neck Surg. 2016; 45(1):41

32 Early Primary Tumor with Advanced Neck Disease

Matthew E. Spector, Jayne R. Stevens, Carol R. Bradford

Abstract

Advanced metastases to the cervical lymph nodes from a small primary cancer is an uncommon pattern of disease in squamous cell carcinoma of the larynx with unique treatment considerations. This pattern is seen more commonly with a supraglottic than a glottic primary cancer, and almost all such patients have a significant smoking history. In accordance with the National Comprehensive Cancer Network (NCCN) guidelines, treatment decisions should be based on the extent of the primary cancer, expected functional outcomes, and patient preferences. Treatment options include surgery to the primary and neck, followed by directed adjuvant therapy, primary concurrent chemoradiation, or chemoselection (neoadjuvant chemotherapy), followed by concurrent chemoradiation for responders and surgery for nonresponders. Oncologic outcomes are similar with all three treatment options. While primary surgical treatment paradigms provide more accurate staging and prognostic information, advanced nodal disease may preclude a modality-sparing approach and all patients will likely still require radiation with or without chemotherapy. As such, functional outcomes may be better in patients treated with concurrent chemoradiation or chemoselection which are the preferred treatment in this patient population. Close monitoring of the neck is important to ensure treatment response, with salvage neck dissection indicated for persistent metastatic cancer in the neck.

Keywords: laryngeal cancer, advanced nodal disease, early primary tumor, organ preservation therapy, functional outcomes, chemoselection

32.1 Introduction

Squamous cell carcinoma of the larynx (LSCC) represents a common subsite of head and neck cancers, and unfortunately has not seen improvement in survival over the past 40 years.[1] The majority of patients who present with cancer of the larynx are male, have a significant history of smoking cigarettes and alcohol, and have advanced cancer at the time of diagnosis.[1,2,3] Staging of LSCC is based on the eighth edition of the American Joint Commission on Cancer TNM (*t*umor size, *n*ode involvement, and *m*etastasis status) staging system.[4] Advanced stage is defined as patients who have advanced T classification (T3–T4) or N classification (N1–N3) and requires multimodality therapy for the best chance of cure.

Patients who have an early primary cancer with advanced cervical lymph node metastases are stage III/IV, and are particularly interesting, because the larynx is typically quite functional because the cancer is low volume and has not invaded in the vital laryngeal structures. The primary cancer is, therefore, amenable to organ-preservation therapies, including partial laryngectomy or radiation paradigms. In this chapter, we present a clinical case and discuss the presentation, evaluation, and treatment options in patients with an early primary cancer and advanced metastases to the neck.

32.2 Case Example

A 55-year-old male with a 25 pack-year history of smoking cigarettes presented with a 3-month history of worsening hoarseness. He reported no dysphagia, odynophagia, or shortness of breath. Examination revealed left palpable cervical lymphadenopathy at the level of the hyoid bone. Flexible laryngoscopy revealed a left glottic mass that extended to the false vocal fold and onto the arytenoid mucosa, without fixation of the vocal cord. A contrast-enhanced CT scan of the neck revealed showed a left glottic lesion extending into the false vocal cord (▶Fig. 32.1a), without definitive pre-epiglottic or paraglottic space involvement, with pathologic nodes in the left neck at the level of the hyoid bone (▶Fig. 32.1b). Chest imaging was negative for metastasis. Biopsies obtained in the operating room were positive for squamous cell carcinoma, assessed as T2N2bM0, stage IV disease.

32.3 Presentation Evaluation

Both glottic and supraglottic cancers can present as early primary cancer with advanced metastases to the cervical lymph nodes. Supraglottic cancers are more common than glottic scancers with this presentation given the readily accessible lymphatic system of the pre-epiglottic and paraglottic spaces.

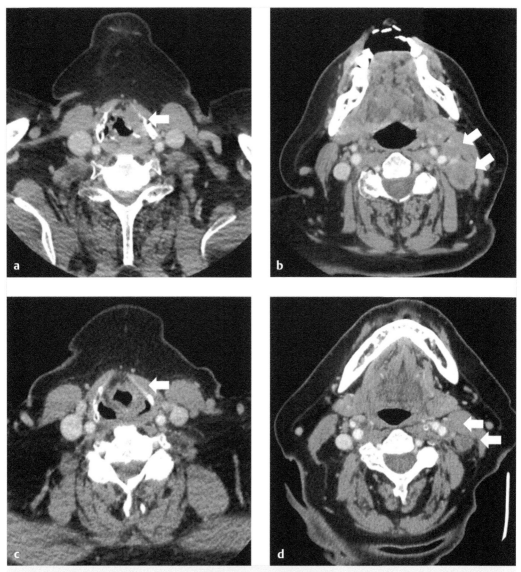

Fig. 32.1 Axial CT images of a patient with an early primary cancer with advanced metastases to the neck treated with chemoselection with an excellent response, followed by concurrent chemoradiation. There is left glottic cancer (**a**, *white arrows*) involving the false cord before chemoselection. There are multiple level 2 lymph nodes (**b**, *white arrows*) in the left neck with associated stranding of adipose tissue (N2b). (**c**) The same left glottic cancer (*white arrow*) 3 weeks after chemoselection with an 80% response. (**d**) The lymph nodes (*white arrows*) after chemoselection with a 50% response.

Glottic cancers typically do not present with neck disease as patients develop hoarseness early in the course of their disease, but growth of the cancer can involve the laryngeal ventricle and subsequent nodal metastasis does occur.[5]

Evaluation of these patients should include a full history and physical examination, supplemented with a fiberoptic examination of the larynx. A thorough assessment of the patient's overall functional status and pulmonary comorbidities is necessary to evaluate surgical candidacy. Vocal fold mobility, speech and swallowing ability, and airway patency should be documented. Patients with lymphadenopathy at presentation have a higher risk of distant metastasis, and imaging should include the neck as well as the chest to evaluate the extent of disease and/or presence of synchronous malignancy.[6] Biopsies taken in the operating room allow for a close examination of the subsites involved by the primary cancer and can aid in surgical and radiation planning.

32.4 Treatment Options

The treatment options for advanced stage LSCC have evolved, with organ preservation protocols favored when compared to total laryngectomy.[5,7,8] Patients who present with early primary cancer of the larynx of the glottis and supraglottis may be amenable to organ-preservation surgery, but the advanced nodal stage drives treatment paradigms that require the need for adjuvant radiation with or without chemotherapy. Consistent with the National Comprehensive Cancer Network (NCCN) guidelines, there are three treatment paradigms that are available to patients with early primary laryngeal cancer with advanced lymph node metastasis: surgery followed by directed adjuvant therapy, concurrent chemoradiation, or chemoselection.[9]

32.5 Surgery Followed by Directed Adjuvant Therapy

Surgery followed by directed adjuvant therapy allows for the most accurate staging and prognostic information as pathology reports are available to keep direct treatment. The presence or absence of adverse pathologic features, such as positive margins or lymphovascular invasion, can be determined from the primary site, as well as the number of positive nodes and the presence of extracapsular spread (ECS) in the neck. These adverse features have consistently been shown to predict survival, and are important in helping to direct adjuvant therapy and counsel patients regarding the risk of recurrence.[10] With the presence of advanced nodal disease, the need for adjuvant therapy is necessary as patients are presenting with stage III or IV metastases requiring multimodality treatment. Therefore, surgery as a primary treatment modality is almost always used in combination with radiation and occasionally the addition of chemotherapy.

Surgery can be performed transorally or via an open approach, with the former being favored to improve the functional outcome. Control rates are similar for both approaches. Zhang et al reviewed their 205 patients treated with a combination of transoral and open approaches, and the 3-year disease-free survival and overall survival were 71.2 and 81. 5%, respectively.[10] The authors reported that while overall stage was prognostic, patients with early primary tumors with advanced nodal disease did not differ in survival than patients with advanced primary tumors (T3–T4 classification).[10]

An important consideration after surgery is the need for adjuvant therapy and the expected functional outcomes following postoperative radiation. The effect of radiation on the larynx is detrimental, and patients who receive adjuvant therapy tend to have worse speaking and swallowing outcomes than patients who undergo surgery alone.[11,12] Lewin et al studied functional outcomes of supracricoid partial laryngectomy after surgical treatment for T2–T4 tumors, including a cohort of patients with previous radiation therapy. Of these patients, 14.8% were partially gastrostomy tube (g-tube) dependent and 3.7% were entirely g-tube dependent.[13] Nakayama et al showed 10-year laryngeal preservation rates of 88.9 and 98.5% in open partial and transoral laser surgery, respectively, with a 10% g-tube rate in the open partial laryngectomy group.[14]

32.6 Concurrent Chemoradiation

Concurrent chemoradiation is the most common treatment for patients with early primary cancer and advanced lymph node metastasis. Beginning with the results of the Radiation Therapy Oncology Group (RTOG) 91–11 study, chemoradiation became the standard of care for advanced laryngeal cancer.[8] The 2-year locoregional control and overall survival in this study were 78 and 75%, respectively. The laryngeal preservation rate was 84% at 3.8 years. Subsequent subset analysis from this original publication has shown improved outcomes and less toxicity in early-stage cancer, suggesting that this population does better than these published rates.[15]

The long-term follow-up from the RTOG 91–11 examining speech and swallowing outcomes using concurrent chemoradiation was published in 2013.[16] Patients were followed for a median of 10.8 years. Speech difficulty, classified as moderate difficulty saying some words, ranged from 4 to 8.5%.

Difficulty swallowing was rated as soft food only or liquids only and occurred in 17 to 24%, respectively. The g-tube rate was 3%, although the authors note this was not collected at the trial onset and may not have complete data.

32.7 Chemoselection

Chemoselection offers a unique paradigm for patients with early primary cancer and advanced cervical lymph node metastases. The benefit of this approach is that the surgical oncologist is able to identify patients who are likely to fail treatment with concurrent chemoradiation and who would require surgical salvage.[17] Patients are given a single cycle of cisplatin and 5-fluorouracil (PF) or docetaxel, cisplatin, and 5-fluorouracil (TPF) and response is assessed at 3 weeks in the operating room. Patients with a greater than 50% response receive concurrent chemoradiation, and patients with less than 50% response receive surgery followed by directed adjuvant therapy.[7,18] This "in vivo" method of selecting patients allows for a personalized approach to therapy.

The results of chemoselection yielded excellent survival in a single-institution phase II trial, with 3-year overall survival and disease-specific survival rates of 85 and 87%, respectively.[18] In addition, the laryngeal preservation rate was 70% at 3 years. The majority of the patients who required laryngectomy for recurrent cancer or a dysfunctional larynx had T3 and T4 primary cancers, suggesting that even early primary tumors treated with chemoselection continue to have long-term laryngeal preservation in addition to cure.

The chemoselection response in the neck was also examined as part of the Veterans Affairs (VA) larynx study.[19] In this study, 92 of 332 patients had advanced lymph node metastases (N2–N3), and 25% had early primary tumors (T1–T2). Chemoselection in this study used three cycles of PF. Patients who achieved a complete response in the neck after induction chemotherapy had improved survival compared to patients treated with surgery and radiation, or patients who achieved less than a complete response in the neck. This finding confirms that even patients who have the poorest prognosis with laryngeal cancer (N2–N3 disease) may benefit from chemoselection approaches.

The speech and swallowing outcomes of patients who underwent chemoselection was published by Fung et al in 2005.[20] With a median follow-up of 40 months, there were no patients with g-tube dependence, and the majority of patients took an oral diet with no need for nutritional supplements (88.9%). Patients with lower T classification had significantly higher voice-related quality-of-life scores.

32.8 Salvage Neck Dissection

The role of salvage neck dissection in the treatment of LSCC requires special consideration. The presence of advanced nodal disease requires careful follow-up in the posttreatment period. Imaging should be obtained 8 to 12 weeks following the completion of radiation therapy, and PET/CT is the most commonly used imaging modality.[21] Patients who have no evidence of cancer on imaging and clinical examination are considered to have a complete response, and the isolated regional failure in this population ranges in studies from 0 to 7.5%.[22,23] Patients with persistent imaging abnormalities after definitive treatment may harbor viable tumor cells up to 20% of the time, and close observation versus salvage neck dissection should be considered based on disease location, imaging findings, and patient preferences.[21,24] If salvage neck dissection is not performed, fine-needle aspiration, repeat imaging, or close clinical follow-up can be used for surveillance.

32.9 Case Conclusion

We discussed treatment options for the patient based on NCCN guidelines, and the patient chose chemoselection. The patient was given a single cycle induction with PF and assessed in the operating room at 3 weeks. There was an 80% response of the primary tumor (▸Fig. 32.1c) and approximately 50% response of the cervical lymph node metastases (▸Fig. 32.1d). The patient underwent concurrent chemoradiation and is currently disease free at 3 years. He reports normal voicing with occasional dryness and takes a regular diet.

References

[1] Siegel RL, Miller KD, Jemal A. Cancer statistics, 2016. CA Cancer J Clin. 2016; 66(1):7–30
[2] Groome PA, O'Sullivan B, Irish JC, et al. Management and outcome differences in supraglottic cancer between Ontario, Canada, and the Surveillance, Epidemiology, and End Results areas of the United States. J Clin Oncol. 2003; 21(3):496–505

[3] Talamini R, Bosetti C, La Vecchia C, et al. Combined effect of tobacco and alcohol on laryngeal cancer risk: a case-control study. Cancer Causes Control. 2002; 13(10):957–964

[4] Amin MB, Edge S, Greene F, et al, eds. AJCC Cancer Staging Manual. 8th ed. New York, NY: Springer; 2017

[5] Sheahan P. Management of advanced laryngeal cancer. Rambam Maimonides Med J. 2014; 5(2):e0015

[6] Birkeland AC, Rosko AJ, Chinn SB, Prince ME, Sun GH, Spector ME. Prevalence and outcomes of head and neck versus non-head and neck second primary malignancies in head and neck squamous cell carcinoma: an analysis of the Surveillance, Epidemiology, and End Results database. ORL J Otorhinolaryngol Relat Spec. 2016; 78(2):61–69

[7] Wolf GT, Fisher SG, Hong WK, et al; Department of Veterans Affairs Laryngeal Cancer Study Group. Induction chemotherapy plus radiation compared with surgery plus radiation in patients with advanced laryngeal cancer. N Engl J Med. 1991; 324(24):1685–1690

[8] Forastiere AA, Goepfert H, Maor M, et al. Concurrent chemotherapy and radiotherapy for organ preservation in advanced laryngeal cancer. N Engl J Med. 2003; 349(22):2091–2098

[9] National Comprehensive Cancer Network. Head and Neck Cancers Version 1.2018. 2018. Available at: https://www.nccn.org/professionals/physician_gls/pdf/head-and-neck.pdf. Accessed April 7, 2018

[10] Zhang SY, Lu ZM, Luo XN, et al. Retrospective analysis of prognostic factors in 205 patients with laryngeal squamous cell carcinoma who underwent surgical treatment. PLoS One. 2013; 8(4):e60157

[11] Cho KJ, Joo YH, Sun DI, Kim MS. Supracricoid laryngectomy: oncologic validity and functional safety. Eur Arch Otorhinolaryngol. 2010; 267(12):1919–1925

[12] Topaloglu I, Köprücü G, Bal M. Analysis of swallowing function after supracricoid laryngectomy with cricohyoidopexy. Otolaryngol Head Neck Surg. 2012; 146(3):412–418

[13] Lewin JS, Hutcheson KA, Barringer DA, et al. Functional analysis of swallowing outcomes after supracricoid partial laryngectomy. Head Neck. 2008; 30(5):559–566

[14] Nakayama M, Okamoto M, Hayakawa K, et al. Clinical outcomes of 849 laryngeal cancers treated in the past 40 years: are we succeeding? Jpn J Clin Oncol. 2014; 44(1):57–64

[15] Machtay M, Moughan J, Trotti A, et al. Factors associated with severe late toxicity after concurrent chemoradiation for locally advanced head and neck cancer: an RTOG analysis. J Clin Oncol. 2008; 26(21):3582–3589

[16] Forastiere AA, Zhang Q, Weber RS, et al. Long-term results of RTOG 91–11: a comparison of three nonsurgical treatment strategies to preserve the larynx in patients with locally advanced larynx cancer. J Clin Oncol. 2013; 31(7):845–852

[17] Vainshtein JM, Wu VF, Spector ME, Bradford CR, Wolf GT, Worden FP. Chemoselection: a paradigm for optimization of organ preservation in locally advanced larynx cancer. Expert Rev Anticancer Ther. 2013; 13(9):1053–1064

[18] Urba S, Wolf G, Eisbruch A, et al. Single-cycle induction chemotherapy selects patients with advanced laryngeal cancer for combined chemoradiation: a new treatment paradigm. J Clin Oncol. 2006; 24(4):593–598

[19] Wolf GT, Fisher SG. Effectiveness of salvage neck dissection for advanced regional metastases when induction chemotherapy and radiation are used for organ preservation. Laryngoscope. 1992; 102(8):934–939

[20] Fung K, Lyden TH, Lee J, et al. Voice and swallowing outcomes of an organ-preservation trial for advanced laryngeal cancer. Int J Radiat Oncol Biol Phys. 2005; 63(5):1395–1399

[21] Hamoir M, Ferlito A, Schmitz S, et al. The role of neck dissection in the setting of chemoradiation therapy for head and neck squamous cell carcinoma with advanced neck disease. Oral Oncol. 2012; 48(3):203–210

[22] Chan AW, Ancukiewicz M, Carballo N, Montgomery W, Wang CC. The role of postradiotherapy neck dissection in supraglottic carcinoma. Int J Radiat Oncol Biol Phys. 2001; 50(2):367–375

[23] Corry J, Peters L, Fisher R, et al. N2-N3 neck nodal control without planned neck dissection for clinical/radiologic complete responders-results of Trans Tasman Radiation Oncology Group Study 98.02. Head Neck. 2008; 30(6):737–742

[24] Strasser MD, Gleich LL, Miller MA, Saavedra HI, Gluckman JL. Management implications of evaluating the N2 and N3 neck after organ preservation therapy. Laryngoscope. 1999; 109(11):1776–1780

33 Targeted Therapy for the Treatment of Advanced Squamous Cell Carcinoma of the Larynx

Dan P. Zandberg

Abstract

In this chapter, systemic agents targeted against the epidermal growth factor receptor and the programed death 1: programed death ligand 1 pathway are discussed. The trials leading to the approval of cetuximab in the first-line setting and nivolumab after platinum failure are highlighted and exploration of predictive biomarkers and future directions are discussed.

Keywords: epidermal growth factor receptor, cetuximab, immunotherapy, PD-1, PD-L1, advanced laryngeal cancer

33.1 Introduction

For patients with squamous cell carcinoma (SCC) of the larynx with a locoregional recurrence not amenable to surgery or radiation, and/or metastatic disease, palliative systemic therapy is the only option for treatment. Traditional cytotoxic chemotherapeutic agents used in SCC of the head and neck (HNSCC) include platinum (carboplatin, cisplatin), taxanes (paclitaxel, docetaxel), and 5-fluorouracil (5FU). In the recurrent/metastatic (R/M) setting, no platinum-based doublet has improved overall survival (OS) in non-nasopharyngeal HNSCC compared to a single agent, although doublets are associated with significantly higher response rates.[1,2] Platinum-based doublet combinations, cisplatin 5FU and cisplatin paclitaxel have been compared in a phase III trial with no difference in efficacy.[3] Outcomes with traditional chemotherapy regimens alone remain poor with median OS between 8 and 9 months.[3] In an effort to improve outcomes for patients with R/M HNSCC including laryngeal SCC, molecular pathways involved in oncogenesis and proliferation, as well as immune co-signaling have been targeted. In this chapter, targeted therapy will be discussed with a focus on the epidermal growth factor receptor (EGFR) and the programed death 1 (PD-1): programed death ligand 1 (PD-L1) pathway, which have shaped our current standard of care approach to patients with advanced SCC of the larynx.

33.2 Case Discussion

A 63-year-old male with a past history of hypertension presented to your clinic with a diagnosis of metastatic SCC of the larynx. The patient was found to have biopsy-proven SCC of the supraglottic larynx with metastasis to the lung and liver on imaging. He is hoarse and has some weight loss but otherwise is active and still working.

33.3 Targeting the Epidermal Growth Factor Receptor in the First-line Setting

The EGFR is a transmembrane receptor that is part of the ErbB family. Stimulation of EGFR leads to activation of downstream pathways including ras/raf/mitogen-activated protein kinase, phosphatidylinositol 3-kinase/v-Akt murine thymoma vial oncogene homolog, and phospholipase-C-y/protein kinase C, resulting in increased proliferation and survival of cells.[4,5,6] EGFR is overexpressed in approximately 90% of HNSCC patients and has been associated with a worse prognosis.[7,8,9] In SCC of the larynx, EGFR has been targeted with both monoclonal antibodies and tyrosine kinase inhibitors.

Cetuximab is an immunoglobulin G1 (IgG1) human-murine monoclonal antibody (mAb) that binds irreversibly to the extracellular domain of the EGFR receptor, blocking EGFR signaling.[10] It has been evaluated in the R/M setting in trials including laryngeal SCC both as a single agent and in combination with chemotherapy. Cetuximab was combined with platinum (cisplatin or carboplatin) and 5-FU in a phase III EXTREME Trial, comparing this regimen to platinum and 5-FU alone in the first-line setting for R/M HNSCC. Those in the experimental arm went on to receive cetuximab alone after six cycles of the triplet regimen. The addition of cetuximab led to a significant increase in response rate (RR; 36 vs. 20%; $p < 0.001$), progression-free survival (PFS; median: 5.6 vs. 3.3 months; hazard ratio [HR] for progression: 0.54; 95% confidence interval [CI]: 0.43–0.67; $p < 0.001$), and OS (median OS: 10.1 vs. 7.4 months; HR for death:

0.80; 95% CI: 0.64–0.99; p = 0.04),[11] resulting in its approval in combination with platinum and 5-FU by the Food and Drug Administration (FDA) and European Medical Agency in November 2011. It is currently the standard of care regimen for front-line treatment of R/M HNSCC including laryngeal SCC for patients who can tolerate a triplet regimen.

Panitumumab, a fully human IgG2 mAb against EGFR, was also combined with platinum and 5-FU in the phase III SPECTRUM trial. While the addition of panitumumab lead to a significant increase in RR and PFS compared to platinum and 5-FU alone, this did not translate into a significant OS benefit (median OS: 11·1 vs. 9.0 months; HR: 0·873; 95% CI: 0·729–1·046; p = 0.1403).[12] One possible reason for a lack of OS benefit with panitumumab as opposed to cetuximab is a longer OS in the control group in SPECTRUM compared to EXTREME (median OS: 9 vs. 7.4 months, respectively), which may have partially been from improved outcomes in patients from the Asia-Pacific geographic region (median OS of 11.7 months in control arm), which were not included in the EXTREME trial. Additionally, there are differences in the immunologic effects of the two antibodies. Cetuximab is an IgG1 mAb, and in contrast to IgG2 mAb panitumumab, cetuximab can induce the innate immune system through natural killer (NK) cell mediated antibody-dependent cellular cytotoxicity (ADCC) and additionally stimulate adaptive immunity, specifically the development of EGFR-specific CD8 T cells via NK cell/dendritic cell crosstalk.[13,14] Whether or not this contributed significantly to the difference in outcomes is not known.

33.4 Case Discussion (Continued)

Based on the EXTREME trial a regimen of cisplatin, 5FU and cetuximab is selected for treating this patient. The patient is treated with 6 cycles with a partial response and then is transitioned to cetuximab alone. Repeat imaging after 2 months of cetuximab alone shows progression of the cancers. The patient is started on nivolumab.

33.5 Targeted Therapy after Failure of Platinum-Based Chemotherapy

The patient has failed platinum-based chemotherapy. Traditional chemotherapeutic agents including taxanes, methotrexate, and gemcitabine have been evaluated in this setting with limited efficacy.[15] Treatment with cetuximab alone yielded a response rate of 13% and disease control rate of 46%; however, control was short lived as the time to progression was only 70 days.[16] Tyrosine kinase inhibitor afatinib, an irreversible ErbB family blocker, which inhibits EGFR, human epidermal growth factor receptor 2 (HER2), HER3, and HER4, was compared to methotrexate in a randomized phase III trial in HNSCC patients who had failed at least two cycles of platinum-based chemotherapy for R/M disease. Approximately 60% of patients had received prior mAb against EGFR in the frontline setting. PFS, the primary endpoint of the trial, was significantly increased with afatinib (median: 2.6 vs. 1.7 months; HR: 0.80; 95% CI: 0.65–0.98; p = 0.03). However, there was no difference in RR (10 vs. 6%; p = 0.10) or OS (median: 6.8 vs. 6 months; HR: 0.96; 95% CI: 0.77–1.19; p = 0.70) between afatinib and methotrexate.[17]

33.5.1 Immune Checkpoint Inhibitors

The immune response involves the complex interplay of immune cells driven by co-signaling molecule interaction and the cytokine/chemokine milieu. Immune checkpoint inhibitors target these co-signaling molecules and blockade of the PD-1:PD-L1 pathway has proven efficacious in multiple solid tumors including HNSCC.[18,19,20] Ligation of PD-1 on cytotoxic T cells by PD-L1 or PD-L2 expressed by tumor cells can result in T-cell anergy and apoptosis, providing protection for the tumor.[21,22,23,24] Anti-PD-1 mAbs block the interaction of PD-1 with PD-L1 and PD-L2, while anti-PD-L1 mAbs block the interaction of PD-L1 with PD-1 and CD80 (▶Fig. 33.1). Ligation of CD80 on effector T cells by PD-L1 can also lead to immune suppression.[25] Nivolumab, a fully human IgG4 anti-PD-1 mAb, was compared to investigators' choice treatment (docetaxel, cetuximab, or methotrexate) in a randomized phase III trial in patients who had failed prior platinum chemotherapy. All patients were included regardless of PD-L1 status. Treatment with nivolumab was associated with a response rate of 13.3% and while there was no difference in PFS, nivolumab led to a significant increase in OS (median: 7.5 vs. 5.1 months; HR: 0.70; 97.73% CI: 0.51–0.96; p = 0.01).[26] This led to the approval of nivolumab in both the United States and Europe for R/M HNSCC, including laryngeal

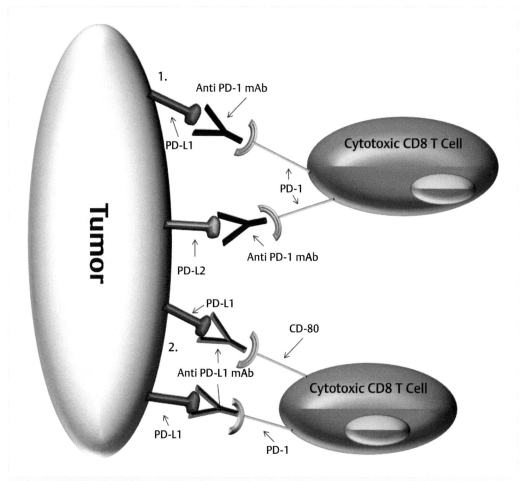

Fig. 33.1 Therapeutic blockade of the PD-1: PD-L1 pathway by anti-PD-1 and anti-PD-L1 monoclonal antibodies. **1.** Anti-PD-1 mAb: anti-PD-1 mAbs block the interaction of PD-1 and PD-L1 and PD-1 and PD-L2. **2.** Anti-PD-L1 mAb: anti-PD-L1 mAbs block the interaction of PD-L1 and PD-1 and PD-L1 and CD80.

SCC, as standard of care treatment for patients with disease progression on or after platinum-based therapy, which includes failure within 6 months of platinum-based chemoradiation given in the upfront locally advanced setting. Another IgG4 anti-PD-1 mAb, pembrolizumab, was evaluated in a similarly designed phase III trial. The primary endpoint was OS in the intention to treat cohort with an efficacy boundary of one-sided α of 0.0175 corresponding to a HR for risk of death of 0.80. Initial analysis showed that patients treated with pembrolizumab had a median OS of 8.4 months compared to 7.1 months in the control arm (HR: 0.81; 95% CI: 0.66–0.99; p = 0.0204); therefore, the improvement in OS with pembrolizumab was not statistically significant. Interestingly, the control arm of Keynote 040 did better than in CheckMate 141 (7.1 vs. 5.1 months, respectively). This may have been partially driven by the receipt of subsequent immune checkpoint inhibitors by patients in the control arm.[27] However, updated analysis of Keynote 040, which included survival data on 11 additional patients, showed a decrease in the hazard ratio for the risk of death to 0.80 (0.65-0.98) with a p value of 0.0161 for the intention to treat cohort who received pembrolizumab. Anti-PD-L1 mAb durvalumab has been evaluated in phase II trials in platinum failure patients both alone and in combination with anti-CTLA4 (cytotoxic T-lymphocyte–associated antigen 4) mAb tremelimumab. In the single-arm phase II HAWK trial, which included R/M HNSCC patients who had failed platinum chemotherapy and were PD-L1 high (≥ 25% tumor cell PD-L1 expression), treatment with single agent durvalumab led to RR of 16.2% and a median OS of 7.1 months (95% CI: 4.9–9.9).[28] A phase III trial is ongoing evaluating durvalumab ± tremelimumab versus investigators' choice chemotherapy in the platinum failure setting.

Treatment with anti-PD-1 or anti-PD-L1 mAbs can be associated with immune-related adverse events (IrAEs), which can affect any organ system including the pituitary (hypophysitis), thyroid (hypothyroid/hyperthyroid), skin (rash), lung (pneumonitis), liver (hepatitis), and colon (colitis). Importantly, these agents have been well tolerated in trials with, for example, less frequent G3/G4 treatment-related adverse events (13%) with nivolumab in CheckMate 141. Pneumonitis was only observed in 2.1% of patients.[26] However, IrAEs can occur at any time with these agents and the treating physician must remain vigilant as prompt treatment with steroids is required to prevent serious adverse events.

33.6 Predictive Biomarkers

Currently, there are no approved predictive biomarkers for EGFR-targeted therapy. Both EGFR copy number by FISH (fluorescence in situ hybridization) and EGFR expression by immunohistochemistry were evaluated retrospectively in patients treated with cetuximab in the EXTREME trial, and both were not predictive of efficacy.[29,30] Presence of the KRAS variant, a germline mutation in micro-RNA-binding site in KRAS, was found to be predictive of benefit with cetuximab combined with cisplatin given concurrent with radiation in the locally advanced setting; however, to date it has not been evaluated in the R/M setting.[31] Subgroup analysis of LUX1 Head and Neck phase III trial with afatinib showed that patients who were both p16 negative and EGFR amplified seemed to derive the most benefit with afatinib compared to methotrexate, especially if they were EGFR monoclonal AB naive.[32] Data as to whether human papillomavirus (HPV) negative patients do better with EGFR-targeted therapy are conflicting. While subgroup analysis of the SPECTRUM trial showed that p16-negative patients had significantly longer OS with the addition of panitumumab, benefit with cetuximab in the EXTREME trial was independent of HPV status.[12,33]

In the CheckMate 141 study, despite a response rate of only 13%, nivolumab significantly improved OS. While only a minority of patients respond to single-agent anti-PD-1 mAb, those who do can have a prolonged duration of response.[26,34] This highlights the importance of biomarkers to select both those patients who will benefit from single-agent therapy and those who would benefit from another therapeutic strategy. The most well-studied biomarker is PD-L1, which across multiple solid tumor types has shown predictive value.[35] Specifically in HNSCC, increased tumor PD-L1 expression was associated with increased RR in both checkmate 141 (PD-L1 > 1% vs. > 5% vs. > 10%) and Keynote 040 (PD-L1 > 50%). In terms of overall survival, patients who were PD-L1 positive (≥ 1% tumor cell expression) in CheckMate 141 had greater benefit from nivolumab versus chemotherapy (HR for death: 0.55; 95% CI: 0.36–0.83) compared to those who were PD-L1 negative (HR for death: 0.89; 95% CI: 0.54–1.45). While this initial analysis showed only an 11% reduction in the risk of death for PD-L1 negative patients, with longer follow up (2 years) a greater reduction in the risk of death (27%) with Nivolumab compared to chemotherapy, was observed (HR for death for PD-L1 negative vs. chemotherapy: 0.73; 95% CI: 0.49–1.09).[26] In terms of overall survival, patients who were PD-L1 positive (≥ 1% tumor cell expression) in CheckMate 141 had greater benefit from Nivolumab. The predictive value of tumor PD-L1 expression can also be enhanced by including PD-L1 expression on tumor infiltrating immune cells as well as PD-L2 expression.[36,37] However, while PD-L1 may be predictive, those who are PD-L1 negative may still benefit, with limitations to PD-L1 as a biomarker including lack of consistent cut point for defining positive as well as heterogeneity in expression in the tumor microenvironment. Both high mutational burden and T-cell-inflamed phenotype based on interferon-gamma gene expression scoring has been associated with improved efficacy with treatment with anti-PD-1 mAb.[38,39] Currently, nivolumab is approved for all patients regardless of PD-L1 status and there is no biomarker testing required for treatment.

33.7 Future Directions

There is still a great need for better outcomes in patients with advanced SCC of the larynx. Work continues to be done to find new and novel molecular pathways to target. The efficacy of single-agent anti-PD-1 or anti-PD-L1 mAbs has led to the development of many trials, including in the frontline setting in R/M laryngeal SCC as well as in combination with radiation in the curative intent setting. Importantly, biomarker discovery and selection strategies continue to be studied. These next-generation trials are poised to continue to improve the treatment of advanced laryngeal cancer.

References

[1] Jacobs C, Lyman G, Velez-García E, et al. A phase III randomized study comparing cisplatin and fluorouracil as single agents and in combination for advanced squamous cell carcinoma of the head and neck. J Clin Oncol. 1992; 10(2):257–263

[2] Forastiere AA, Metch B, Schuller DE, et al. Randomized comparison of cisplatin plus fluorouracil and carboplatin plus fluorouracil versus methotrexate in advanced squamous-cell carcinoma of the head and neck: a Southwest Oncology Group study. J Clin Oncol. 1992; 10(8):1245–1251

[3] Gibson MK, Li Y, Murphy B, et al; Eastern Cooperative Oncology Group. Randomized phase III evaluation of cisplatin plus fluorouracil versus cisplatin plus paclitaxel in advanced head and neck cancer (E1395): an intergroup trial of the Eastern Cooperative Oncology Group. J Clin Oncol. 2005; 23(15):3562–3567

[4] Sacco AG, Worden FP. Molecularly targeted therapy for the treatment of head and neck cancer: a review of the ErbB family inhibitors. Onco Targets Ther. 2016; 9:1927–1943

[5] Egloff AM, Grandis JR. Targeting epidermal growth factor receptor and SRC pathways in head and neck cancer. Semin Oncol. 2008; 35(3):286–297

[6] Moreira J, Tobias A, O'Brien MP, Agulnik M. Targeted therapy in head and neck cancer: an update on current clinical developments in epidermal growth factor receptor-targeted therapy and immunotherapies. Drugs. 2017; 77(8):843–857

[7] Santini J, Formento JL, Francoual M, et al. Characterization, quantification, and potential clinical value of the epidermal growth factor receptor in head and neck squamous cell carcinomas. Head Neck. 1991; 13(2):132–139

[8] Rubin Grandis J, Melhem MF, Gooding WE, et al. Levels of TGF-alpha and EGFR protein in head and neck squamous cell carcinoma and patient survival. J Natl Cancer Inst. 1998; 90(11):824–832

[9] Ang KK, Berkey BA, Tu X, et al. Impact of epidermal growth factor receptor expression on survival and pattern of relapse in patients with advanced head and neck carcinoma. Cancer Res. 2002; 62(24):7350–7356

[10] Goldstein NI, Prewett M, Zuklys K, Rockwell P, Mendelsohn J. Biological efficacy of a chimeric antibody to the epidermal growth factor receptor in a human tumor xenograft model. Clin Cancer Res. 1995; 1(11):1311–1318

[11] Vermorken JB, Mesia R, Rivera F, et al. Platinum-based chemotherapy plus cetuximab in head and neck cancer. N Engl J Med. 2008; 359(11):1116–1127

[12] Vermorken JB, Stöhlmacher-Williams J, Davidenko I, et al; SPECTRUM investigators. Cisplatin and fluorouracil with or without panitumumab in patients with recurrent or metastatic squamous-cell carcinoma of the head and neck (SPECTRUM): an open-label phase 3 randomised trial. Lancet Oncol. 2013; 14(8):697–710

[13] Ferris RL, Lenz HJ, Trotta AM, et al. Rationale for combination of therapeutic antibodies targeting tumor cells and immune checkpoint receptors: harnessing innate and adaptive immunity through IgG1 isotype immune effector stimulation. Cancer Treat Rev. 2018; 63:48–60

[14] Srivastava RM, Lee SC, Andrade Filho PA, et al. Cetuximab-activated natural killer and dendritic cells collaborate to trigger tumor antigen-specific T-cell immunity in head and neck cancer patients. Clin Cancer Res. 2013; 19(7):1858–1872

[15] Argiris A, Harrington KJ, Tahara M, et al. Evidence-based treatment options in recurrent and/or metastatic squamous cell carcinoma of the head and neck. Front Oncol. 2017; 7:72

[16] Vermorken JB, Trigo J, Hitt R, et al. Open-label, uncontrolled, multicenter phase II study to evaluate the efficacy and toxicity of cetuximab as a single agent in patients with recurrent and/or metastatic squamous cell carcinoma of the head and neck who failed to respond to platinum-based therapy. J Clin Oncol. 2007; 25(16):2171–2177

[17] Machiels JP, Haddad RI, Fayette J, et al; LUX-H&N 1 investigators. Afatinib versus methotrexate as second-line treatment in patients with recurrent or metastatic squamous-cell carcinoma of the head and neck progressing on or after platinum-based therapy (LUX-Head & Neck 1): an open-label, randomised phase 3 trial. Lancet Oncol. 2015; 16(5):583–594

[18] Motzer RJ, Escudier B, McDermott DF, et al; CheckMate 025 Investigators. Nivolumab versus everolimus in advanced renal-cell carcinoma. N Engl J Med. 2015; 373(19):1803–1813

[19] Borghaei H, Paz-Ares L, Horn L, et al. Nivolumab versus docetaxel in advanced nonsquamous non-small-cell lung cancer. N Engl J Med. 2015; 373(17):1627–1639

[20] Larkin J, Chiarion-Sileni V, Gonzalez R, et al. Combined nivolumab and ipilimumab or monotherapy in untreated melanoma. N Engl J Med. 2015; 373(1):23–34

[21] Wilke CM, Wei S, Wang L, Kryczek I, Kao J, Zou W. Dual biological effects of the cytokines interleukin-10 and interferon-γ. Cancer Immunol Immunother. 2011; 60(11):1529–1541

[22] Barber DL, Wherry EJ, Masopust D, et al. Restoring function in exhausted CD8 T cells during chronic viral infection. Nature. 2006; 439(7077):682–687

[23] Topalian SL, Drake CG, Pardoll DM. Targeting the PD-1/B7-H1(PD-L1) pathway to activate anti-tumor immunity. Curr Opin Immunol. 2012; 24(2):207–212

[24] Badoual C, Hans S, Merillon N, et al. PD-1-expressing tumor-infiltrating T cells are a favorable prognostic biomarker in HPV-associated head and neck cancer. Cancer Res. 2013; 73(1):128–138

[25] Park JJ, Omiya R, Matsumura Y, et al. B7-H1/CD80 interaction is required for the induction and maintenance of peripheral T-cell tolerance. Blood. 2010; 116(8):1291–1298

[26] Ferris RL, Blumenschein G, Jr, Fayette J, et al. Nivolumab for recurrent squamous-cell carcinoma of the head and neck. N Engl J Med. 2016; 375(19):1856–1867

[27] Cohen EEHK, Le Tourneau C, et al. Pembrolizumab (pembro) vs standard of care (SOC) for recurrent or metastatic head and neck squamous cell carcinoma (R/M HNSCC): Phase 3 KEYNOTE-040 trial. Presented at ESMO 2017 Congress; September 8–12, 2017; Madrid, Spain

[28] Zandberg AA, Jimeno A, Good JS, et al. Durvalumab for recurrent/metastatic (R/M) head and neck squamous cell carcinoma (HNSCC): preliminary results from a single-arm, phase 2 study. Ann Oncol. 2017; 28:v372–v394

[29] Licitra L, Mesia R, Rivera F, et al. Evaluation of EGFR gene copy number as a predictive biomarker for the efficacy of cetuximab in combination with chemotherapy in the first-line treatment of recurrent and/or metastatic squamous cell carcinoma of the head and neck: EXTREME study. Ann Oncol. 2011; 22(5):1078–1087

[30] Licitra L, Störkel S, Kerr KM, et al. Predictive value of epidermal growth factor receptor expression for first-line chemotherapy plus cetuximab in patients with head and neck and colorectal cancer: analysis of data from the EXTREME and CRYSTAL studies. Eur J Cancer. 2013; 49(6):1161–1168

[31] Weidhaas JB, Harris J, Schaue D, et al. The KRAS- variant and cetuximab response in head and neck squamous cell cancer: a secondary analysis of a randomized clinical trial. JAMA Oncol. 2017; 3(4):483–491

[32] Cohen EEW, Licitra LF, Burtness B, et al. Biomarkers predict enhanced clinical outcomes with afatinib versus methotrexate in patients with second-line recurrent and/or metastatic head and neck cancer. Ann Oncol. 2017; 28(10):2526–2532

[33] Vermorken JB, Psyrri A, Mesía R, et al. Impact of tumor HPV status on outcome in patients with recurrent and/or metastatic squamous cell carcinoma of the head and neck receiving chemotherapy with or without cetuximab: retrospective analysis of the phase III EXTREME trial. Ann Oncol. 2014; 25(4):801–807

[34] Seiwert TY, Burtness B, Mehra R, et al. Safety and clinical activity of pembrolizumab for treatment of recurrent or metastatic squamous cell carcinoma of the head and neck (KEYNOTE-012): an open-label, multicentre, phase 1b trial. Lancet Oncol. 2016; 17(7):956–965

[35] Carbognin L, Pilotto S, Milella M, et al. Differential activity of nivolumab, pembrolizumab and MPDL3280A according to the tumor expression of programmed death-ligand-1 (PD-L1): sensitivity analysis of trials in melanoma, lung and genitourinary cancers. PLoS One. 2015; 10(6):e0130142

[36] Yearley JH, Gibson C, Yu N, et al. PD-L2 expression in human tumors: relevance to anti-PD-1 therapy in cancer. Clin Cancer Res. 2017; 23(12):3158–3167

[37] Chow LQM, Haddad R, Gupta S, et al. Antitumor activity of pembrolizumab in biomarker-unselected patients with recurrent and/or metastatic head and neck squamous cell carcinoma: results from the phase Ib KEYNOTE-012 expansion cohort. J Clin Oncol. 2016; 34(32):3838–3845

[38] Ayers M, Lunceford J, Nebozhyn M, et al. IFN-γ-related mRNA profile predicts clinical response to PD-1 blockade. J Clin Invest. 2017; 127(8):2930–2940

[39] Haddad RIST, Chow L, Gupta S, et al. Genomic determinants of response to pembrolizumab in head and neck squamous cell carcinoma (HNSCC). J Clin Oncol. 2017; 35(15):6009

[40] Ferris RL, Blumenschein G, Jr., Fayette J, et al. Nivolumab vs investigator's choice in recurrent or metastatic squamous cell carcinoma of the head and neck: 2-year long-term survival update of CheckMate 141 with analyses by tumor PD-L1 expression. Oral Oncol. 2018; 81:45-51.

34 Laryngeal Transplantation

D. Gregory Farwell, Arnaud F. Bewley

Abstract

Laryngeal transplantation is an exciting option for replacing laryngeal function. There have been three human larynx transplants that have been successful and fully reported. The surgical procedure has been well developed and variations have been described that include transplantation of skin, esophagus, and pharynx. Organ transplantation has several known associated risks and side effects including immune suppression–associated malignancies. These become increasingly important for non–life-sustaining transplants, especially in the setting of prior malignancies such as larynx cancer. Understanding these risks and placing them in the context of quality-of-life goals for patients is important. This chapter will describe the current state of the field and summarize the results of the three transplants previously performed.

Keywords: larynx, trachea, pharynx, esophagus, thyroid, transplant, immunosuppression, function, risks, rejection

34.1 Case Report

A 51-year-old female presented with a 10-year history of a tracheotomy-dependent, benign, and complete laryngotracheal stenosis. The stenosis was the result of a prolonged hospitalization for renal failure during which time, she required prolonged intubation and sustained multiple traumatic extubations. She underwent a kidney–pancreas transplantation 4 years prior to her larynx transplant presentation and was maintained on lifelong immunosuppression consisting of tacrolimus and leflunomide.[1]

Endoscopic attempts had been unsuccessful in reestablishing an airway. At the time of her presentation, endoscopy demonstrated a fused glottis with absence of any air passage from the trachea through the larynx. CT with 3D reconstruction of her airway demonstrated that the complete stenosis extended from the level of the glottis to below the second ring of the trachea. She was completely aphonic and tracheostomy dependent.

After extensive counseling and testing, the decision was made to offer the patient a larynx transplant. A 2-year preparatory period commenced involving psychological evaluation, technical preparation using a porcine model and cadaveric specimens, team building with transplant support, and patient preparation.[2,3] Pretransplant, the patient underwent percutaneous gastrostomy tube placement and botulinum toxin (Allergan, Irvine, CA) injection into her bilateral submandibular and parotid glands in an effort to reduce salivary flow and potential aspiration. The procedure followed closely after the 2001 Cleveland Clinic publication describing the only comprehensively reported transplant. Significant modifications were made in the approach to the vascular and neural anastamoses.[4] In 2010, we performed our transplant at the University of California, Davis (UC Davis) over 18 hours in adjacent operating rooms with simultaneous organ procurement and recipient laryngectomy and transplant preparation occurring simultaneously.

The donor was a healthy, well-matched 38-year-old female who had suffered an anoxic arrest and had only been intubated for 3 days. Pretransplant evaluation included ABO blood group that was compatible with the recipient. Human leukocyte antigen alleles were tested and the recipient expressed a low level of sensitization against human leukocyte antigens (HLAs) despite her prior transplantation. While we avoided donor HLAs that our recipient had antibodies against, we did not limit the donor to minor loci match as we prioritized the donor's anatomic and functional factors. Of note, a positive cytomegalovirus result was detected on her infectious panel.

The organ retrieval included the larynx, pharynx, esophagus, thyroid, and parathyroid glands, with all of the nourishing great vessels of the neck and mediastinum. After perfusion with University of Wisconsin perfusate, the transplant was procured at the same time as the liver and kidneys for other transplant recipients. The larynx transplant was prepared by isolating the dominant arterial flow that happened to be from the right side, which was prioritized for the first revascularization anastomoses. The mucosa was removed from the esophagus, but the muscular esophagus was opened and used as a secondary blood supply to the membranous trachea. Additionally, the superior laryngeal nerves bilaterally, right recurrent laryngeal nerve, and left adductor branch of the recurrent nerve were isolated. The left adductor branch was divided from the recurrent laryngeal nerve leaving abductor fibers still in continuity with the stump of the recurrent laryngeal nerve.

The transplantation was performed after laryngectomy by anastomosing the right recipient transverse cervical artery to the right inferior thyroid artery of the transplant and the right recipient jugular vein to the donor brachiocephalic vein. Successful reperfusion of the entire transplant was confirmed with an ischemia time of 300 minutes. Additional microvascular anastomoses were made between the recipient right superior thyroid artery and the donor right superior thyroid artery, the recipient left transverse cervical artery to the donor left inferior thyroid artery, and the recipient left internal jugular vein and the recipient left superior thyroid vein. Microneurorrhaphies were performed between the donor and recipient superior laryngeal nerves bilaterally and recurrent laryngeal nerve on the right side. An attempt at selective reinnervation was performed on the left side with an end-to-side microneurorrhaphy from the recipient phrenic nerve to the donor recurrent laryngeal nerve (abductor fibers) and the ansa cervicalis of the recipient to the adductor branch of the donor recurrent laryngeal nerve. Eight rings of transplanted trachea were used to reconstruct the trachea. Pharyngeal anastomoses were performed and the larynx was suspended to the hyoid bone.

Perioperatively, the patient was immunosuppressed with rabbit antithymocyte globulin, methylprednisolone, and mycophenolate. She was ultimately maintained on her renal transplant regimen of tacrolimus and leflunomide. Despite some minor perioperative complications such as transient infections of her trachea, lung and central line, mucosal candidiasis, and diarrhea, she did well postoperatively.

Her function posttransplant has been remarkable. She unequivocally professes a significant improvement in her quality of life and social engagement. While she remains cannulated with a tracheostomy, she has a widely patent airway and a strong voice. Acoustic analysis demonstrated normal parameters except for a lower fundamental frequency for her conversational voice. She is able to take a normal oral diet despite having some delay in initiation of her diet in the posttransplant period and requiring several dilations of an upper esophageal stricture. To date, after several biopsies up to 4 years after her transplant, she has not manifested any signs of rejection and it is now 7 years since the surgery.

34.2 Discussion

The field of vascularized composite allotransplantation has expanded significantly in the last decade. Transplantation of non–life-saving organs and structures such as larynx, hand, face, abdominal wall, and uterus, among others, has offered new options for reconstructing previously untreatable traumatic and functional defects. The advantages of replacing tissue of identical composition and anatomic form hold promise to bring us closer to our goal of being able to completely replace form and function from these challenging defects. Multiple successes have been reported in the lay and scientific press with remarkable benefits to patient function and quality of life.[5,6]

Laryngeal function is arguably one of the most complex and coordinated of any organ in the body. The ability to manage the airway, vocalization, and safe swallowing centers on the function of the larynx and surrounding tissues. Many attempts have been made with local tissues and vascularized free flaps to reconstruct defects and functional deficiencies of the larynx with varying results.[7,8,9] However, when these options are not appropriate or have failed, laryngeal transplant may be considered.

To date, there have been three comprehensive reports of single successful cases of laryngeal transplantation.[1,4,10] Additionally, there is a technical report of a series of purported laryngeal transplants from Medellin, Colombia.[11] This report describes a cohort of laryngeal transplants but unfortunately without significant details or subsequent publications to provide information on indications or outcomes of these procedures.

In 2001, the Cleveland Clinic described the initial laryngeal transplant in a patient who suffered a crush injury.[12] Over the 14 years of his transplant, he benefitted from an outstanding voice quality and swallowing function. When he had to undergo explantation for chronic rejection, he requested another transplant. Much has been learned by the experience of his case, which demonstrated multiple bouts of rejection manifest by mucosal lesions in the postcricoid area and vocal fold edema. Despite medical attempts to counter the rejection, chronic rejection, manifest by scar and atrophy, resulted in aspiration prompting explantation. Prior to explantation, the transplanted thyroid was inspected with a I-123 uptake scan, which demonstrated no uptake, confirming rejection of the entire transplant.

A recent publication describes the most recent laryngeal transplantation occurring in Poland in 2015. The patient was a 6-year cancer survivor who had undergone salvage laryngectomy for a T3N1 squamous cell carcinoma. His procedure involved transplantation of anterior neck skin, larynx, 8 cm of trachea, pharynx, esophagus, thyroid and four parathyroid glands, hyoid bone, and anterior digastric muscles. Now 2 years posttransplant, the patient is without evidence of rejection.[10]

Our patient, here at UC Davis, is now 7.5 years posttransplant and has done extremely well with restoration of voice, and patent airway. Despite some posttransplant dysphagia and stricture that required dilation, she is able to swallow a full oral diet.

Both the UC Davis patient and the Polish patients were unique in that they had previously undergone transplantation with a kidney/pancreas for the UC Davis patient and a kidney transplant for the Polish patient. As such, both patients were already immunosuppressed and the additional requirement of immunosuppression for the larynx transplant was not an additional risk. It is well known that immunosuppression carries significant risks for the patient both acutely and in the long term. Infection including atypical fungal infections may be life-threatening and are one of the most significant risks of immunosuppression. In the longer term, the development of posttransplant malignancies is a significant source of morbidity and mortality in the transplant population. Posttransplant lymphoproliferative disorders and non-Hodgkin's lymphomas are the most common hematologic malignancies and may be related to loss of immunosurveillance, direct toxicities of immunosuppressant medications, or Epstein–Barr virus–related oncogenic properties. The incidence of solid organ malignances are increased by twofold to threefold in transplant recipients[16]. When these cancers occur, the outcomes for treatment are poorer and the complications associated with treatment are more significant[17]. As such, the largest population of larynx transplant candidates, having undergone laryngectomy for larynx cancer, have historically been considered ineligible for transplantation. Interestingly, the Polish patient was a cancer survivor, having undergone salvage laryngectomy for T3N1 squamous cell carcinoma 6 years prior to his transplant. While he is doing well, there is concern in the community that even long-term cancer survivors are at increased risk for additional tumors, especially for carcinogen-induced tumors such as cancer of the larynx.

The research on quality of life and patients' willingness to undergo larynx transplant in an effort to regain laryngeal function is compelling. Several studies have demonstrated a significant portion of eligible patients would undergo transplantation with patients having undergone prior transplantation being the most risk tolerant.[13,14,15] As immunosuppressant regimens improve, it is hoped that the number of candidate patients will increase.

34.3 Tips

- Laryngeal transplantation has been shown in three well-reported cases to offer an additional option for replacing laryngeal function in patients with severe injuries or after laryngectomy.
- The candidacy is limited by the significant ethical concerns over the risks of lifelong immunosuppression.
- Two out of the three reported cases were already on lifelong immunosuppression for prior transplants. Careful examination of this patient population, where the risks of immunosuppression have been already assumed, may provide more opportunities to advance the field and better understand the limitations and possibilities of transplanting the larynx.
- Working closely with a team of dedicated transplant physicians is key to success as it is likely that laryngeal transplant surgeons may not routinely have the knowledge and skill of managing the immunosuppression and associated risks.

34.4 Traps

- Given the wealth of literature demonstrating an increased risk of both solid and hematologic malignancies in transplant patients, great care should be taken in considering transplantation in larynx cancer survivors, despite the fact that this is the largest group of candidate patients.
- In an era of value-based medical decisions, careful consideration must be taken to balance the financial cost of a "nonvital" organ transplantation against the demonstrated desire of patients and the documented improvement in quality of life after transplantation.

References

[1] Farwell DG, Birchall MA, Macchiarini P, et al. Laryngotracheal transplantation: technical modifications and functional outcomes. Laryngoscope. 2013; 123(10):2502–2508

[2] Birchall MA, Ayling SM, Harley R, et al. Laryngeal transplantation in minipigs: early immunological outcomes. Clin Exp Immunol. 2012; 167(3):556–564

[3] Macchiarini P, Lenot B, de Montpreville V, et al; Paris-Sud University Lung Transplantation Group. Heterotopic pig model for direct revascularization and venous drainage of tracheal allografts. J Thorac Cardiovasc Surg. 1994; 108(6):1066–1075

[4] Strome M, Stein J, Esclamado R, et al. Laryngeal transplantation and 40-month follow-up. N Engl J Med. 2001; 344(22):1676–1679

[5] Aycart MA, Kiwanuka H, Krezdorn N, et al. Quality of life after face transplantation: outcomes, assessment tools, and future directions. Plast Reconstr Surg. 2017; 139(1):194–203

[6] Chełmoński A, Kowal K, Jabłecki J. The physical and psychosocial benefits of upper-limb transplantation: a case series of 5 polish patients. Ann Transplant. 2015; 20:639–648

[7] Cheng OT, Tamaki A, Rezaee RP, Zender CA. Laryngotracheal reconstruction with a prefabricated fasciocutaneous free flap for recurrent papillary thyroid carcinoma. Head Neck. 2016; 38(11):E2512–E2514

[8] Gilbert RW, Goldstein DP, Guillemaud JP, Patel RS, Higgins KM, Enepekides DJ. Vertical partial laryngectomy with temporoparietal free flap reconstruction for recurrent laryngeal squamous cell carcinoma: technique and long-term outcomes. Arch Otolaryngol Head Neck Surg. 2012; 138(5):484–491

[9] Loos E, Meulemans J, Vranckx J, Poorten VV, Delaere P. Tracheal autotransplantation for functional reconstruction of extended hemilaryngectomy defects: a single-center experience in 30 patients. Ann Surg Oncol. 2016; 23(5):1674–1683

[10] Grajek M, Maciejewski A, Giebel S, et al. First complex allotransplantation of neck organs: larynx, trachea, pharynx, esophagus, thyroid, parathyroid glands, and anterior cervical wall: a case report. Ann Surg. 2017; 266(2):e19–e24

[11] Duque E, Duque J, Nieves M, Mejía G, López B, Tintinago L. Management of larynx and trachea donors. Transplant Proc. 2007; 39(7):2076–2078

[12] Lorenz RR, Strome M. Total laryngeal transplant explanted: 14 years of lessons learned. Otolaryngol Head Neck Surg. 2014; 150(4):509–511

[13] Reynolds CC, Martinez SA, Furr A, et al. Risk acceptance in laryngeal transplantation. Laryngoscope. 2006; 116(10):1770–1775

[14] Jo HK, Park JW, Hwang JH, Kim KS, Lee SY, Shin JH. Risk acceptance and expectations of laryngeal allotransplantation. Arch Plast Surg. 2014; 41(5):505–512

[15] Buiret G, Rabilloud M, Combe C, Paliot H, Disant F, Céruse P. Larynx transplantation: laryngectomees' opinion poll. Transplantation. 2007; 84(12):1584–1589

[16] Chapman JR, Webster AC, Wong G. Cold Spring Harb Perspect Med 2018; 3(7). Pii:a015677

[17] Dharnidharka VR. Comprehensive review of post-organ transplant hematologic cancers. Am J Transplant 2018; 18(3):537–549

Index

Note: Page numbers set in **bold** or *italic* indicate headings or figures, respectively.